ELECTROCARDIOGRAPHY
The Monitoring Lead

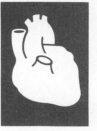

ELECTROCARDIOGRAPHY
The Monitoring Lead

Richard Wiederhold

W.B. SAUNDERS COMPANY
A Division of Harcourt Brace & Company
Philadelphia   London   Toronto   Montreal   Sydney   Tokyo

W.B. SAUNDERS COMPANY
A Division of
Harcourt Brace & Company

The Curtis Center
Independence Square West
Philadelphia, Pennsylvania 19106

ISBN: 0-7216-2979-2

Library of Congress Catalog Card Number: 87–80980

Printed in the United States of America

The Wiederhold Algorithm © 1985 by Richard Wiederhold.

Last digit is the print number: 9 8 7 6 5

I dedicate this book
to my wonderful wife, Marietta,
to my son, Erich,
and to the Leaders of the Band.

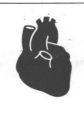

No man can reveal to you aught
but that which already lies half
asleep
in the dawning of your knowledge.

The teacher who walks
in the shadow of the temple,
among his followers, gives not of his
wisdom
but rather of his faith and his
lovingness.

If he is indeed wise
he does not bid you enter the house
of his wisdom,
but rather leads you to the threshold
of your own mind.

KAHLIL GIBRAN

Preface

This textbook is written for the non-cardiologist and is intended as a resource for physicians in office practice, paramedics, nurses, medical students, monitoring technicians in intensive-care and cardiac-care units, and other health care professionals and students. What distinguishes the book from other electrocardiographic books in the field is that it limits itself to the purview of *monitoring* and *dysrhythmia* recognition, rather than attempting to address the whole field of electrocardiography. Its primary objective is to enable the clinician to interpret electrocardiograms and to recognize major dysrhythmias on monitoring leads.

The book creates a bridge from the known to the unknown for the student clinician. It approaches electrocardiogram analysis on a systematic basis, starting with normal sinus rhythm and proceeding through a study of ectopy and dysrhythmias. A number of criteria apply to each dysrhythmia. Many dysrhythmias share one or more of these criteria, which tends to contribute to confusion for the student clinician. Each dysrhythmia is unique. Each criterion is a piece of a puzzle that makes up the dysrhythmia. While one puzzle piece may fit more than one dysrhythmia, the combination of the three or four puzzle pieces for each dysrhythmia is unique. That should become clear to students as they read and study the book. Skill at interpretation will come only with practice, practice, and more practice.

The book concentrates on *dysrhythmia recognition*. It does not address patient management or the patient's clinical symptomology. Many dysrhythmias relate to serious medical problems, such as myocardial infarction. The electrocardiogram is only one aspect of patient assessment. Patient symptomology may or may not be related to the dysrhythmia. The clinician should always bear in mind that *interpretation of an electrocardiogram without an associated patient case history and physical examination is valuable only as an academic exercise.*

I have presented, at the end of this book, an algorithmic procedure of electrocardiograph analysis, titled the Wiederhold Algorithm, that will facilitate the clinician's rapid recognition of major forms of dysrhythmia. This algorithm will direct the clinician's attention to dysrhythmia possibilities (or even probabilities), but it should not exclude evaluation of the general rules of each dysrhythmia. The clinician using this algorithmic procedure should formulate a tentative interpretation and apply the criteria of that dysrhythmia to the electrocardiogram being considered for confirmation of the interpretation. The algorithm considers only the possibility of one major dysrhythmia being present and does not include consideration of ectopy. The clinician should recognize that ectopy or multiple dysrhythmias may be present in any underlying rhythm or dysrhythmia.

This book is for a first course in electrocardiography, addressing techniques for interpreting major dysrhythmias from a monitoring lead. The author has made every effort to assure that material contained in this book is accurate and in accord with the standards in effect at the time of its publication and that students will learn a procedure that collates dysrhythmia criteria into a format that facilitates evaluation. This book is not a manual of procedure but a learning instrument. The state of knowledge of the art of evaluating criteria changes constantly, and new research may result in changes in procedures and techniques. The author and the publisher cannot be responsible for misuse of this book, including use as a source of specific procedures, instructions, or techniques of diagnosis.

The role of an educator is not to teach but to invite the student to learn. Learning is an active role on the part of the student. No educator can "teach" anyone anything. Your success in your field of study is to your credit and is equally your responsibility. I invite you to learn electrocardiography. Good reading!

Acknowledgments

No textbook is a solitary effort. The assistance of many people made this one possible. My family deserves my deepest love and appreciation, especially my wife, the computer widow. I would also like to thank the staff members at Harcourt Brace Jovanovich for their many contributions: Cathleen Petree and Jeff Holtmeier, sponsoring editors; Zanae Rodrigo, manuscript editor; Cheryl Solheid, designer; Cindy Robinson, art editor; Anthony Maddela and Karen Davidson, production editors; and Lesley Lenox, production manager.

A very special thank-you goes to the reviewers, who offered excellent advice and encouragement: Jim Beck, San Joaquin Delta College; Rosie Bolenbaucher, Houston Community College; Dan Finley, Austin Community College; Meg Kilgore, Johnson County Community College; and Richard Osgood, Oakland Community College, Auburn Hills Campus.

I also would like to thank Dr. Ricardo Ramos, a kind and considerate medical authority, and my many students and friends who collected literally thousands of EKG rhythm strips for my evaluation. Dr. Bruce Bickley provided encouragement and support for many years and had an important hand in this text. You have all made this project work!

Richard Wiederhold

You can find in a text whatever you bring,
if you will stand between it
and the mirror of your imagination.
You may not see your ears,
but they will be there.

Mark Twain

Contents

List of Figures

List of Tables

ELECTROCARDIOGRAPHY

The Monitoring Lead

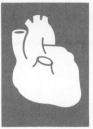

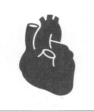

The white rabbit put on his
spectacles.
"Where shall I begin,
please your majesty?" he asked.
"Begin at the beginning,"
the King said gravely,
"and go on till you come to the end:
then stop."

LEWIS CARROLL

1

Introduction

OBJECTIVES

■ Form an expectation of the format and purpose of the text.

■ Identify the components of competency-based instruction, as used in the text.

■ Identify the purpose and clinical application of electrocardiography and the role of monitoring and dysrhythmia recognition.

■ Define the limitations of the monitoring electrocardiogram.

KEY TERMINOLOGY

algorithm
arrhythmia
dysrhythmia

The field of electrocardiography is an exciting one that may be confusing. At times a clinician will determine that a given electrocardiogram is a particular dysrhythmia, although it does not meet all the established criteria. At other times the same clinician will determine that a given electrocardiogram is not a particular dysrhythmia, because it does not meet all the established criteria. What appears to be mystic, cabalistic intuition is merely a logical deduction based on a knowledge of the criteria for dysrhythmia recognition and experience with applying it.

It is most important to recognize that electrocardiographic analysis is a technique of patient assessment that is (in this text) out of the context of the patient. Electrocardiogram interpretation is a skill used to more effectively manage the patient clinically. The most important aspect of any dysrhythmia is its impact on the patient. The symptomology and management of dysrhythmias are not within the scope of this text. Reference to the American Heart Association's *Textbook of Advanced Cardiac Life Support* is recommended for the most current medical standard of care in patient management.

No good workman will approach his appointed task without the tools needed to complement his skills. The electrocardiographic clinician also needs the tools of his trade. These tools include, in addition to the obvious machinery, an open inquiring mind, a basic knowledge of cardiovascular anatomy and physiology, a thorough acquaintance with the criteria of each dysrhythmia, a good pair of calipers, and patience.

This text will review the anatomy and physiology of the cardiovascular system, comprehensively address the criteria of dysrhythmia recognition from a monitoring EKG, and introduce an **algorithmic method** of electrocardiogram analysis.

The student-reader will benefit most by reading with comprehension, an activity best achieved with a thorough knowledge of the terminology used in the field. The lack of a thorough knowledge of medical terminology may be compensated for by researching the terminology during reading. This is not always convenient; therefore, a glossary with phonetic pronunciations has been incorporated.

The term **arrhythmia** literally defined means *without rhythm*. The term **dysrhythmia** is defined as *difficult (or abnormal) rhythm*. The term dysrhythmia is the most appropriate application for the dysrhythmias in this text. Most clinicians entering the field for the first time are acquainted with it. Many of these clinicians have false expectations. The only diagnostic capacity of the *monitoring* EKG is for diagnosis of major dysrhythmias. It is, therefore, used only to monitor the patient's rhythm pattern and observe for the development of dysrhythmia.

Acute myocardial infarction and other medical emergencies may be diagnosed on a complete electrocardiogram. The complete EKG is a diagnostic tool. It may be able to diagnose such medical emergencies, but cannot be used to rule them out conclusively. Medical emergencies may be present in the patient with a completely normal electrocardiogram. These medical emergencies, including problems such as myocardial ischemia, bundle branch block, pulmo-

> **A competent clinician must always be aware that electrocardiogram analysis must be considered only a component of a thorough patient assessment.**

nary embolism, pulmonary infarction, cardiac tamponade, valvular stenosis, and so on, *cannot be diagnosed on a monitoring EKG.*

This text is competency based. The concepts of competency-based instruction applied in this text include advising the reader of the objectives to be accomplished in each chapter and provision of self-study questions and procedures to enable the reader to make a self-determination of accomplishment of objectives. It also provides electrocardiographic rhythm recordings for practice interpretation and reference evaluations of them for self-checking. If your interests stimulate you to skip ahead, by all means, do so. The nature of the text is that it progressively builds on preceding chapters and assumes the reader has completed those chapters. The reader will benefit most by a cohesive course of instruction matched by attention to the text, working with the self-study questions, defining the terminology, and mastering the objectives stated at the beginning of each chapter.

Practice with electrocardiogram interpretation is essential. Strong electrocardiographic interpretative skills can only be achieved with practice! The reader is encouraged to practice as much as possible. Remember that medicine is an art that is practiced as a science and there are as many correct interpretations as there are informed opinions.

Self-Study Questions

1. Identify the most important aspect of any dysrhythmia.
2. Identify the appropriate reference text for the most current medical standard of care in patient management of the cardiac emergency.
3. Explain the purpose and limitations of the monitoring EKG and the complete electrocardiogram.

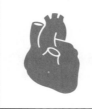

The leader of the band is tired
and his eyes are growing old
but his blood runs through
my instrument
and his song is in my soul.
My life has been a poor attempt
to imitate the man
I'm just a living legacy
to the leader of the band.

DAN FOGELBERG

2
Cardiovascular Anatomy

OBJECTIVES

■ Identify and define the function of each structure of the heart, including tissues, chambers, valves, vessels, circulatory patterns, cardiac output, stroke volume, and blood pressure.

■ Identify and define the structure of the electrical properties of the heart, including innervation, receptor sites, depolarization, repolarization, automaticity, and conduction.

■ Identify and list the function of the components of the conduction system.

KEY TERMINOLOGY

absolute refractory period
action potential
adrenergic influence
adrenergic receptor sites
   alpha
   beta
   dopaminergic
afterload
atria
atrial kick

automaticity
bifurcate
bradydysrhythmia
bundle branch
bundle of His
cardiac cycle
cardiac output
cardiac oxygen need
catecholamine
cholinergic effect
chordae tendineae
chronotropic effect
chronotropy
conduction system
conductivity
contractility
coronary artery
coronary sinus
coronary sulcus
depolarization
electrocardiogram
electrolyte
electromechanical activity
electrophysiology
endocardium
epicardium
Frank-Starling effect
innervation
inotropy
junction
myocardium

node
   atrioventricular
   sinoatrial
pacemaker
parasympathetic influence
pericardium
polarized
preload
propagated action potential
pulmonary circulation
Purkinje fibers
refractory period
relative refractory period
repolarization
resting membrane potential
septum
stroke volume
sympathetic hormonal influence
systemic circulation
systole
tachydysrhythmia
threshold potential
valves
   aortic
   mitral
   pulmonic
   tricuspid
vascular compartment
vasomotor tone
ventricles

The heart is a hollow, muscular organ. An organ, by definition, functions as part of a *system*. The system in which the heart functions is the **cardiovascular system.**

The Cardiovascular System

The cardiovascular system has three related aspects that function to provide circulation of oxygenated blood, nutrients, endogenous secretions, injected substances, and waste products. The components of the system, in addition to the heart, include the vascular compartment and the blood.

    The function of the heart within the system is that of a pump. Like most pumps, the heart has fluid to pump (blood) and a pathway (the vascular compartment). Every pump also has the hydraulic concepts of volume and pressure. Simply put, the pump output provides a given volume of material (blood) within a given compartment (the vascular system). This system exists at a pressure. A change of any individual component of the system (such as, pump output, the quantity of material, or the size of the system) will result in a change in the pressure. Slightly more complicated, any combination of changes will usually result in a change of pressure.

    The pressure of the cardiovascular system is the individual's blood pressure. It is determined by the two factors of **cardiac output** and **vasomotor tone.**

FIGURE 2-1
Components of the Circulatory System

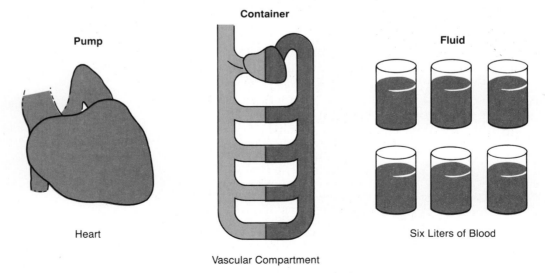

Pump

Container

Fluid

Heart

Vascular Compartment

Six Liters of Blood

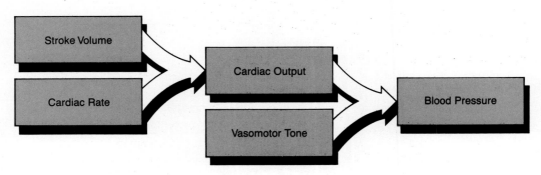

FIGURE 2-2
Blood Pressure, Cardiac Output, and Vasomotor Tone

Cardiac output (cardiac rate times stroke volume) is the amount of blood pumped by the heart per minute. **Stroke volume** is the amount of blood pumped with each *stroke*. The equation may be deduced as follows:

$$\text{cardiac output} \times \text{vasomotor tone} = \text{blood pressure}$$
$$\text{cardiac rate} \times \text{stroke volume} = \text{cardiac output}$$
$$\text{therefore}$$
$$[\text{cardiac rate} \times \text{stroke volume}] \times \text{vasomotor tone} = \text{blood pressure}$$

Vasomotor tone refers to the size of the vascular compartment or, more specifically, the resistance the muscular tone of the blood vessels offers to the circulation of blood. If vasomotor tone is poor, resistance is low, and the blood vessels are dilated. This allows the size of the compartment to increase with a resultant decrease in blood pressure. If vasomotor tone is excessive, resistance is high, the blood vessels are constricted, and hypertension exists.

All three factors of cardiac rate, stroke volume, and vasomotor tone are directly proportional. An increase in any one will result in an increase in blood pressure. A decrease in any one will result in a decrease in blood pressure. This assumes that the other factors remain constant.

The heart is a marvelously efficient device. It contracts and pumps, in adults at rest, approximately 70 milliliters of blood per stroke, about 72 strokes per minute, for an average resting cardiac output of five liters every minute of our lives. This is enough force to lift roughly a one-ton automobile or pickup truck over one's head about every two and one-half hours. It moves about 7,250 liters a day through our cardiovascular system. It responds to increased need during activity and compensates for hypotension to a point. That is quite an accomplishment for a 250 to 350 gram muscle, when one considers that the muscle does this for about 80 years uninterrupted (hopefully).

Cardiac Anatomy

The anatomy of the heart appears fairly simple (see Figure 2-3). There are four chambers, two **atria** (plural for atrium), and two **ventricles.** The atria are separated from the ventricles by the **junction. Valves,** which prevent the back-flow of blood, are located in the junction between the atria and the ventricles. The **tricuspid valve** is on the right side and the **mitral valve** is on the left.

Brachiocephalic Trunk

Superior Vena Cava

Ascending Aorta

R. Pulmonary
Artery

R. Pulmonary
Veins

Aortic Valve

Pulmonary Valve

R. Atrium

Tricuspid Valve

Chordae Tendineae

R Ventricle

Papillary Muscle

Inferior Vena Cava

L. Subclavian Artery

L. Common Carotid Artery

Aortic Arch

L. Pulmonary
Artery

L. Pulmonary
Veins

L. Atrium

Mitral Valve

L. Ventricle
(contracted)

Endocardium

Myocardium

Epicardium

Pericardium

Intraventricular
Septum

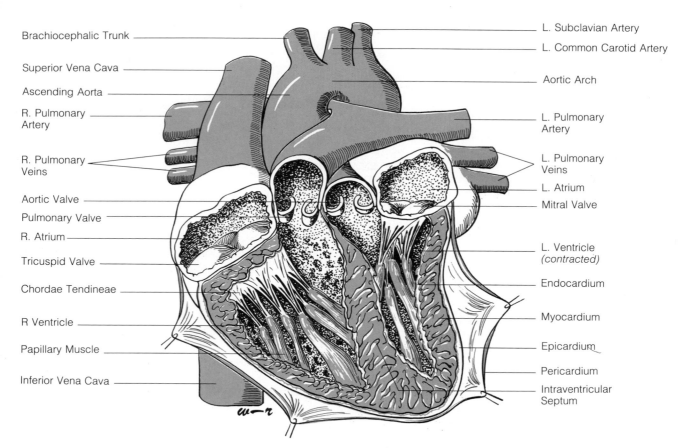

FIGURE 2-3
Cardiac Anatomy

Anatomical structures, called **chordae tendineae,** anchor these valves. The chordae tendineae attach inside the ventricles to muscles called **papillary bodies.** These anchors prevent the valves from turning inside out and allowing the force of ventricular contraction to cause backflow of blood. A valve with one or more of the leaflets turned backwards (or inside out), allowing blood to regurgitate from the ventricle into the atrium, is a **prolapsed valve.** Prolapse may occur because of stretching or rupture of the chordae tendineae or because of a variety of valve diseases.

Other valves are located at the articulation of the ventricles with the pulmonary artery (at the right ventricle) and the aorta (at the left ventricle). These are the pulmonic and aortic valves, respectively, and prevent the backflow of blood. The left and right halves of the heart (each containing one atrium and one ventricle) are separated by the **septum.**

The wall of the heart is composed of three layers: the outer **epicardium,** the mid-layer **myocardium,** and the inner **endocardium.** The myocardium (or muscle layer) of the heart is thickest in the left ventricle because the left ventricle does more work (pumping against systemic diastolic pressure) than any other chamber. The left ventricle is frequently called the *workhorse of the heart.*

The entire heart is surrounded by the **pericardium,** a membranous sac which is attached to adjacent surrounding structures such as the sternum, pleura, trachea, esophagus, bronchi, and great vessels. The pericardial sac contains a serous lubricating fluid, which eases the friction of the heart moving within it.

Coronary Circulation

The heart itself is perfused with oxygenated blood through **coronary circulation.** Coronary circulation involves two main **coronary arteries** that branch off the aorta where it joins the heart, the coronary veins, and the coronary sinus.

These coronary arteries are the left coronary artery and the right coronary artery. The coronary arteries **bifurcate** into other branches and supply the heart. The left coronary artery branches more than the right because the left side of the heart is more muscular. The first major branches of the left coronary artery are the left anterior descending artery and the circumflex artery.

The arteries and the main coronary vein run across the heart in a fissure

FIGURE 2-4
Coronary Circulation

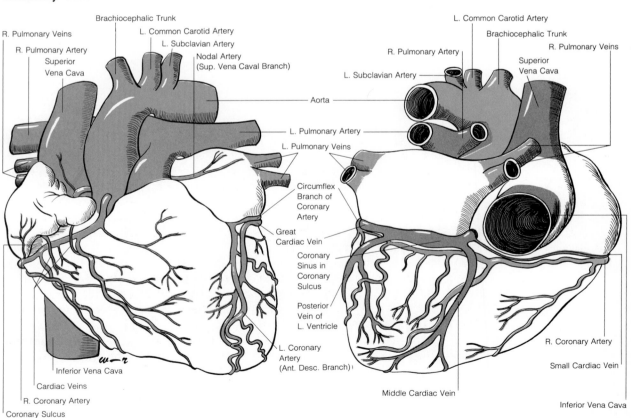

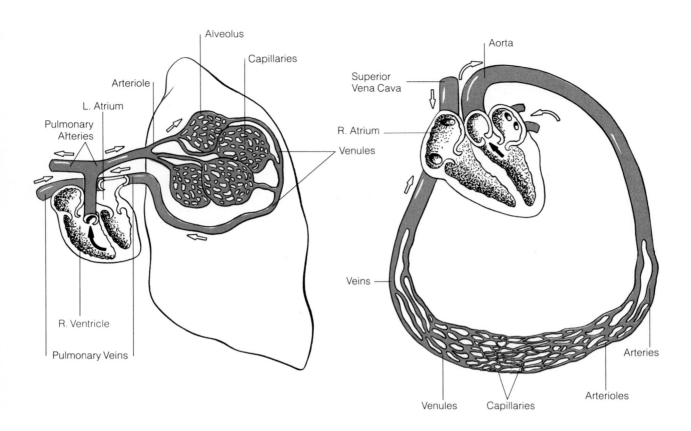

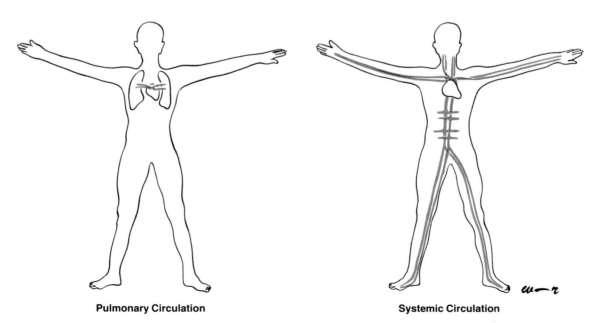

Pulmonary Circulation

Systemic Circulation

FIGURE 2-5
Systemic and Pulmonary Circulation

called the **coronary sulcus.** The vessels terminate in a cavity called the **coronary sinus.** This venous blood then is emptied directly into the right atrium.

The atrium then has three sources of venous blood: the superior vena cava, the inferior vena cava, and the coronary sinus.

Systemic and Pulmonary Circulation

The existence of a left atrium and ventricle in addition to the right atrium and ventricle points out a division in the circulatory system between the **systemic circuit** and the **pulmonary circuit.** The heart is commonly perceived as a double pump, the left heart and the right heart being the two pumps (see Figure 2-5).

Blood enters the pulmonary circuit through the right atrium into the right ventricle which is the starting point of the pulmonary circuit. After the right atrium has filled (and the right ventricle has filled about 80 percent), by venous pressure, the atrium contracts, engorging the ventricle with the **atrial kick.** This atrial kick completes the filling (the remaining 20 percent) of the ventricle. The right ventricle then contracts and pumps blood through the **pulmonic valve** into the pulmonary artery. The blood, even though it is in an artery at this point, is unoxygenated. The pulmonary artery carries blood to the lungs where external gas exchange with environmental air occurs. As the blood circulates through the pulmonary circuit into the four pulmonary veins it returns to the left atrium (which is the end point of the pulmonary circuit), and then into the left ventricle, where the systemic circuit begins.

The left atrium fills by venous pressure (and 80 percent of ventricular filling occurs as well). The atrium contracts and engorges the ventricle supplying the left-sided atrial kick. The left and right atrial contractions (or systoles) normally occur simultaneously. The left ventricle contracts (almost simultaneously with the right ventricle) and pumps blood through the **aortic valve** into the aorta. The aorta provides the pathway for blood to circulate throughout the entire cardiovascular system (other than the pulmonary circuit). Internal gas exchange occurs at the cellular level and blood flow returns from the system to the heart through the veins and specifically to the right atrium through the superior and inferior vena cava.

Afterload and Preload

The blood pressure that exists in the arteries (either pulmonary or systemic) during diastole is the pressure the heart must pump against to push blood out of the heart. This pressure is **afterload.** If afterload is high, the heart must work harder to pump the blood out against it.

TABLE 2-1   Afterload/Preload Areas

Circuit	Preload Vessel	Afterload Vessel
Pulmonary	Vena Cava	Pulmonary Artery
Systemic	Pulmonary Vein	Aorta

The pressure of the venous blood entering the heart is **preload.** If preload is high, the heart must pump harder against it to cause a cardiac stroke output.

The pulmonary and systemic circuits both have preload and afterload pressures; however, a general reference to cardiac workloads refers to systemic values.

Cardiac Cycle

The **cardiac cycle** is composed of a complete phase of atrial contraction and ventricular contraction, followed by relaxation. This all occurs about 60 to 100 times a minute. Contraction of the heart muscle is **systole.** There is an atrial systole and a ventricular systole. Ventricular systole follows atrial systole by about two-tenths of a second, allowing atrial systole to pump blood into the ventricle to supply the atrial kick.

When a clinician refers to systole generically, without specifying atrial or ventricular, one may assume that the reference is to the output producing ventricular systole. The mitral and tricuspid valves close during ventricular systole to prevent backflow of blood into the atria. The pulmonic and aortic valves close during ventricular diastole (relaxation) to prevent backflow of blood from the aorta and pulmonary arteries into the ventricles. A clinician should be able to, when presented with a diagram of the heart, discern by the positions of the valves the stage of the **cardiac cycle.**

A phenomena called the **Frank-Starling effect** contributes to maintaining stroke volume. This effect is the greater a muscle is stretched (to a point), the more effective its contraction will be. The atrial kick stretches the ventricle and enables its contraction to be more forceful than it could possibly be without an atrial chamber. This points out the marvelous economy of engineering of the heart. Two chambers accomplish a much more effective stroke volume than one chamber with the equivalent muscle mass could accomplish.

Any change in cardiac rate is a **chronotropic effect.** A number of factors govern the cardiac rate. The heart's unique **automaticity** (the inherent ability of the heart's cells to initiate impulses) contributes to the heart's ability to regulate itself. Other regulatory influences include innervation from the sympathetic and parasympathetic nervous systems.

Sympathetic Nervous System Influence

Sympathetic hormonal influence originates from the adrenal glands. This is a response to stimuli from the cardiac center in the medulla oblongata portion of the brain. The adrenal glands located in the kidneys secrete a group of hormones known as **catecholamines.** Catecholamine influence is categorized as **adrenergic influence.** It serves to *stimulate* heart rate and the force of the heart beat. Any change in the *contractility* or strength of the heart beat is an **inotropic effect.**

Sympathetic nervous system stimulation also causes direct stimulation via sympathetic nerve fibers. The hormonal influence has an indirect, but powerful, effect on the heart. The catecholamines circulate to the heart through the blood stream. Upon arriving at the heart, they act on **adrenergic receptor sites** to exert a stimulatory influence on the heart. Adrenergic receptor sites are also located in other areas of the body (the vascular system, the lungs, and the renal

TABLE 2-2 Sympathetic Receptor Sites and Effects

Receptor Site	Heart	Lungs	Vasculature
Alpha	No Sites	No Sites or Very Small Effect	Vasoconstriction
Beta	+ Chronotropic + Inotropic	Bronchodilation	No Sites or Very Small Effect
Dopaminergic	No Sites	No Sites	Selective Vasodilation

mesentery). Catecholamines also have an effect on those adrenergic receptor sites. Excessive sympathetic stimulation tends to result in **tachydysrhythmia,** which is an abnormally fast heart rate.

Receptor sites are labeled according to effect. They are arbitrarily called **alpha, beta,** or **dopaminergic** receptor sites. Some agents exert a combination of effects and have both alpha and beta properties (or any combination of the three properties). Others are purely alpha (phenylephrine) or purely beta (isoproterenol). Please refer to Table 2-2 for a list of agents and effects. Some researchers believe other types of receptor sites are undiscovered. They should make the study of pharmacokinetics more stimulating.

Sympathetic Effects

The sympathetic nervous system exerts a stimulatory effect on the heart by direct innervation and indirect secretion of hormones. These effects include a positive chronotropic effect (an increase in rate), a positive inotropic effect (an increase in force of contraction), and an increase in automaticity (the inherent ability of the heart's cells to initiate and conduct impulses). These effects increase *cardiac oxygen need* and demand, by increasing cardiac workload.

The sympathetic effect can be compared to using an accelerator in an automobile which has a cruise control set at 55 miles per hour. (The heart's cruise control is set at 60 to 100 beats per minute.) The accelerator (without the brake) can only have a stimulatory effect, and increase the rate above its normal (cruise control) setting.

Removing the sympathetic stimulation (releasing the accelerator) will allow it to coast down to its normal rate (cruise control setting of 55 mph). It cannot reverse its effects to depress the heart's (engine's) function and cause a slower rate than normal, like the accelerator (without the brake) of a car cannot cause the car to go slower than the rate the cruise control is causing. The *cruise control* in this sense is the inherent *normal* cardiac rate.

Parasympathetic Effects

Stimulation of the **parasympathetic influence** exerts a depressant effect on the heart by direct innervation through the vagus nerve. Parasympathetic involvement is the **cholinergic effect** as opposed to the sympathetic adrenergic effect.

It delays impulse formation and conduction within the heart, resulting in a slowing of cardiac rate. The vagus nerve is the major nerve of the parasympathetic system exerting an effect on many of the body organs. It is the tenth cranial nerve and is widespread throughout the body.

This can be compared to the application of a brake in that same car with the cruise control set at 55 mph. *Stimulation* of the vagus nerve (the primary parasympathetic influence on the heart) therefore actively *slows* the heart (in the same way applying the brake slows the car). It is confusing to think in terms of stimulating a nerve as depressing a function, but that is how the parasympathetic effect works (like a brake). Excessive parasympathetic stimulation frequently results in **bradydysrhythmia,** which is an abnormally slow heart rate.

Depression of the parasympathetic influence (cholinergic blockade) via the vagus nerve allows the heart to return to normal rate (removing the brake and allowing the automobile to accelerate to its cruise control setting). This gives the *appearance* of stimulating the heart while in effect it is really only preventing the continued action of parasympathetic (brake) effect.

The *effects* of stimulating one system and blocking the other appear similar. That is, stimulating one has similar effects to blocking the other. That is a slight oversimplification. Please refer to Table 2-3 for a list of effects.

FIGURE 2-6
Sympathetic and Parasympathetic System Effects

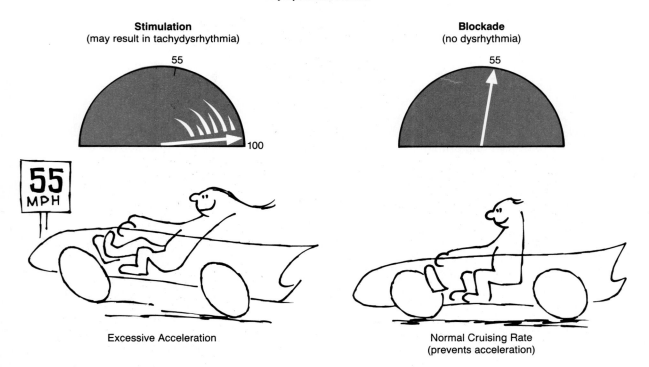

Sympathetic Effects

Stimulation
(may result in tachydysrhythmia)

Blockade
(no dysrhythmia)

Excessive Acceleration

Normal Cruising Rate
(prevents acceleration)

TABLE 2-3   Sympathetic and Parasympathetic Effects

Effect on Heart	Blockade	Stimulatory
Sympathetic	*Indirectly* "slows" the heart to normal. *Blockade* of sympathetic stimulation. Results in prevention of sympathetic stimulation. This allows a return to normal rate, and *appears* to exhibit a slowing effect. Agents include Inderal®, Corgard®, and Tenormin®.	*Stimulation directly* results in increases in chronotropic, inotropic, and automatic effects. Agents include epinephrine, isoproterenol, norepinephrine, and many others.
Parasympathetic	*Blockade indirectly* allows prevention of slowing. Resulting in a return to normal rate and *appears* to exhibit a positive inotropic effect. Blocking agent is atropine sulfate.	*Stimulation directly* delays impulse formation and conduction, slowing cardiac rate from fast → normal or normal → slow. Stimulating agent is Tensilon®.

®registered trademark

Parasympathetic Effects

Stimulation
(may result in bradydysrhythmia)

Blockade
(no dysrhythmia)

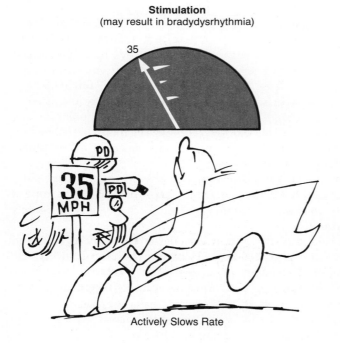

Actively Slows Rate

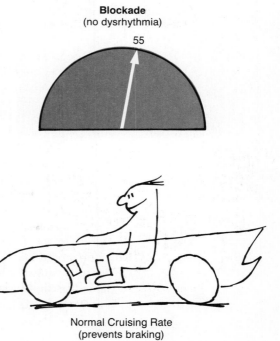

Normal Cruising Rate
(prevents braking)

Electrophysiology of the Heart

It is necessary, prior to entering a study of electrocardiography, to review the anatomy of the heart at the cellular level. It is the unique aspect of the heart's *electrophysiology* that makes electrocardiography possible. The two major electrical aspects of the heart are automaticity and conductivity.

Automaticity refers to the heart's ability to generate its own electrical stimulus. Each cell of the heart, like every cell in the body, is bathed in **electrolytes** (positively or negatively charged ions) on the inside and on the outside. These electrolytes, by their charge and location, cause the resting cardiac cell to have a net charge of negative 90 millivolts. This causes the cell to exist in a **polarized state.** This charge is the **resting membrane potential.**

When the heart cell is stimulated sufficiently to evoke a reaction, the **threshold potential** has been achieved. An **action potential** is created and specific pores (sometimes called "channels" or "gates") in the cell open and allow the intracellular and extracellular electrolytes to permeate the cellular membrane. This causes a reversal of electrical charge known as **depolarization.** Depolarization starts at one spot in the cell and spreads throughout the cell in a wavelike action.

Each of the cells in the conduction system has the ability to generate its own action potential, but some do so more rapidly than others (the significance of this will become clear later in this text). When a heart muscle cell depolarizes, the outside becomes negative and the inside becomes positive and the cell contracts. Fortunately the cell is able to recover from depolarization, otherwise our hearts would only function for one beat, significantly affecting our life expectancies.

Recovery from the depolarized state to the polarized resting state is **repolarization.** The electrolytes return to their original resting locations during repolarization. Repolarization spreads, just as depolarization did, in a wavelike motion throughout the cell. Depolarization, repolarization, and their pathways are represented in Figure 2-7.

The heart cell will not respond normally to a second stimulus until it is fully repolarized. Its capacity to depolarize is exhausted, a situation similar to the Queen's comment to Alice in Lewis Carroll's novel, "Now, here, you see, it takes all the running you can do, to keep in the same place. If you want to get somewhere else, you must run at least twice as fast as that!" It is fairly obvious that a completely contracted muscle is unable to contract any more, just as Alice could run no faster. A depolarized cell is equally unable to depolarize any more. The time during which the cell will not respond normally is the **refractory period.** The refractory period includes the period of depolarization and the period of repolarizing.

It is divided into two categories. The first is a period during which the cell will not respond to a repeated action potential, regardless of how strong it is. The first period is an **absolute refractory period** because it is absolutely refractory to additional stimuli.

The second is a period during which the cell will respond to a second action potential, but the action potential must be stronger than usual because the cell is not yet fully repolarized. The second period is a **relative refractory period** because it is relatively refractory, but will respond to stronger than normal stimuli.

The second electrical aspect of the heart is **conductivity.** The cells of the heart are not only able to generate their own stimuli, but are also able to re-

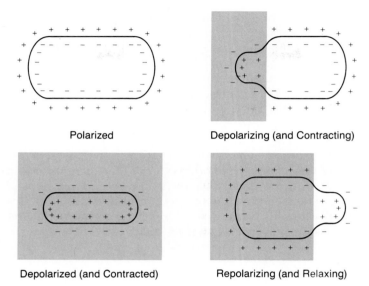

Polarized

Depolarizing (and Contracting)

Depolarized (and Contracted)

Repolarizing (and Relaxing)

FIGURE 2-7
Cellular Depolarization-Repolarization

ceive a stimulus from a neighboring cell, pick it up, depolarize, and pass the stimulus on to the next cell, similar to the manner in which a falling domino will cause the next domino, in a row of dominoes, to tumble. This simulates the passage of an electrical stimulus through a nerve cell and is frequently confused with nerve cell activity by the new student. These cells are specialized cardiac cells and, unlike nerve cells, are able to contract when they depolarize.

This spread of depolarization through the heart occurs, as within the cell, in a wavelike motion. Just as some cells had greater automaticity (the ability to repolarize and generate their own impulses more rapidly than other cells), some cells also have greater conductivity.

FIGURE 2-8
Action Potential of Myocardial Working Cell

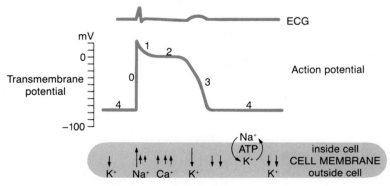

A stimulus capable of generating depolarization in one cell creates an action potential. An action potential, picked up by adjacent cells causing them to depolarize and carry the impulse on (to other cells), is a **propagated action potential.**

Electrical activity is occurring in muscle cells. This is normally associated with the cardiac muscle cell's contraction, and is **electromechanical activity.**

The flow of electrical energy follows the path of least resistance. The cardiac electrical activity flows through the cells of least resistance (or greater conductivity), more easily than others, just as it flows through copper wire more easily than through wood. The cardiac electrical activity is generated in cells that have greater automaticity than others. A cell that "fires" more rapidly than an adjacent cell will cause depolarization in the second cell by a propagated action potential. The second cell never gets an opportunity to initiate its very own spontaneous stimulus because it is forever capturing the action potential of the first cell. This is **"overdrive suppression."**

The Conduction System

These areas of greater automaticity and conductivity are fixed (they do not move) in the heart. The electrical activity routinely starts in the most automatic cells and conducts through the most conductive cells to the least conductive cells. These particular cells make up a regular pathway for electrical activity called the **conduction system.**

Naturally these areas of the conduction pathway have been identified and named. These areas are formed of specialized cardiac tissues that have electrical properties that make them unique. They are named for those properties and their physiological location in the heart.

A **pacemaker** is a site of impulse formation. Any cardiac conduction system cell can potentially function as a pacemaker. There is a consistent trend in the degree of automaticity of a cell dependent on its location within the heart. The automaticity progressively increases in the cells located along an imaginary line from the apex, low in the ventricles to the superior aspect, high in the

FIGURE 2-9
Electric Conduction System of the Heart

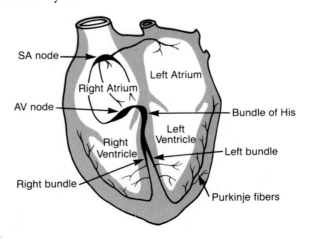

right atrium, where the sinoatrial node is located. Each region therefore has an *intrinsic firing rate*. The intrinsic firing rates are

1. less than forty (40) per minute for cells in the region of the ventricles.
2. forty (40) to sixty (60) per minute for cells in the myocardial junction.
3. sixty (60) to one hundred (100) per minute for cells in the atria.

The **sinoatrial node** is in the superior aspect of the right atrium. It is the dominant pacemaker, because its intrinsic firing rate (rate of depolarization) is the fastest (most automatic) of the heart.

The conduction system begins at the sinoatrial node and carries the propagated action potential along **intra-atrial pathways** through the atrium, allowing depolarization, and arrives at the **atrioventricular node** which is in the septum at the junction.

The atrioventricular node delays the conduction of the impulse. This permits a time delay between atrial depolarization (and contraction) and ventricular depolarization (and contraction) which allows atrial kick to occur.

The impulse then passes through the junction to the **bundle of His** which is a network that rapidly conducts the impulse down through the ventricles to the area of the apex of the heart. The bundle of His branches immediately into two main branches. One main branch rapidly branches into two sub-**bundle branches** supplying the left ventricle with conduction pathways. The other main branch supplies the right ventricle.

The impulse spreads from the bundles of His via the **Purkinje fibers,** which supply a pathway to the individual cells of the ventricles, resulting in ventricular depolarization.

Electrical activity that is generated (by automaticity) and spread (by conduction) through the heart, creates an electrical change in each cell. This results in the generation of an electrical wave. This electrical wave can be measured. The measurement of the electrical activity of the heart is the **electrocardiogram.**

Summary

The heart is the pump of the cardiovascular system, which also includes the blood and the vascular compartment. The cardiovascular features of stroke volume and cardiac rate make up cardiac output. The Frank-Starling effect contributes to the efficiency of the cardiac muscle.

Blood pressure is a component of vasomotor tone and cardiac output.

The anatomical structure of the heart includes four chambers and four major valves. These function to provide separate circuits, pulmonary and systemic, to the circulatory system. The heart itself, like any other muscle, is also provided a circulatory system, known as coronary circulation. The heart is surrounded by a fibrous sac, the pericardium.

Contraction of the heart muscle is systole and relaxation is diastole. There is both a ventricular and an atrial systole and diastole. Left and right atrial systoles occur simultaneously, slightly before ventricular systoles, which also occur together. Ventricular filling occurs during ventricular diastole and is accomplished by venous pressure and atrial kick.

Cardiac afterload refers to arterial diastolic pressure and preload refers to venous pressure. Afterload and preload are major determinants of cardiac workload and oxygen consumption.

Major influence on the heart is exerted by the autonomic nervous systems, both the sympathetic adrenergic and parasympathetic cholinergic. Their effects are inversely similar (but not the same). The sympathetic nervous system works through direct innervation and through endocrinic secretions and receptor sites in the organs affected. The parasympathetic nervous system works primarily via direct innervation.

The major electrical aspects of the heart that make the study of electrocardiography (and our lively status) possible are automaticity and conductivity. Automaticity enables the cardiac muscle cells to depolarize on their own initiative. Conduction enables the cells to pass the depolarization along to other cells to effect a rhythmic cardiac muscle contraction. The cells then repolarize in preparation for the next depolarization. During the repolarization period, the cells cannot normally respond to a second stimulus and are refractory.

Specialized cells are more automatic and conductive than others and these make up the conduction system. The conduction system includes the sinoatrial node, the intra-atrial pathways, the atrioventricular node, the bundle of His, and the Purkinje fibers. There is a consistent trend to the degree of automaticity of the parts of the conduction system with the most distal being the slowest. This trend gives rise to intrinsic firing rates for pacemakers from each region. The fastest (and most proximal aspect) component of the conduction is the sinoatrial node and by overdrive suppression it dominates the automaticity of the entire conduction system.

The electrical activity of the heart can be measured. This measurement is called the electrocardiograph.

Self-Study Questions

1. Identify and define the tissue layers of the heart.
2. Identify the chambers of the heart, the anatomical structures separating them, the valves between them, the sources of blood flow for each, and the vessel into which they pump.
3. Trace the pathway of blood circulating through the pulmonary and systemic circuits.
4. List the two components of cardiac output.
5. List the two major components of blood pressure.
6. What structures prevent the *prolapse* (turning inside out) of valves? What do these structures attach to, and where?
7. What is the Frank-Starling effect? Why is it important to circulation and blood pressure?
8. What three major factors govern cardiac rate?
9. Identify the effect on the heart of each of the following: sympathetic nervous system stimulation, sympathetic nervous system blockade, parasympathetic nervous system stimulation, and parasympathetic nervous system depression. List three types of sympathetic receptor sites.
10. Discuss valve positions during ventricular systole and diastole.
11. Describe the electrical change, in the cell and in the heart, that occurs during depolarization and repolarization.

12. List and define the two major electrical properties of the heart.
13. List five components of the conduction system in the order in which impulses generate and pass through them.
14. Discuss why the sinoatrial node is the dominant pacemaker of the heart.
15. What is the function of the atrioventricular node in the conduction system?
16. Identify the inherent firing rates for the cardiac regions of the atria, junction, and ventricles.
17. Discuss "overdrive suppression" and how it contributes to regulating cardiac rate.

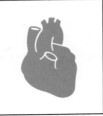

**And now here is my secret,
a very simple secret:
It is only with the heart that one
can see rightly; what is essential
is invisible to the eye.**

ANTOINE DE SAINT-EXUPÉRY

3

The Electrocardiogram

OBJECTIVES

■ Identify and define the function of the electrocardiograph and its components, including cathode ray tube monitors, strip writers, calibration settings, rate settings, marking devices, power switches, and associated devices, such as defibrillators, electrodes, conduction improving mediums, and so on.

■ Explain how the electrocardiograph measures cardiac electrical activity.

■ Discuss the three basic laws of electrocardiography.

■ Identify the anatomical locations for electrode placement in performing 12-lead electrocardiographic determinations and monitoring lead placements for monitoring lead II and MCL 1.

■ Differentiate between bipolar and unipolar lead configurations.

■ Identify the clinical applications of electrocardiography.

■ Identify and define the representative functions of the cardiac cycle and its components, including waves, segments, baseline, intervals, and complexes.

■ Recognize and identify the common causes for artifact in the electrocardiogram.

■ Relate the waves and deflections to electrode monitoring and directional travel of the cardiac impulses, and their normally associated mechanical activity.

KEY TERMINOLOGY

aVF
aVL
aVR
amplitude
anode

axis
bipolar lead
bipolar limb lead
blind defibrillation
calibration
cathode
CRT
defibrillation
defibrillator
ECG
EKG
electrode
false negative
false positive
graph paper
ischemia
leads
    I, II, & III
    V1 through V6
limb leads
MCL 1
net deflection
precordial leads
strip chart recorder
stylus
unipolar lead
unipolar limb lead
wave

The electrocardiogram is a measurement of the electrical activity of the heart. This measurement is frequently abbreviated as **EKG,** to avoid confusion, in conversation, with similar terms such as EEG (electro-encephalogram). It is also the original Dutch spelling in recognition of the technique's Germanic origin. The abbreviation **ECG** is also used.

Electrodes

A measurement is made of electrical flow between two *poles* of an electrically sensitive machine. These poles are the **electrodes** of an electrocardiographic monitor. One pole is the **anode** or positive terminal; the other is the **cathode** or negative terminal. The third contact commonly used with a monitor is a ground electrode designed to provide a circuit "to ground" for any extraneous electrical current present in the body. The third electrode is not a pole. The body is a good conductor of electricity and an electrocardiogram can be taken between any two points on it. However there are a number of preferred pre-established locations, called **leads.**

FIGURE 3-1
Electrodes

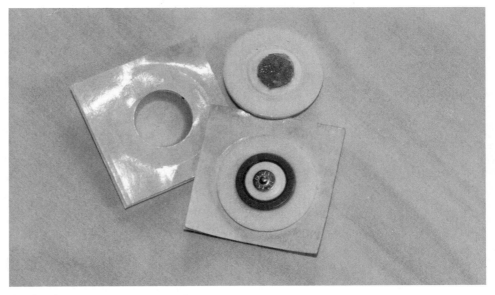

Photo by author

Electrodes come in a number of sizes and shapes. Most are small round adhesive pads containing a conductive gel to improve electrical contact. Others are metal contacts attached to rubber tubing or suction cups which hold them to the patient's body. If the latter is used, a tube of conductive medium or small pads dampened with saline are used to improve electrical conduction through the skin to the electrodes.

Cables attach the electrodes to the monitoring device. The monitoring device measures the electrical impulses of the cardiac conduction system, amplifies the measured electrical activity, and displays it in a manner the clinician can observe and interpret.

Display Devices

A number of display devices are used. The most common is a **cathode ray tube.** This is the same kind of tube that is found in the common television set, and is commonly referred to as the picture tube. The cathode ray tube (CRT for short) displays the electrocardiogram as a bright line on the gray or green background of the tube. This enables the clinician to continuously observe the patient's EKG without the necessity of continuously recording and replacing expensive electrocardiograph paper. The disadvantage of the CRT is that it is a dynamic monitoring device with a line that continually moves, making it difficult for the clinician to interpret. Some of the more sophisticated units on the market do have the capacity to "freeze" action if something attracts the clinician's attention. A more significant problem may be that there is also no graphic background to facilitate measurement of the electrocardiogram. There is also no *documentation* of activity which, in our legal theater of medicine, can be a real disadvantage.

Recording the EKG

Most monitors that have a cathode ray tube also have a **strip chart recorder.** A strip chart recorder is a device that produces a written representation of the electrocardiogram on a narrow strip of graph paper. The graph paper is drawn past a heated **stylus** at a standard rate of 25 millimeters per second. The stylus is a point of metal (something like the tip of a ballpoint pen except that it contains no ink and is more finely designed) that moves up and down in response to the measured electrical activity of the myocardium. The **graph paper** is heat sensitive so that when it moves horizontally under the stylus, an impression is imprinted in the graph by the heated stylus. As it is driven past the stylus, the graph paper is imprinted and then passes through the machine.

The standard rate of marking the graph paper at 25 millimeters per second produces a consistent, measurable, timed recording of the electrocardiographic activity of the heart. The graph paper used for strip writing is also standardized. The graph paper is marked off in one millimeter blocks with each five square blocks indicated by a darkened line (see Figure 3-2). Horizontal measurements on the graph represent time while vertical measurements represent **amplitude.** At the rate of 25 millimeters per second, each one milli-

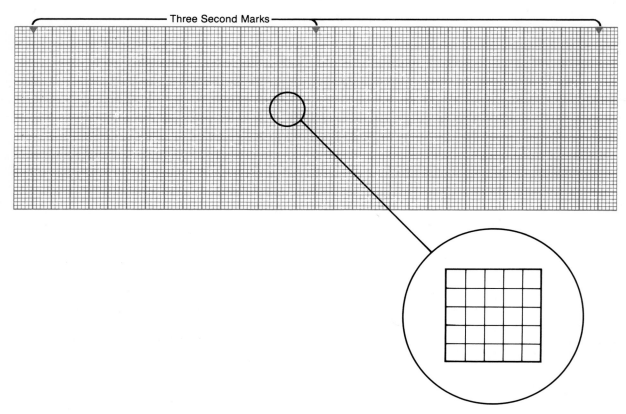

FIGURE 3-2
EKG Graph Paper

meter square on the graph paper represents a four-hundredths (0.04) second interval, and each darkened five millimeter block represents (5 millimeters × 0.04 seconds/millimeter = 0.2 seconds) two-tenths of a second. This enables the clinician to evaluate the rate and regularity of the electrocardiogram.

The graphs usually have indicators in the border of the graph paper that mark the paper in three-second intervals. Some indicators are vertical marks. Some are circles or wedges. Whatever the mark, it is provided to enable the clinician to determine rapidly, without counting each block, a time segment from the EKG. (Please refer to Figure 3-2.)

EKG Machines

Many EKG machines have switches to change the print rate from 25 millimeters per second to 50 millimeters per second when desired. This can be useful in cases of fast rhythms to give a more defined complex. It allows the fast EKG to be recorded in a kind of slow motion. It records twice as fast as usual, and the recorded complex is twice as wide as usual.

All EKG devices share some common characteristics such as a power

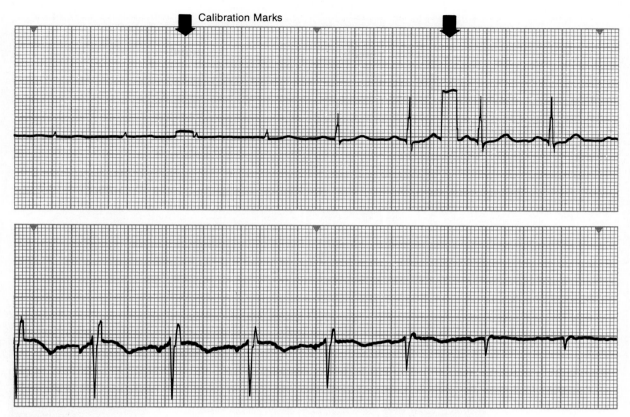

FIGURE 3-3
Calibration and Amplitude Adjustment

In the top EKG, the calibration mark shows the size adjustment of the EKG machine. The standard is exactly 10 mm tall. Adjustments should be made to the monitoring EKG as necessary to provide an easily recognizable cardiac complex. This rhythm started with a low adjustment and was turned up during recording. The first calibration mark is about 1 mm. The second is about 12.5 mm. This rhythm resulted from the calibration being turned down while it was being recorded, as shown in the bottom EKG.

switch, a switch which selects the lead, an adjustment for stylus heat (to make the marking on the paper darker or lighter), a calibration mechanism, and a device for adjustment of amplitude.

Amplitude, which is the height of the EKG measurements, is measured in millimeters. It has no special significance in dysrhythmia recognition and is normally calibrated at ten millimeters which represents one millivolt. **Calibration** enables the exact voltage of cardiac conduction to be evaluated. A more practical application of calibration for the monitoring lead is to enlarge small complexes, which may be difficult to read because of their size, or to turn down complexes which are so large, they have become difficult to read also.

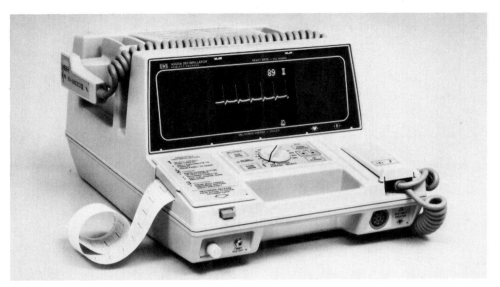

Photo courtesy of Hewlett-Packard Company

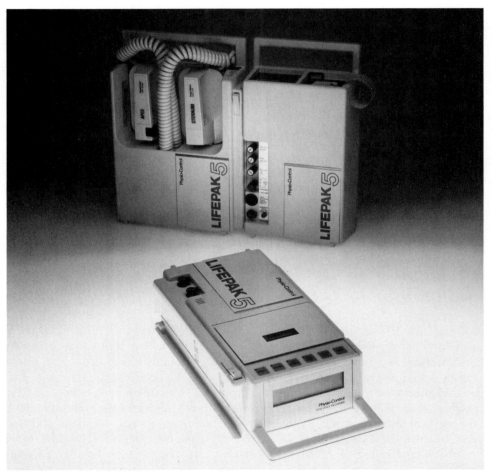

Photo courtesy of Physio-Control Corporation

FIGURE 3-4
Popular Monitor-Defibrillators
Top photo is an HP 43120A Defibrillator. Bottom photo is a Lifepak 5 Monitor Defibrillator.

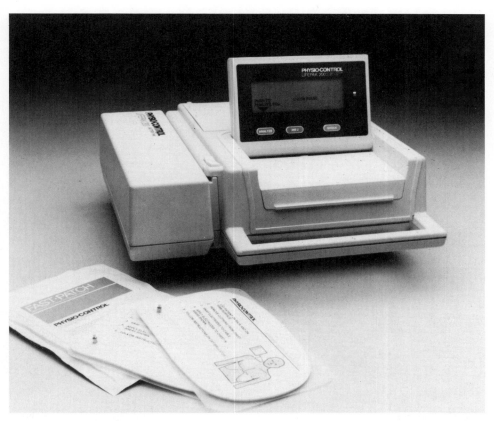

Photo courtesy of Physio-Control Corporation

FIGURE 3-5
Automatic Defibrillators
Physio-Control Lifepak 200 Automatic Advisory Defibrillator

Many EKG devices have a button or switch which records a mark on the upper border of the printed strip. This enables the clinician to indicate on the written EKG which of the various leads was recorded.

Defibrillators

A **defibrillator** is an electrical device with terminals called paddles which are hand held by the clinician and applied to the chest of a patient in ventricular fibrillation (an abnormal life-threatening cardiac dysrhythmia) and used to discharge electrical energy through the chest wall into the heart. The purpose of **defibrillation** is to simultaneously depolarize all cardiac cells in order to allow them to resume normal conduction activity after repolarization. Many EKG devices have ancillary defibrillators. All defibrillators have EKG monitoring devices.

Some defibrillators are designed to have sensing devices which can recognize ventricular fibrillation. After recognizing ventricular fibrillation the automatic defibrillator delivers a defibrillating shock automatically. This tech-

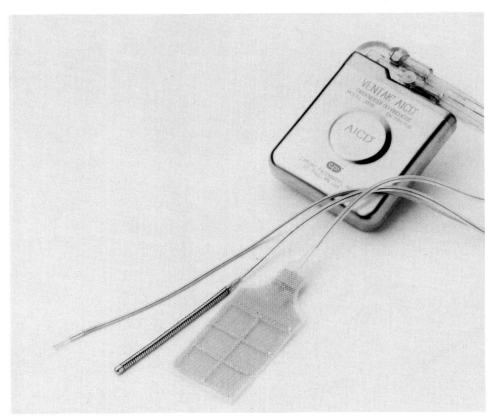

Photo courtesy of CPI, Inc.

FIGURE 3-6
The Ventak® Automatic Implantable Cardioverter Defibrillator

nique is sometimes referred to as **blind defibrillation** because it may be performed without an EKG interpretation by the clinician. Blind defibrillation may be most useful in prehospital cardiac arrest situations when fully trained Advanced Cardiac Life Support clinicians are not available.

One type of automatic defibrillator is surgically implantable, as a result of miniaturization available with electronic (integrated circuit) technology. The device is an automatic implantable cardioverter defibrillator (AICD) and is implanted in the abdomen of patients who are at high risk of ventricular fibrillation. A disadvantage of the device is current techniques require open heart surgery to insert two sensing electrodes and attach two cardioverting electrical pads to the epicardium. The advantage is a dramatic increase in long-term survival rates for patients at high risk of ventricular fibrillation.

The Monitoring Leads

Electrical flow in the heart is measured by externally applied electrodes in relationship to a direct line, called an **axis,** between the two poles. The locations of a set (one negative pole, one positive pole, and one ground) of electrodes is

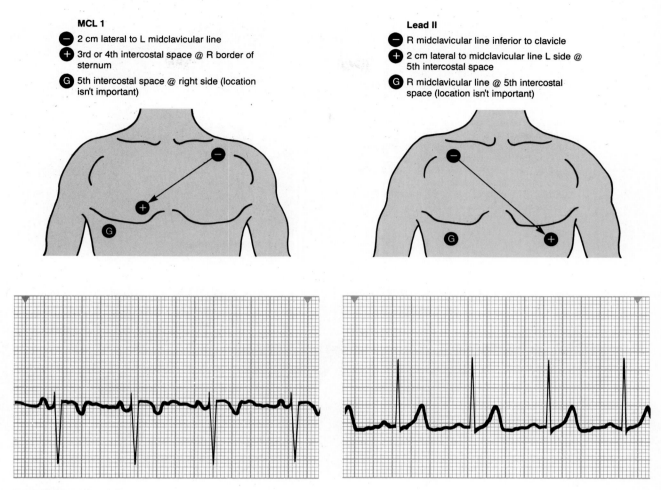

MCL 1
- ⊖ 2 cm lateral to L midclavicular line
- ⊕ 3rd or 4th intercostal space @ R border of sternum
- Ⓖ 5th intercostal space @ right side (location isn't important)

Lead II
- ⊖ R midclavicular line inferior to clavicle
- ⊕ 2 cm lateral to midclavicular line L side @ 5th intercostal space
- Ⓖ R midclavicular line @ 5th intercostal space (location isn't important)

FIGURE 3-7
Modified (Marriott's) Chest Lead 1 and Lead 2 Monitoring Leads

a lead. There are 12 established leads, each of which has a unique individual axis. Any lead may be used to continuously observe or *monitor* cardiac activity for the occurrence of dysrhythmias. Some leads are more popular for monitoring than others.

Limb lead II and a **modified chest lead I (MCL 1)** are the two most commonly used monitoring leads. Limb lead II is the most traditional monitoring lead but has the disadvantage of being in the way if defibrillation is required. MCL 1, also known as Marriott's chest lead, is an acceptable lead that does not interfere with defibrillation or auscultation but produces an EKG complex slightly different from the traditional lead II complex.

Lead V₁   The electrode is at the fourth intercostal space just to the right of the sternum.
Lead V₂   The electrode is at the fourth intercostal space just to the left of the sternum.
Lead V₃   The electrode is at the line midway between leads V₂ and V₄.
Lead V₄   The electrode is at the midclavicular line in the fifth interspace.
Lead V₅   The electrode is at the anterior axillary line at the same level as lead V₄.
Lead V₆   The electrode is at the midaxillary line at the same level as lead V₄.

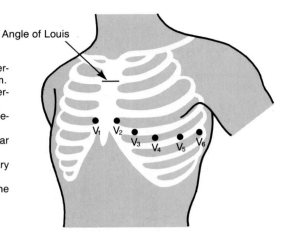

Chest Lead Placement

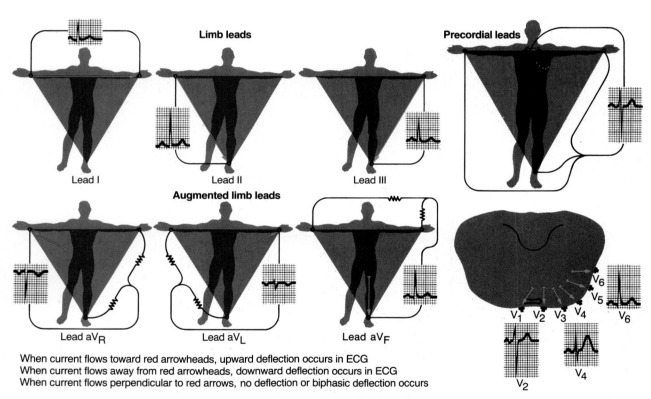

When current flows toward red arrowheads, upward deflection occurs in ECG
When current flows away from red arrowheads, downward deflection occurs in ECG
When current flows perpendicular to red arrows, no deflection or biphasic deflection occurs

FIGURE 3-8
Electrode Placement for the 12-Lead EKG

The Twelve Leads

Six of the 12 established leads are called **limb leads.** Three limb leads (1, 2, and 3) measure the cardiac electrical activity between two of the patient's extremities. These are called **bipolar limb leads** because each one measures from one pole (the negative electrode) to the second pole (the positive electrode).

Three other limb leads, aVR, aVL, and aVF, measure electrical activity between the patient's heart and one extremity. These latter are called **unipolar limb leads** because each measures from the posterior heart (electronically a combination of three extremity leads) to the positive pole (the positive electrode) on the anterior chest. The combination of the three extremity leads is done within the EKG device electronically.

A **bipolar lead** will require three electrodes, a positive pole electrode, a negative pole electrode, and a ground. A **unipolar lead** will require five electrodes, one positive pole electrode, one negative pole (a mathematical, electronic combination of three extremity electrodes), and a ground electrode.

Limb lead electrodes are applied to the patient's extremities. They are applied in some cases, for convenience of monitoring, to the chest on the axis that leads to the extremity. It appears to be a contradiction in terms to apply a limb lead to the chest, but for monitoring purposes it is the axis that is significant, not the location of the electrode on the axis.

The six chest leads (V1 through V6) are called **precordial leads.** They, like the aV leads, are unipolar and also require a combination of electrodes from the extremities to be electronically evaluated together to represent one pole (at the posterior heart). The positive electrode is then attached to the anterior chest in six specified locations. They have very specific axes and electrode locations. Locations of the electrodes for all 12 leads are listed in Figure 3-8.

Analysis of 12-lead electrocardiography is a sophisticated diagnostic technique which will not be addressed in this text.

Three Basic Laws of Electrocardiography

Evaluation of the electrical activity of the heart in the EKG will be greatly facilitated by keeping in mind the *three basic laws of electrocardiography.*[1] These three laws indicate how the propagated action potential wave (the cardiac conduction cycle) is interpreted by the electrodes of any lead. The three laws are as follows:

1. A positive deviation will be recorded in any lead if the wave of depolarization spreads toward the positive electrode on the axis of the lead.
2. A negative deviation will be recorded in any lead if the wave of depolarization spreads toward the negative electrode on the axis of the lead.
3. A biphasic (both positive and negative) deflection will be recorded in any lead if the wave of depolarization spreads away from the axis of the lead.

---

[1]A. L. Goldberger and E. Goldberger, *Clinical Electrocardiography,* 2nd ed. (St. Louis: The C. V. Mosby Co., 1981).

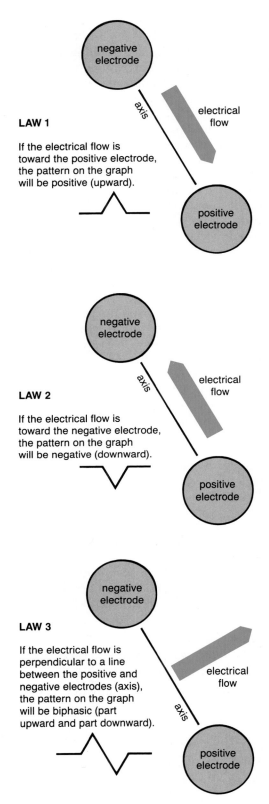

LAW 1

If the electrical flow is toward the positive electrode, the pattern on the graph will be positive (upward).

LAW 2

If the electrical flow is toward the negative electrode, the pattern on the graph will be negative (downward).

LAW 3

If the electrical flow is perpendicular to a line between the positive and negative electrodes (axis), the pattern on the graph will be biphasic (part upward and part downward).

FIGURE 3-9
Goldberger's Three Laws Graphically Represented

Law one means cardiac conduction traveling through the heart along the lead axis toward the positive electrode is interpreted as a deflection upwards (positively) from the isoelectric baseline. The deflection will return to baseline as the wave of depolarization ends. Any deflection from and return to baseline is a **wave.**

Law two says a downward (negative) wave will result from a cardiac conduction pathway that moves along the lead axis away from the positive electrode toward the negative electrode.

Law three is a combination of laws one and two. A cardiac conduction pathway that does not travel along the lead axis will result in a partially positive (upward from baseline) and partially negative (downward from baseline) wave. This is a biphasic wave. A wave pathway exactly perpendicular to the axis will be equally negative and positive.

Biphasic conduction, which is more towards the negative electrode than towards the positive one, will have greater amplitude downward than upward and the wave is said to have a *net deflection* which is negative. The negative portion of the EKG complex will deviate negatively from the baseline farther than the positive portion deviates positively from the baseline.

A net positive wave results from a conduction pathway that is more positive (more toward the positive electrode end of the lead axis) than negative.

Combined positive and negative waves may be compared like vectors. The sum of their differences will indicate a net deflection of positive or negative.

Electrocardiographic analysis of the heart can reveal a great deal of information, but cannot quantitatively rule out any medical emergency because of its normalcy.

False Negatives and False Positives

A **false negative** is an apparently normal EKG in a patient undergoing a medical problem, when that medical problem usually has an abnormal sign or symptom. An example is a patient having a myocardial infarction with no chest pain. Chest pain is associated with heart attack in 80 percent of all cases, so its absence in the patient with a heart attack is a false negative. It is negative because it is absent when it is normally present. It is false because the patient really is having a heart attack despite the absence of chest pain.

Many clinicians make the mistake of reading too much into a monitoring lead EKG and attempt to diagnose subtle electrocardiographic features such as **ischemia,** a pattern of injury, or the presence of block. Attempts to evaluate these subtleties in the monitoring lead may be frustrated by electronic devices within the monitor that affect the complex, mild irregularity in conduction or in electrode placement, and the possibility of false positives. A **false positive** is an apparently abnormal EKG without underlying pathology or disability.

Features which may be indicated by analysis of the 12-lead electrocardiogram include, but are not limited to, acute myocardial infarction, bundle branch block, valvular disease, pulmonary embolism, cardiac tamponade, aneurysm, hypothyroidism, acute electrolyte imbalance, chronic obstructive pulmonary disease, and so on.

A normal 12-lead EKG in a patient who is suffering a medical emergency, which is usually reflected in electrocardiographic analysis, is a false negative.

Analysis of the monitoring lead can reveal only major dysrhythmias.

Summary

Electrocardiograms are measured between two poles—the positive anode and the negative cathode. The poles are electrodes and have a variety of styles and shapes. These poles may be placed anywhere on the body, but preestablished locations called leads are most commonly used.

The electrodes are attached to a monitoring device by cables. The monitoring device amplifies and displays the EKG. The monitor usually contains a cathode ray tube and may have ancillary devices such as a strip writer or defibrillator.

The disadvantages of the cathode ray tube as the only display device for a monitor are that it is dynamic and does not provide a "still" EKG for evaluation and does not have a graphic background for detailed evaluation.

Heat sensitive EKG graph paper is marked by a heated stylus as the paper is drawn by it at a rate of 25 millimeters per second.

All electrocardiographs have a number of controls in common, such as a power switch, a calibration device, a stylus heat adjustment, a marking device, and a lead selector.

The 12 established leads each have an axis. Bipolar leads measure electrical activity on an axis between a negative electrode and a positive electrode. Unipolar leads measure electrical activity on an axis between a position at the posterior heart and the positive electrode. The position at the posterior heart is electronically established as a combination of three extremity leads. Limb leads may be applied to the torso of the patient if they are on the correct limb lead axis. The six chest leads are the precordial leads.

Goldberger's three laws of electrocardiography govern evaluation of electrical activity of the heart.

Twelve-lead electrocardiography may reveal a great deal of information about the heart, while monitoring lead electrocardiography is useful only for major dysrhythmia recognition.

Self-Study Questions

1. How many electrodes are used for a monitoring lead and what does each electrode represent?
2. What is conductive gel used for in recording an electrocardiogram?
3. List an advantage and three disadvantages to using the CRT as the primary monitoring device.
4. Explain how the electrocardiogram is recorded on EKG paper.
5. Discuss amplitude in terms of what it represents—to what amplitude is it calibrated and what advantages does adjustment of it offer to the technician?
6. How are each of multiple leads identified on the EKG?
7. If the EKG is switched to 50 millimeters per second, the three-second indicators actually represent what time increment?
8. What is the purpose of the ground electrode?
9. List the locations for electrodes for a 12-lead electrocardiogram.
10. List at least eight problems which may be diagnosed or confirmed by 12-lead electrocardiography.

11. Discuss the diagnostic limitations of monitoring lead electrocardiography.
12. Name the two most common monitoring leads and identify the locations of the electrodes for each.
13. List two advantages to using a strip writer to record an EKG.
14. What is the purpose of defibrillation?
15. Why can limb leads be applied to the patient's chest, and why are the leads attached to the chest?

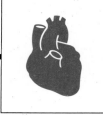

"We are plain quiet folk and have
no use for adventures.
Nasty disturbing uncomfortable
things!
Make you late for dinner!
I can't think what anybody
sees in them. . . ."

J. R. R. TOLKIEN

4

Normal Sinus Rhythm

OBJECTIVES

■ Identify and define the representative functions of the cardiac cycle and its components, including baseline, segments, waves, complexes, and intervals.

■ Relate the waves and deflections to electrode monitoring and directional travel of the cardiac impulses, and their normally associated mechanical activity.

■ Identify the characteristics of the normal cardiac cycle and of normal sinus rhythm, including rate, regularity, shape and deflection of waves, complexes and intervals.

■ Recognize and identify the common causes for artifact in the electrocardiogram.

KEY TERMINOLOGY

artifact
  60-cycle interference
baseline
block rule
cardiac contraction
cardiac cycle
  electrical
  mechanical
deflection
  negative
  positive
interval
  abbreviated
  elongated
  PP
  PR
  prolonged
  QRS
  RR
inversion
isoelectric
J point
normal sinus rhythm (NSR)

perfusion
QRS complex
rate
segment
  ST
six-second rule
spike
wave
  biphasic
  double prime
  P
  prime
  Q
  R
  S
  T
  U

Electrical activity of the heart is conducted by a propagated action potential in a wave-like manner through the heart. The electrocardiogram also records the electrical activity in wave-like patterns. That wave is recorded as a positive wave if the conduction travels toward the positive electrode and as a negative wave if it travels away from it.

The Cardiac Cycle

Each phase of the mechanical **cardiac cycle** is represented on the electrocardiographic cardiac cycle. The clinician must bear in mind that EKG activity alone is not evidence of cardiac contraction. **Cardiac contraction** is normally associated with electrical activity but exceptions may occur.

The **baseline** is a horizontal isoelectric line usually at the vertical midline of the graph paper. **Waves** are deflections away from and a return to the baseline. Waves may have a rounded or pointed form. A deflection away from the baseline which usually does not return is a **spike.** Spikes are not found on the normal EKG.

Deflections upward are positive, indicating a travel of conduction toward the positive electrode. A deflection downward is negative, indicating a conduction pathway away from the positive electrode. A wave which is partially positive and partially negative is said to be **biphasic.**

A **segment** is a portion of baseline between two waves. Segments are **isoelectric** and contain no waves. Segments may be elevated above or depressed

Pulses or blood pressures are the only valid criteria for perfusing cardiac contractions and must be checked and continually evaluated in the emergent patient regardless of electrocardiographic monitoring.

FIGURE 4-1
A Biphasic Wave
A biphasic wave, P wave, or QRS complex.

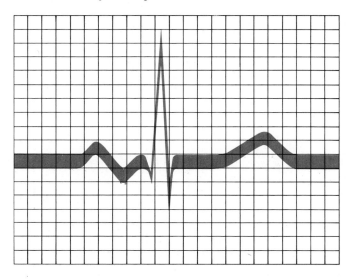

below the normal baseline. Any measurement of an EKG, containing one or more segments and one or more waves, is an **interval.**

Right and left atrial impulse formation and conduction (depolarization) is represented by one wave which is the **P wave.** The P wave is small (compared to the other waves of the EKG), rounded, and the first wave of the normal electrocardiographic complex.

There is a delay of conduction in the junction. This delay is not active conduction, but is actually an interruption of conduction. This delay has no depolarization or repolarization wave and therefore is represented by a lack of a wave (the baseline segment between the P wave and the QRS complex) during the cardiac cycle. Please refer to Figure 4-2.

The QRS Complex

Ventricular impulse conduction (depolarization) quite naturally follows the atrial depolarization and the atrioventricular node delay. The ventricles contract from the apex upwards. In order to do this the conduction must pass from the atrioventricular node through the bundle of His (without muscular contraction) downward to the apex of the heart and into the Purkinje fibers where muscular depolarization begins. As a result, within a very short time frame, the propagated action potential travels in different directions. This is represented on the EKG by a number of pointed waves. Because the waves occur so fast, they are measured together and form a complex of waves rather than a series of single waves. The waves are the Q, R, and S waves. The complex is the **QRS complex.** The complex is always called the QRS complex even if only one or two of the Q, R, or S waves are present. The QRS complex may normally be either positive, negative, or biphasic in the monitoring leads.

The **Q wave** is the first negative wave in the QRS complex which precedes the first positive wave. It represents the conduction of the stimulus through the septum. It is not unusual or abnormal for a QRS complex to have no Q wave.

FIGURE 4-2
The Normal Electrocardiographic Cycle
The normal electrocardiographic cardiac cycle of the P, QRS, T, and U waves.

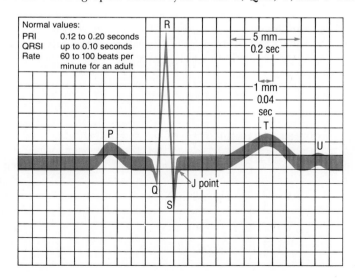

Normal values:	
PRI	0.12 to 0.20 seconds
QRSI	up to 0.10 seconds
Rate	60 to 100 beats per minute for an adult

The **R wave** is the first positive wave. It represents the conduction of the stimulus toward the left ventricle. Occasionally an EKG may have two R waves. The second R wave is called the **R prime wave.**

The **S wave** is the first negative wave after the R wave. It represents the conduction of the stimulus through both ventricles and (normally) mechanical muscular contraction of the ventricles.

Repolarization

The repolarization of the ventricles may also be measured electrocardiographically. Naturally the repolarization wave follows the depolarization wave. It is represented on the EKG as the rounded **T wave** (see Figure 4-2). A general rule is the T wave deflections, in any lead, usually follow the same direction as the net deflection of the QRS complex. The T wave, unlike the symmetrical P wave, tends to be mildly asymmetrical, looking like a small mountain with one sloping side.

The *atrial repolarization* generally is not strong enough to be read on the standard EKG. One possible explanation assumes the wave is lost in the much stronger QRS complex. This is something like having an explosion occur with a window breaking at the same time. An observer hears the explosion but not the breaking window because the explosion is so much louder. The electrocardiogram records only the strongest impulse it measures.

A small wave called the **U wave** may occasionally follow the T wave. It is not significant to monitoring electrocardiography and neither its presence nor its absence is considered abnormal. It is smaller than the P wave and represents a portion of ventricular repolarization. It is important to recognize it in order to avoid confusing it with other possible waves (see Figure 4-2).

The P, Q, R, S, T, and U designations for these waves are arbitrary and have no special significance.

Intervals

An **interval** is a measurement of time and can be from any point on the graph to any other horizontal point. Common intervals and segments are identified by these points, such as the PR interval, QRS interval, RR interval, PP interval, and the ST segment. Measurement of two intervals, the PRI and the QRSI, are essential to evaluating the EKG.

TABLE 4-1   Representative Portions of the EKG Complex

	Depolarization	Repolarization
	(stimulation)	(recovery)
Atrial	P wave	None
Ventricle	QRS complex	ST segment
		T wave
		U wave

The **PR interval** is measured from the start of the P wave to the start of the QRS complex and includes the PR segment. Normal values for the PR interval vary (from one EKG to another) within a normal range of twelve-hundredths (0.12) seconds to twenty-hundredths (0.20) seconds. PR intervals less than twelve-hundredths (0.12) seconds are **abbreviated** and values greater than twenty-hundredths (0.20) seconds are **prolonged** or **elongated.** PR intervals on any single EKG are normally consistent.

The **QRS interval** is measured from the start of the QRS complex to the end of the QRS complex. Normal values for the QRS interval vary, from one EKG to another, up to one-tenth (0.10) second. Any QRS interval longer than one-tenth (0.10) second is *wide*. QRS intervals on any EKG are also normally consistent.

The **R to R interval** is a measurement from the start of a QRS complex in a rhythm to the start of the next adjacent QRS complex. The RR interval may be measured from R wave to R wave in the regular rhythm with uniformed complexes (which are shaped alike). The pointed R waves form a clearly defined point of measure. This may be easier to rapidly identify and measure than the start of the complex.

The **P to P interval** is a measurement from the start of a P wave to the start of the next P wave in a rhythm. P waves are rounded and do not provide a more clearly defined point of measure as the R waves do. The PP interval, in a regular rhythm, should be the same measurement as the RR interval.

ST Segment

The **ST segment** is the short portion of baseline between the end of the S wave and the start of the T wave. Changes in the elevation of the ST segment throughout the complete 12-lead EKG may be a diagnostic tool. ST changes are not considered diagnostic in the single monitoring lead.

One last feature of the normal EKG which is neither a wave, segment,

FIGURE 4-3
J Point, Segments, and Intervals

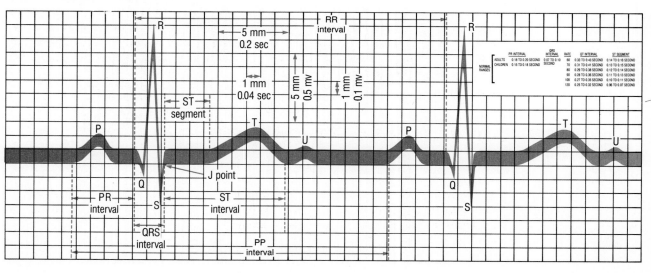

nor interval is the point at the conclusion of the QRS complex. This is the *junction* of the QRS interval and ST segment and is the **J point** (please refer to Figure 4-3).

Extra Waves

Any extra waves, such as a second positive wave, are identified as **prime** or if there are two extra waves **double-prime**. A second positive wave in the QRS complex would be an R prime wave. A third positive wave in the QRS complex would be an R double prime.

Inversion

An **inversion** is a conduction pathway opposite from what is normal for a particular lead. It is frequently confused with negative deflections, but an inversion is not always negative. Any normally positive wave, which is negatively deflected, is inverted. Any normally negative wave, which is positively deflected, is also inverted.

Rate

Rate is the single most important determinant in identifying the rhythm or dysrhythmia of an EKG. There are a variety of methods of determining rate. The most accurate is to count the number of cardiac cycles in a 60-second period. Most clinicians prefer a more rapid method.

FIGURE 4-4
Electrocardiographic Cycle with R Prime Wave
The R prime (R′) wave sometimes appears as a "notch" in the R wave because the R wave doesn't have time to return fully to baseline before the R prime (R′) wave is recorded.

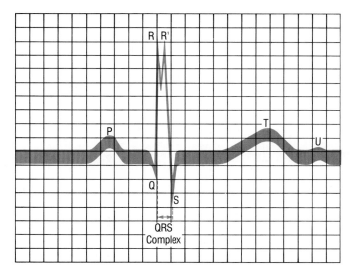

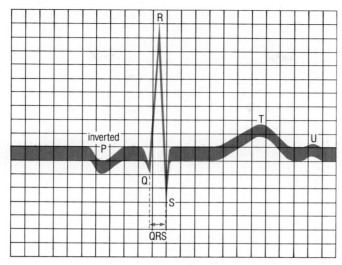

FIGURE 4-5
An Inverted P Wave
In this example the P wave is inverted (opposite from normal) and negative. However, not all inversions are negative.

The Six-Second Rule

The **six-second rule** is probably the most popular. Most EKG graph papers are marked in three second intervals. A count is taken of the number of cardiac complexes which are *completely within* a period of six seconds on the graph paper. This is multiplied by ten and a minute rate is quickly determined.

FIGURE 4-6
Six-Second Rule
Six complexes (within 6 seconds) times 10 yields 60 complexes in 60 seconds or a rate of 60 beats per minute. Pulses should always be confirmed clinically!

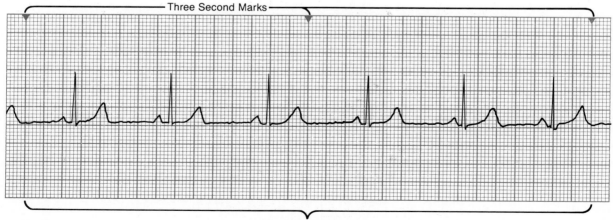

$$\text{(N beats/6 seconds)} \times \text{(60 seconds/minute)} = \text{N beats/minute}$$

Any complex in which the complete P, QRS, and T are not within the six-second markers is not counted. Many students have a tendency to see a number of full complexes, and one-half of another and estimate the rate at a value between the two whole numbers. This is inaccurate. For example, six full complexes and one-half of a seventh complex would be a rate of 60, not 65. Another common mistake is to count six full complexes with one-half complex at the start of the strip and a second one-half complex at the end of the strip and calculate this as a rate of 70. This also is inaccurate. An alternative to this kind of estimation (with half complexes) is to select another six-second EKG which is more clearly defined.

The Block Rule

A second method which allows an even more rapid determination of rate involves counting the number of boxes on the graph paper between any two cardiac complexes. This text shall address this rule, for the sake of convenience, as the **block rule.**

Each one millimeter box on the graph paper represents 0.04 seconds. There are fifteen hundred (1500) boxes in one minute [60 seconds/minute ÷ four-hundredths (0.04) seconds/box = 1500 boxes/minute].

The cardiac rate between any two adjacent complexes may be calculated. This is done by first counting the boxes (X boxes/beat) between any two complexes next to each other in a regular rhythm. This is the number of boxes per

FIGURE 4-7
Block Rule
The block rule is most easily applied by selecting a cardiac complex on a darkened line and counting the five millimeter blocks to the next complex. If the next complex isn't conveniently on a darkened line (a whole number of five mm blocks), its rate can be determined within a range of the darkened lines on either side of it. A second complex in this EKG rhythm, falling anywhere in range A, is tachycardic (>100 BPM); falling anywhere in range B, is normocardic (60 to 100 BPM); and falling anywhere in range C, is bradycardic (<60 BPM). For example the rate for a second complex falling at the asterisk would be between 60 and 75 beats per minute.

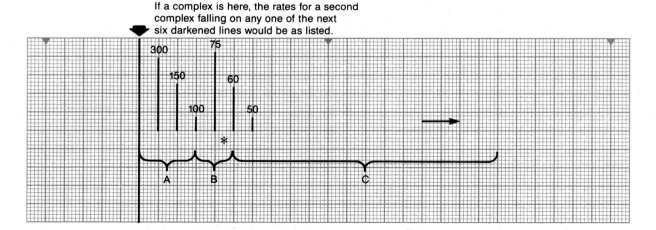

TABLE 4-2   Measurement of R to R Interval

Large Boxes	Seconds	Cardiac Rate/Minute
1	0.2	300
2	0.4	150
3	0.6	100
4	0.8	75
5	1.0	60
6	1.2	50

beat. Then the number of boxes per minute (1500 boxes/minute) is divided by the number of boxes per beat (X boxes/beat) to get a number of beats per minute (N beats/minute).

$$(1500 \text{ boxes/minute}) \div (X \text{ boxes/beat}) = N \text{ beats/minute}$$

There are disadvantages to this method. The rule is only applicable for determining the rate between two complexes. If the rhythm is regular, one may determine the rate of the rhythm in this manner. However, if the rhythm is irregular, one can only compare rates between different couplets of complexes. Counting several dozen boxes between beats may also defeat the purpose of using the method as a rapid method of rate determination. A more useful application of the rule is to count the boxes by fives, which are marked by darkened lines on the graph paper. Since a regular factor of five is used, it is convenient to memorize a number of rates so the rule may be quickly applied without mathematical operations. The clinician can look for a complex that is on a darkened line and count the boxes to the next complex for a reasonable estimate of cardiac rate.

The block rule, based on large squares, may not give you a precise rate if the two complexes are not an exact multiple of five boxes apart. It is generally accurate enough to differentiate tachydysrhythmia and bradydysrhythmia from normal rate.

FIGURE 4-8
Rate Calibrated Rule

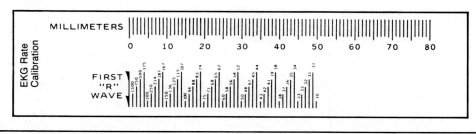

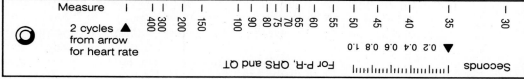

Top: Gail Walraven, Basic Arrhythmias, 2nd ed. rev. 1986. Reprinted by permission of Prentice-Hall, Inc., Englewood Cliffs, New Jersey.
Bottom: Courtesy of Aldomet

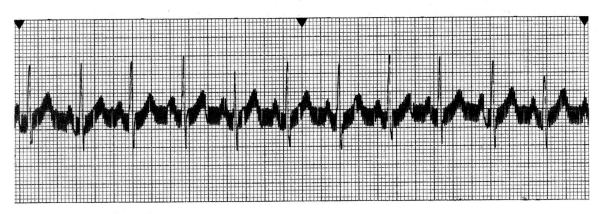

FIGURE 4-9
Sixty-Cycle Artifact

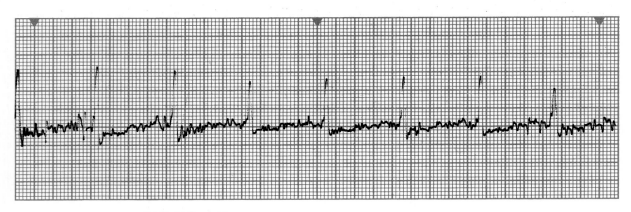

FIGURE 4-10
Baseline Artifact

Another method using an EKG rate calibrated ruler is popular. A ruler may be calibrated to measure between any two or any three complexes and express the measurement in units of complexes per minute. Again this method is accurate only if the rate is regular.

Artifact

The evaluation of the normal EKG is sometimes complicated by the recording of extraneous electrical activity resulting from causes such as poor electrode contact, interference by other electrical devices in the immediate vicinity, and even by patient movement. This kind of interference is **artifact.** Some types of artifact are readily identifiable by their shapes, such as **60-cycle interference** (interference from electrical appliances—commonly fluorescent lighting).

Artifact may mimic a number of dysrhythmias, especially atrial and ventricular fibrillation. This is another reason why *the clinician should confirm his interpretation of the EKG clinically, by checking pulses, pressures, and mental*

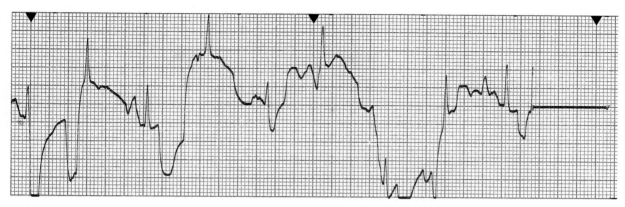

FIGURE 4-11
Patient Movement Artifact

status. Defibrillation of a stable patient suffering only from artifact is usually most unpopular with the patient. An old rule in the profession is do not perform CPR or defibrillation on any patient who must be restrained for the procedure.

Normal Sinus Rhythm

The **normal sinus rhythm (NSR)** is the most desired and most common EKG rhythm. It is a rhythm which has a perfusing rate of 60 to 100 complexes per minute. It is regular, with a normal PRI and QRSI for each beat. Each cardiac complex has one P wave, one QRS complex, one T wave, and possibly a U wave. The rhythm is called sinus, because it originates from the sinoatrial node.

> The clinician must remember, whatever method of rate determination is used, that the EKG rate must always be confirmed clinically with a check of the patient's pulse rate.

FIGURE 4-12
Normal Sinus Rhythm

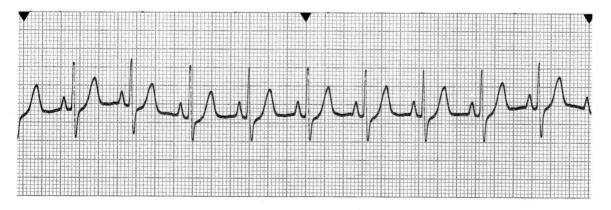

Summary

Electrical activity of the heart is recorded on the EKG. The electrical cardiac cycle is composed of a series of waves superimposed on an electrical neutral isoelectric baseline. Each portion of the electrical cycle normally represents an equivalent portion of the mechanical cardiac cycle.

The waves include the P, Q, R, S, T, and U waves. The P wave represents atrial depolarization. The Q, R, and S waves form the QRS complex and represent ventricular depolarization. The T wave, and any U waves which may be present, both represent ventricular repolarization. Atrial repolarization is not measured on the normal EKG. Additional waves are identified by their position in relation to the first R wave as either Q, R, or S waves and are designated as "prime" or even "double prime" (if there are two extra) waves.

Factors evaluated on an EKG include waves, shape of waves, complexes, segments, intervals, and rate. Inversion occurs when any wave in any lead is deflected in a direction opposite from its normal direction.

The major determinant of normalcy on the EKG is rate. Cardiac rate may be determined from the EKG in a number of ways, but must be clinically confirmed. Different methods include the 60-second count, the six-second rule, the block rule, and use of a calibrated ruler.

Evaluation of rate in portions of the cardiac cycle are time intervals. The two most important intervals are the PR and QRS intervals. The normal range for the PR interval is twelve-hundredths (0.12) to two-tenths (0.20) seconds. A range shorter than normal is considered "abbreviated" and longer is considered "elongated or prolonged." The normal QRS interval is up to one-tenth (0.10) second. Any interval longer than one-tenth second (0.10) is considered "wide."

The point at which the QRS complex returns to baseline is the junction of the S wave and the ST segment and is the "J point."

Normal sinus rhythm is the most desirable, "normal" rhythm. It is determined as a regular rhythm which has a rate of 60 to 100 beats per minute. The PR and QRS intervals are regular and within normal limits. There is one P and one T wave per QRS complex. There may be one U wave per complex. The U wave may or may not be present.

Artifact is interference in the EKG. There are several types including 60 cycle, patient movement, and poor electrode contact. Artifact must be considered in clinical and electrocardiographic evaluations of the patient.

Self-Study Questions

1. How does the clinician determine if the cardiac cycle is a perfusing cardiac contraction?
2. Differentiate between the mechanical and electrical cardiac cycle.
3. List the two major criteria by which cardiac perfusion is evaluated.
4. Identify the waves, complexes, segments, and intervals of the normal EKG and identify what each one represents on the mechanical cardiac cycle.
5. Which waves on the EKG are rounded and which are pointed?
6. What rule applies to evaluation of the T wave?
7. Discuss the preprinted markings on the EKG paper and what each portion of the graph represents.

8. Discuss the electrocardiographic evaluation of positive, negative, and biphasic wave forms.

9. List the acceptable ranges for rates, PRI, and QRSI for normal sinus rhythm.

10. List and discuss four methods of rate determination and the advantages or disadvantages of each.

11. Discuss inversion and differentiate it from negative deflection.

12. List and discuss three forms of artifact and how it can be identified and differentiated from similar dysrhythmias.

13. Identify and label the various waves of the normal cardiac complex.

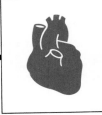

A house divided against itself
cannot stand.
I do not expect the Union
to be dissolved—
I do not expect the house
to fall—
But I do expect
it will cease to be divided.

ABRAHAM LINCOLN

5

Ectopy

OBJECTIVES

■ Identify the characteristics and significance of premature atrial, junctional, and ventricular contractions.

■ Define the characteristics of an escape beat. Differentially diagnose escape beats, PACs, PJCs, and PVCs.

■ List the criteria by which the clinical significance of ectopy is determined.

■ Identify indications for therapeutic intervention.

KEY TERMINOLOGY

bigeminy
bradycardia
cardiac irritability
cardiogenic shock
close coupled beats
compensatory pause
couplet
coupling interval
ectopic focus
ectopy
escape beat
   atrial
   junctional
   ventricular
fibrillation
focus
fusion beat
interpolated beat
multifocal
myocardial infarction
nodal contraction
non-compensatory pause
overdrive suppression
premature atrial contraction
   (PAC)
   aberrant PAC
premature junctional contraction
   (PJC)
premature ventricular contraction
   (PVC)
prognosis
quadrigeminy
retrograde
run
sinus rhythm
tachycardia
trigeminy
unifocal
ventricular premature beat (VPB)

The most common abnormality in an EKG is the presence of one or more extra cardiac cycles. These extra beats may occur in the otherwise normal sinus rhythm or in a dysrhythmia.

Extra contractions occur when conduction cells outside the sinoatrial node develop an abnormally increased automaticity. The sinoatrial node is unable to suppress the increased automaticity by normal **overdrive suppression.** The most automatic cell generates a stimulus which causes a contraction, and the cell becomes an abnormal pacemaker. Increased automaticity, resulting in extra heartbeats, is considered **cardiac irritability** because it is undesirable. Extra heartbeats are undesirable because they may negatively affect cardiac output, precede more serious dysrhythmias, or cause discomfort to the patient.

Another cause for extra beats occurs when the sinoatrial node becomes depressed, resulting in the cardiac rate slowing. Overdrive suppression weakens or fails because the sinoatrial node is no longer the most automatic site in the conduction system. The normal automaticity of another site in the conduction system may compete to overdrive the failing sinoatrial node and cause a conducted impulse.

An **ectopic focus** is a site of impulse formation located somewhere other than the sinoatrial node. Extra contractions are identified by the location of their foci and are known as **ectopic beats** or **ectopy** for short. Additional nomenclature indicates the physical site of the **focus,** defining the contraction as atrial, junctional, or ventricular.

Premature Ectopy

Ectopic beats are also categorized by their timing in the EKG. Premature contractions are beats that occur early, or "prematurely" in the rhythm. These premature beats occur in the EKG before the next regular beat can occur. Premature contractions are either **premature atrial contractions (PACs), premature junctional contractions (PJCs),** or **premature ventricular contractions (PVCs).** These are easily identifiable by their waves of conduction recorded on the EKG. Their ectopic origin results in an abnormal conduction pathway which is measurable on the EKG.

The primary difference between escape beats and premature contractions is the rate of the underlying rhythm.

Escape Ectopy

The other major form of ectopy is the contraction which occurs because the underlying rate is abnormally slow. These contractions are a compensatory mechanism of the heart for a **bradydysrhythmia.** Bradydysrhythmia is any abnormally slow cardiac rhythm. The lower range of a normal rate is 60 beats per minute. **Bradycardia** is any rhythm with a rate slower than 60. The **sinus rhythm** is depressed in bradydysrhythmia. The normal automaticity of the

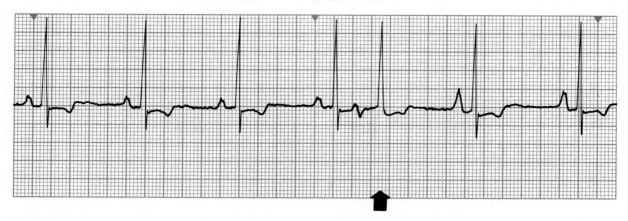

FIGURE 5-1
Premature Contraction
The fifth contraction is "premature" or early in the rhythm.

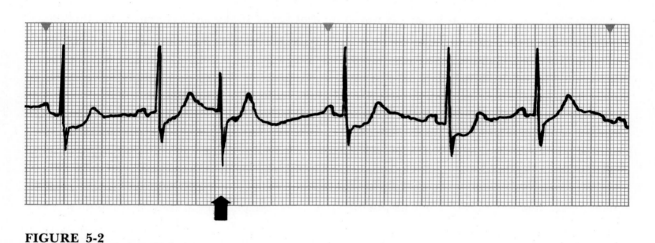

FIGURE 5-2
Bradycardia with Escape Beat
The third beat is an ectopic beat. It is considered an escape beat because its ectopic focus escaped normal overdrive suppression of the sinoatrial node.

other conduction cells of the heart competes with the overdrive suppression of the slowed sinus rhythm. This allows an ectopic focus to *escape* (normal overdrive suppression) to cause a contraction. Any ectopics in a bradycardic rhythm are classified as escape beats, even though they are generally premature in the rhythm. **Escape beats** are identified as **atrial escape beats, junctional escape beats,** or **ventricular escape beats,** depending on the location of their foci.

The difference between escape ectopy and premature ectopy is slight, but clinically important. Escape ectopy is a compensatory mechanism for a slow rate. The premature ectopy indicates cardiac irritability. Management of the patient must consider the underlying pathology. Escape ectopy is generally managed by addressing the bradycardia, while premature ectopy is managed directly with antidysrhythmic therapies.

An old cliché states that "Rules are made to be broken." In the case of evaluating ectopy and dysrhythmia, this appears to be too frequently true. Criteria are stated for each form of ectopy. Sometimes we forget to state them to the ectopics themselves. This gives rise to the occasional funny little beat (FLB) that does not seem to fit the criteria. The clinician should recall there are exceptions to every rule. A methodical approach should permit differential diagnosis of ectopy and dysrhythmia by comparing criteria and ruling out the most exceptional possibilities. In the case of doubt, it is wise to manage ectopics in a conservative manner as if they are ventricular and err on the margin of safety.

PACs

A **premature atrial contraction** has a pacemaker stimulus which arises from an ectopic focus (somewhere other than the sinoatrial node) within the two atria. The PAC depolarizes the atria prematurely in a mildly abnormal pattern, but is conducted normally from the atrioventricular node through the ventricles. It has a normal P, QRS, and T cardiac cycle.

The P wave is within normal limits. It may be different from the other P waves of the "regular" beats, but still within normal limits. For example, the PR interval of the regular rhythm may consistently be an eighteen-hundredths (0.18) second interval and the PAC can have a sixteen-hundredths (0.16) or twenty-hundredths (0.20) second interval.

The QRS complex and T wave are within normal limits and very similar to the QRS complexes and T waves of the regular beats.

There is a slight pause after the PAC before the regular rhythm resumes. The rhythm does not resume in its original timetable as if no ectopic beat had occurred. The pause is not long enough to compensate for the premature contraction and the entire timetable is moved forward slightly. The rhythm resumes in a regular fashion from its new beginning. This type of pause is called a **non-compensatory pause.**

FIGURE 5-3
Premature Atrial Contraction
The fifth beat is a premature atrial contraction.

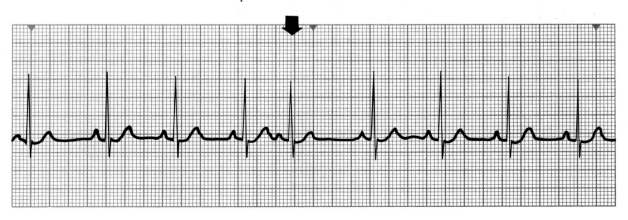

Any premature complex with a P wave within normal limits is a PAC. If it fails to meet the other criteria of atrial ectopy, it is classified as an **aberrant PAC.** For example, a premature complex with a normal P wave with a wide QRS complex is still a PAC, even though the QRS complex should be identical to the regular complexes.

Atrial ectopy is common. While it does not rule out the presence of significant heart disease, it is less malignant and has a less severe prognosis than ventricular ectopy. Premature atrial contractions (PACs) may result from many causes, including caffeine, alcohol, stress, emotional extremes, sympathetic nervous system stimulation, and heart disease or **myocardial infarction.**

PACs may contribute to **tachydysrhythmia.** Tachydysrhythmia includes any rhythm with a rate faster than the normal upper range of 100 beats per minute. Any tachydysrhythmia may compromise cardiac output by reducing the ventricular filling time and stroke volume. It is unusual for PACs to cause such compromise of cardiac output. They may be more significant in patients with underlying health problems, such as congestive heart failure, myocardial infarction, angina, or hypotension. Patients with PACs frequently report a sensation of *palpitations* or of having "skipped a heart beat."

PJCs

The **premature junctional contraction** has a pacemaker stimulus which arises from an ectopic focus (somewhere other than the sinoatrial node) within the junction. The PJC, also known as premature nodal contraction (PNC), depolarizes the atria prematurely in an abnormal pattern. The P wave is abnormal or may be buried in the QRS complex and absent. The stimulus originating in the junction may be conducted away from the junction toward the sinoatrial node resulting in an inversion of the P wave. The P wave may be abbreviated or less than the normal twelve-hundredths seconds. This occurs because the stimulus, starting from the junction, is conducted through the ventricles before it is fully conducted through the atria. It may also be **retrograde,** following the QRS complex, because the atria are depolarizing in reverse fashion (retro, meaning behind) and after the ventricles have depolarized.

If the P wave is within normal limits, the beat is not a PJC. The P wave in a PJC may be

1. inverted
2. absent
3. abbreviated
4. retrograde (follows the QRS)
5. retrograde, or abbreviated *and* inverted

The QRS complex and T wave are within normal limits. The PJC, like the PAC, is followed by a pause. The pause with a PJC is occasionally compensatory.

A **compensatory pause** is a pause (after a premature contraction) allowing the regular rhythm to resume with the next normal beat at its projected *original timing,* as if no ectopy had disrupted the sequence. A compensatory pause occurs when the interval between the regular beat preceding the ectopic to the regular beat following the ectopic is exactly twice the regular RRI and the orig-

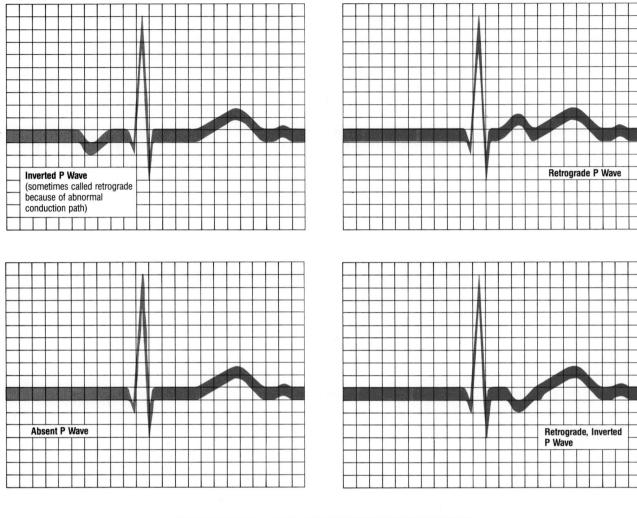

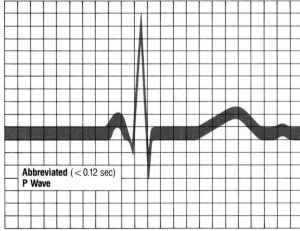

FIGURE 5-4
Abnormal P Waves Associated with Junctional Contractions

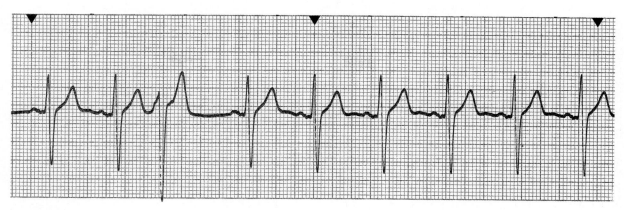

FIGURE 5-5
Premature Junctional Contraction

inal timetable is not upset. A pause always follows a premature contraction. If the pause is not long enough to allow the rhythm to resume in its original track, it is a non-compensatory pause. The pause after a PJC may be compensatory or non-compensatory.

PJCs may contribute to **tachycardia,** but most commonly are escape ectopy. Junctional contractions are more ominous than atrial ectopy and suggest an underlying pathology. The underlying bradycardia of junctional escape beats is slower than 60 beats per minute. This compromises the cardiac rate portion of the cardiac output equation and may reduce cardiac output to dangerous levels. Other major causes of PJCs are myocardial infarction and drug toxicity, especially digitalis. Patients suffering PJCs may report the same sensations as the patient with PACs. They may also present in **cardiogenic shock** from an underlying bradydysrhythmia or myocardial infarction.

> The primary differential characteristic between a PJC and a PAC is the abnormality of the P wave.

PVCs

The **premature ventricular contraction** has a pacemaker stimulus which arises from an ectopic focus within the ventricles. The PVC depolarizes the ventricles prematurely in an abnormal pattern. The P wave is absent. The QRS complex is always wide and equal to or greater than twelve hundredths (0.12) second. It is frequently bizarrely shaped with extra (or prime) waves. The T wave is usually deflected in the opposite direction to the net deflection of the QRS complex. There is a compensatory pause with ventricular ectopy (please see Figure 5-4).

PVCs are the most ominous of all ectopic beats. It is the ventricle which produces the cardiac output. Premature ventricular contractions indicate increased ventricular irritability. They may cause a non-perfusing beat by causing the ventricles to contract before they have adequately filled. They indicate a variety of causes, including myocardial infarction, ischemia, electrolyte imbalance, drug toxicity (especially digitalis), acidosis, pain, chronic obstructive pulmonary disease, gall bladder involvement, and sympathetic nervous system stimulation.

PVCs are usually premature ectopy, but can occur as escape ectopy. They

> The primary differential characteristic between a PVC and a PAC is the absence of the P wave and the width of the QRS complex.

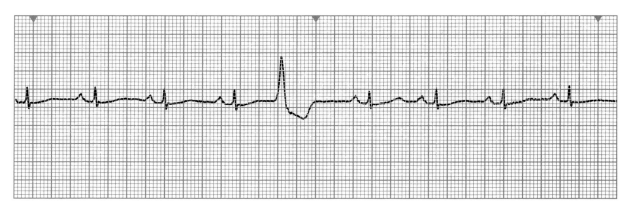

FIGURE 5-6
Premature Ventricular Contraction

may also occasionally exist in the healthy patient from benign causes. Most people have a premature contraction from time to time without serious impact. Many clinicians choose to preventively treat the presence of any ventricular ectopy coupled with medical symptoms until underlying pathology can be ruled out.

The American Heart Association has established the following *criteria for warning dysrhythmias* that require antidysrhythmic therapy.[1] These include

1. five or more premature ventricular complexes (PVCs) per minute.
2. PVCs which are close coupled (QR/QT less than 0.85).
3. those which fall on the T wave of the preceding beat.
4. or PVCs which occur in pairs, in runs (i.e., ventricular tachycardia).
5. or which are multiformed.

The primary differential characteristic between a PVC and a PJC is the width of the QRS complex.

Close coupled refers to the R wave of a PVC falling on the T wave of the preceding normal beat. The **R on T phenomena** is thought to be dangerous because it causes an action potential (QRS complex of the PVC) to occur during ventricular repolarization (T wave). The cardiac cells are in different stages of repolarization. Some are repolarized. Some are in the absolute refractory period, and some are in the relative refractory period. A stimulus occurring before repolarization is complete may cause a disorganized response which can set in motion a life-threatening dysrhythmia, such as **ventricular fibrillation. Fibrillation** is the totally random irregular response of myocardial cells. The danger of ventricular fibrillation is that no effective muscle contraction occurs. No cardiac output can occur, and the patient suffers cardiac arrest. Additional discussion of ventricular fibrillation may be found in Chapter 9, which provides an overview of ventricular dysrhythmia.

A **pair** or **couplet** is two ectopic beats in a row. A **run** is three or more ectopic beats together.

---

[1]Kevin M. McIntyre and A. James Lewis, eds., *Textbook of Advanced Cardiac Life Support* (Dallas, Texas: American Heart Association, 1983), p. 104.

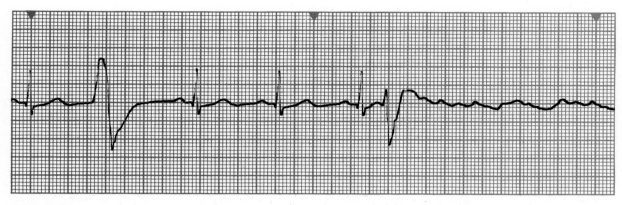

FIGURE 5-7
Close Coupled PVCs
The second of the two PVCs above is close coupled and falls on the T wave of the preceding beat.

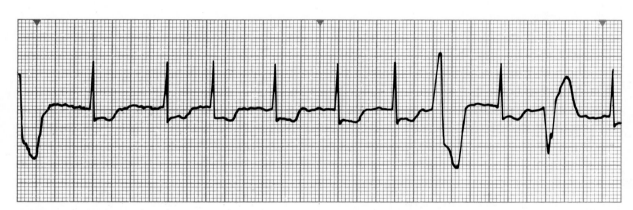

FIGURE 5-8
Multifocal PVCs

Multiformed or **multifocal** means the ectopic beats have more than one shape form, indicating there are multiple ectopic foci. PVCs that originate from one ectopic foci are shaped alike and are **unifocal** (or uniform). The presence of multiple ectopic foci is most ominous because it indicates the myocardium is very irritated and is subject to life-threatening **ventricular dysrhythmias.**

The **coupling interval** is the interval between the preceding regular beat and the ectopic beat. It is usually regular with unifocal PVCs. It may vary, like the shape varies, with multiformed (or multifocal) PVCs.

A PVC may occur about halfway between two normal beats. This is an **interpolated beat.** It is already compensatory in the overall rhythm and has no pause following it. The first regular beat after the interpolated beat occasionally has a prolonged PR interval.

An interpolated PVC occurs approximately on time in a regular rhythm and has no pause following it.

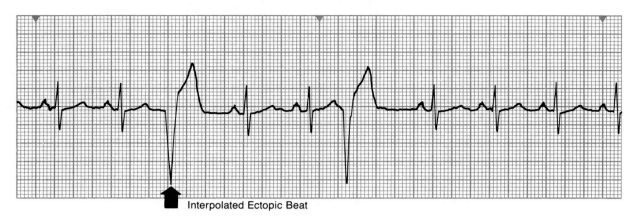

Interpolated Ectopic Beat

FIGURE 5-9
Interpolated Beat

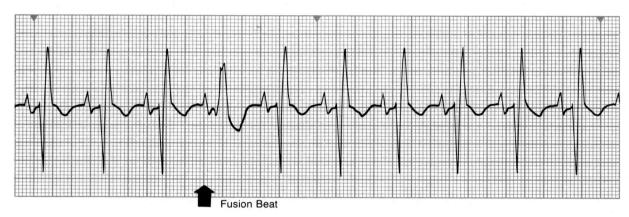

Fusion Beat

FIGURE 5-10
Fusion Beat

Another kind of rare premature ventricular contraction is the **fusion beat,** which occurs when the atria are depolarizing at the same time a ventricular contraction occurs. The resulting beat is a fusion of the normal beat that should have occurred (and was starting in the atria) and the premature ventricular contraction. It is on time and shares characteristics of a PVC and a normal beat. It is wide and bizarre, like a premature ventricular contraction. It usually has a P wave, like a normal complex. It may be difficult to distinguish between a PAC with aberrancy and a fusion beat. The presence of other ventricular or atrial ectopy in the rhythm may provide a clue to diagnosis. Management should be conservative (as if the beat is ventricular) if differentiation from a PAC cannot be made.

The following table compares the characteristics of premature contractions:

TABLE 5-1   Differentiation of Ectopy

	PAC	PJC	PVC
P Wave	Within Normal Limits	Absent or Abnormal	Absent
QRS Interval	Within Normal Limits (≤.10)	Within Normal Limits (≤.10)	Wide and Bizarre (≥.12 sec)
Pause	Non-Compensatory	← Either/Or →	Compensatory
T Wave	Same as Rhythm	Usually Same as Rhythm	Opposite to QRS Complex
Frequency	Most Common in Benign Dysrhythmia	Common in Pathology	Most Common in Pathology
Cause	Anxiety "Stimulants" Stress	Cardiac Irritability/ Escape Rhythm	Cardiac Irritability

Ectopy always must be assessed in regard to its clinical impact on the patient. Unusually fast or unusually slow dysrhythmias may compromise cardiac output and negatively affect the patient.

Any ectopy occurring every other beat is specifically identified as a bigeminal rhythm or as **bigeminy.** Ectopy occurring every third beat is trigeminal or **trigeminy.** Every fourth beat is quadrigeminal or **quadrigeminy.** Quadrigeminal ectopy is rare, because it usually does not remain regular. It is still important to identify the rhythm as atrial, junctional, or ventricular. For example, PVCs occurring every third beat would be trigeminal PVCs or ventricular trigeminy.

FIGURE 5-11
Regular Sinus Rhythm with Bigeminal PVCs

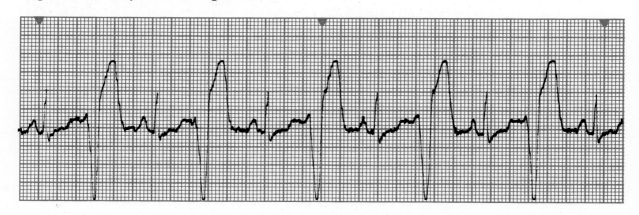

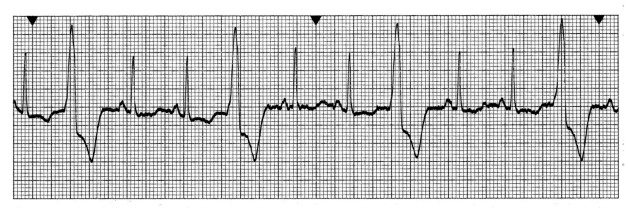

FIGURE 5-12
Regular Sinus Rhythm with Trigeminal PVCs

Summary

Premature ectopic beats are the most common abnormality in the EKG. Ectopy occurs when conduction cells other than the sinoatrial node have increased automaticity (cardiac irritability) or when the sinoatrial node has decreased automaticity.

The focus of an ectopic beat is the physical site of its formation. Ectopic beats are identified by their foci as premature atrial contractions (PACs), premature junctional contractions (PJCs), or premature ventricular contractions (PVCs).

Ectopy may be premature or escape. Premature ectopy contributes to faster than normal rhythms. Escape ectopy is compensating for an abnormally slow rhythm. Fast rhythms are tachydysrhythmias. Slow rhythms are bradydysrhythmias.

The difference between premature ectopy and escape ectopy is clinically important in determining management. Escape ectopy is managed by addressing the causal bradydysrhythmia. Premature ectopy is managed directly by addressing the increased cardiac irritability with antidysrhythmic therapies.

PACs are beats which are normally shaped. The PR interval may be irregular in comparison to the rest of the rhythm, but it is within normal limits. A PAC that is not normally shaped is considered aberrant. It is followed by a non-compensatory pause.

The PJC has an absent or abnormally shaped P wave. The rest of the beat is normally shaped. It may have a non-compensatory or compensatory pause following it. PJCs frequently are escape ectopy.

The PVC has no P wave. Its QRS complex is 0.12 seconds or wider. It is usually bizarre in shape. A compensatory pause follows the T wave. The T wave is usually deflected in a direction opposite to the net deflection of the QRS complex. While PVCs may be benign, they are the most serious of the premature beats. The PVC may be treated preventively with antidysrhythmic therapy or under the five indications provided by the American Heart Association.

Rhythms with ectopic beats occurring every other beat are bigeminal. Rhythms with ectopics occurring every third beat are trigeminal.

Self-Study Questions

1. What is the most common abnormality in an EKG?
2. Discuss and differentiate between the three major types of ectopy.
3. Discuss and differentiate between premature ectopy and escape ectopy. Include concepts of management in the discussion.
4. How do bradycardia and tachycardia compromise cardiac output?
5. What is an aberrant ectopic beat?
6. Differentiate between non-compensatory and compensatory pauses. List the type of ectopy in which each may occur.
7. List five types of abnormality of the P wave associated with PJCs.
8. Rank the three kinds of premature ectopy in descending order of severity (worst to least ominous).
9. Identify five criteria the AHA has established to indicate when therapy is needed for PVCs.
10. What is the significance of multifocal PVCs?
11. What is ventricular bigeminy?

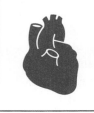

It's not far down to paradise
At least it's not for me
And if the wind is right
you can sail away
And find tranquility
The canvas can do miracles
Just you wait and see.

CHRISTOPHER CROSS

6

Sinus and Atrial Dysrhythmias

OBJECTIVES

■ Identify the characteristics and clinical significance of all major sinus and atrial dysrhythmias, including regular sinus rhythm, sinus bradycardia, sinus tachycardia, atrial tachycardia, sinus arrhythmia, atrial flutter, atrial fibrillation, sinus arrest, wandering atrial pacemaker, and electromechanical dissociation.

■ Perform an electrocardiogram analysis and differentially diagnose these dysrhythmias.

■ Identify indications for therapeutic intervention.

KEY TERMINOLOGY

atrial fibrillation
atrial flutter with variable block
atrial tachycardia
benign
capture
cardiotonic medication
electromechanical dissociation
fibrillatory wave (f wave)
flutter wave (F wave)
hypertrophy
ischemia
paroxysm
paroxysmal atrial tachycardia
regular sinus rhythm with PVC
sinus arrest
sinus arrhythmia
sinus bradycardia
sinus tachycardia
supraventricular dysrhythmia

Dysrhythmia, like ectopy, is identified by the origin of its foci or abnormality. Sinus and atrial dysrhythmias are in the general category of **supraventricular dysrhythmia.** Supraventricular identifies an origin anywhere above (supra) the ventricles. Rate is the single most important criterion of dysrhythmia recognition.

Sinus rhythms originate at the sinus (the sinoatrial) node. Normal sinus rhythm is the most desired of the sinus rhythms. Ectopy is not normal. The overall rhythm of any normal sinus rhythm (NSR) with occasional ectopy is classified **regular sinus rhythm** and the type of ectopy is identified. The term regular identifies the *normal* characteristics of the underlying sinus rhythm. For example, a normal sinus rhythm that contains a PVC would be identified as a **regular sinus rhythm with PVC.**

A number of dysrhythmias originate in the atria, at or near the sinus node and differ from normal sinus rhythm only in rate. The cardiac complexes are identical to those of NSR. These include sinus bradycardia, sinus tachycardia, and atrial tachycardia. Sinus rhythms originate at the sinoatrial node. Atrial rhythms originate from ectopic foci in the atria.

Sinus Bradycardia

Sinus bradycardia results when automaticity of the sinoatrial node is depressed resulting in a slowing of the cardiac rate to any rate below 60 beats per minute. It has classic sinus cardiac complexes, with normal waves and intervals. The only abnormality is rate. Some possible causes include parasympathetic stimulation, myocardial infarction, drug intoxications, especially digitalis or beta receptor site blocking agents, and many more.

Some persons have a normal bradycardiac rate. Many athletes typically develop cardiac athletic **hypertrophy.** The strong heart muscle has a powerful stroke volume and perfuses well with a resting cardiac rate of 60 or fewer beats per minute. This reinforces the need to clinically evaluate the patient.

FIGURE 6-1
Sinus Bradycardia

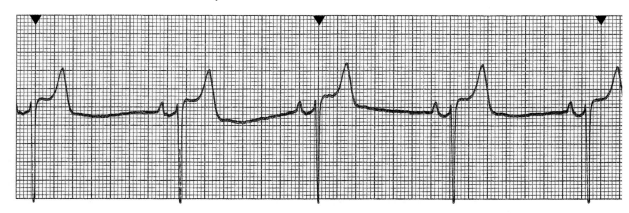

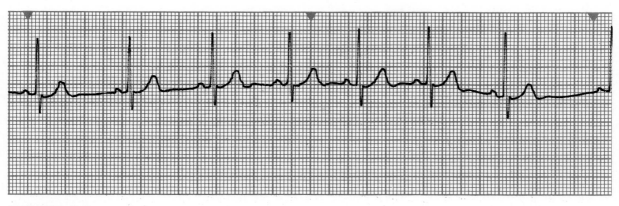

FIGURE 6-2
Sinus Arrhythmia

The bradydysrhythmic patient who is perfusing poorly will demonstrate shock symptoms as a result of decreased cardiac output. These symptoms include dizziness, mental confusion, fainting, fatigue or weakness, slumped posture, and, in the later stages, hypotension, especially when changing position from lying or sitting to standing (orthostatic hypotension). The only classic shock sign missing is tachycardia.

Compromise of cardiac output may occur with any bradydysrhythmia due to a decrease of the cardiac rate part of the cardiac output equation (discussed in Chapter 2).

Sinus Arrhythmia

The sinoatrial node is responsive to a variety of internal regulatory factors. Sympathetic and parasympathetic influences were discussed in Chapter 2. Another normal influence is its response to changing thoracic pressures. Thoracic pressures change slightly in response to respiration. This is a normal, mild parasympathetic vagal influence.

Sinus arrhythmia is the name for the **benign** dysrhythmia associated with respiratory influence of cardiac rate. It is considered benign because it does no harm to the individual and is rarely associated with underlying pathology. It occurs most commonly in young healthy individuals.

Sinus arrhythmia is a sinus rhythm with normal P, QRS, and T waves. It is slightly irregular. The rate slows slightly with respiratory expiration. The irregular effect occurs on a regular cycle. It occurs with each respiration. The EKG will be *regularly irregular*. A regularly irregular rhythm has an abnormality of some kind which is repeated on a regular cycle.

The effect on the EKG is a slight elongation of RR intervals during respiratory expiration. It is repeated throughout the rhythm. The elongation of the RR interval should not be confused with the pauses associated with ectopy. An easily distinguishable difference is that the cardiac complex of sinus arrhythmia does not fall prematurely (early) in the rhythm.

Sinus Arrest

Sinus arrest (or sinus pause) occurs when the sinoatrial node fails to function. The complete cardiac complex is absent from the rhythm. The dysrhythmia usually occurs with the absence of one (but sometimes more) complete cardiac

> Many sinus or atrial dysrhythmias may exist in the healthy patient and must be evaluated as a component of a thorough clinical assessment.

> Sinus arrhythmia may be easily distinguished from the pauses associated with ectopy because its complexes are not premature.

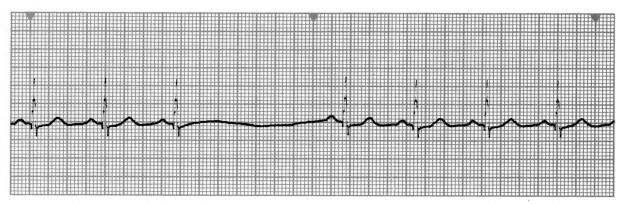

FIGURE 6-3
Sinus Arrest

Sinus arrest may be easily distinguished from the pauses associated with ectopy because its complexes are not premature. Sinus arrest may be easily distinguished from sinus arrhythmia because its occurrence is not cyclical.

complex from an otherwise regular sinus rhythm. The rhythm then returns to its regularity.

Sinus arrest may be the mechanism of sudden death syndrome whereby the patient goes from an apparently normal sinus rhythm into a rhythm, known as asystole, which has no electrical activity. Usually such a total failure of the sinoatrial node would be compensated with an ectopic escape rhythm.

Sinus arrest may be differentiated from sinus arrhythmia by its irregularity. It usually occurs with no association to other stimuli such as respiration. It is also a completely omitted complex as opposed to an elongation of R to R interval.

Sinus Tachycardia

Sinus tachycardia results when automaticity of the sinoatrial node is increased, resulting in speeding up the cardiac rate to anything between 100 and 150 beats per minute. A variety of causes include sympathetic stimulation; emotional extremes; exercise; drug intoxications, especially parasympathetic blocking agents, cocaine, or amphetamine abuse; pain; compensation for hypovolemia; myocardial infarction; and many more.

Like sinus rhythm and sinus bradycardia, sinus tachycardia has normal complexes. The only major abnormality is rate. Sinus tachycardia may become

FIGURE 6-4
Sinus Tachycardia

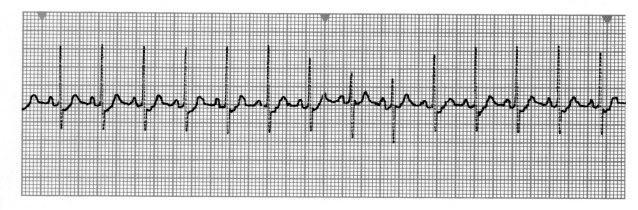

so fast that the P wave of each cardiac complex is actually backing up onto the T wave of the preceding complex. The rate increases cardiac workload and oxygen demand. An increase in oxygen demand, especially in the sick heart, frequently causes ischemia. Ischemia can cause mild changes in the cardiac complex, but it will still be within normal limits for the monitoring lead. Ischemia may also contribute to any existing myocardial infarction.

Atrial Tachycardia

Atrial tachycardia is a tachydysrhythmia that may be associated with a normal heart in a healthy adult. It frequently occurs in stress syndromes and with the use of caffeine, tobacco, and alcohol. It results when the automaticity of the atria is increased. The atria are forming ectopic pacemakers which contribute to or overdrive the sinus rate. This causes a cardiac rate of 150 to 250 beats per minute. The shape of the QRS complex is within normal limits. Three or more PACs in a row may constitute a run of atrial tachycardia. Atrial tachycardia usually responds well to vagal stimulation or cardioversion.

The P wave of the complex in atrial tachycardia may be on the T wave of the preceding complex. This may make the rhythm difficult to identify. If this occurs, the major criteria of identification are the rate and duration of the QRS complex.

If the P waves are hidden and the QRS complexes are aberrantly widened, the dysrhythmia may be indistinguishable from ventricular tachycardia.

Atrial tachycardia is frequently called **paroxysmal atrial tachycardia (PAT)** because of its tendency to occur transiently in **paroxysms.**

Atrial Flutter

Atrial flutter is an ectopic atrial tachydysrhythmia that usually indicates an underlying disease state of the heart. It has a well-defined atrial pacemaker rate of 250 to 350 beats per minute. The QRS complexes are within normal limits. The direct physiological cause is that multiple foci in the atria are competing to drive the heart. Some of the disease-related causes include valvular heart disease, right heart failure, myocardial infarction, and coronary artery disease.

Each ectopic stimulus results in an atrial depolarization **flutter wave.** This is frequently called an F wave (the uppercase form of the "F" is important).

> If the P wave of atrial tachycardia is buried on top of the T wave of the preceding complex, the major identifying criteria are rate and QRS complex duration.

> Sinus and atrial dysrhythmias that have normal EKG cardiac complexes and have only an abnormal rate include:
> 1. sinus bradycardia <60 beats per minute (bpm)
> 2. sinus tachycardia >100 bpm and ≤150 bpm
> 3. atrial tachycardia >150 bpm and ≤250 bpm.

FIGURE 6-5
Atrial Tachycardia

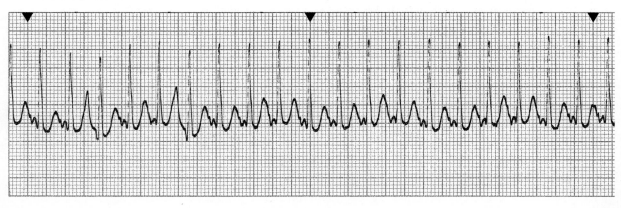

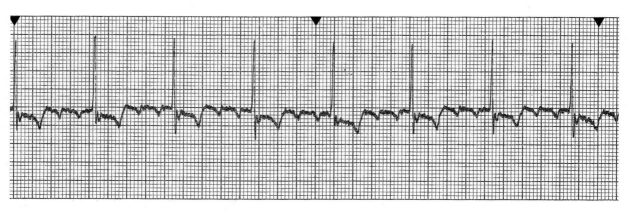

FIGURE 6-6
Atrial Flutter Without Buried F Wave

These waves are slightly more pointed than the normal P wave and form a *saw-toothed pattern* (referring to their similarity to the teeth of a carpenter's saw blade) on the EKG. The waves are clear, rounded with a slight point, well defined, and repeated without a segment of baseline between them.

Flutter waves are clear, rounded, slightly pointed, well-defined and repeated. They form a saw-toothed pattern.

The atria are depolarizing so fast the atrioventricular node and the rest of the conduction system cannot keep up with and respond to each atrial stimulus. There are, as a result, more atrial beats than ventricular beats. It is rare for an atrial flutter to have the same atrial and ventricular rates. The ventricular response may be tachycardic, but is usually in the normal range of 60 to 100 beats per minute.

The QRS complexes of the ventricular responses are within normal limits and are usually regular. There will be a ratio of two, three, four, or even more flutter waves to each QRS complex. The flutter waves are regular and can be measured with a caliper. The rate occasionally results in a flutter wave being buried in the QRS complex. Any buried waves can be discovered by comparing the waves' regularity with a caliper and predicting if one will fall in the QRS complex.

The ratio of F waves to QRS complexes is referred to as a **block,** meaning there is more than one F wave to each QRS complex. The term block is commonly used because it is descriptive of the P (atrial) to R (ventricular) ratio being two or more to one. This may be misleading in relationship to the dys-

FIGURE 6-7
Atrial Flutter with Buried F Wave

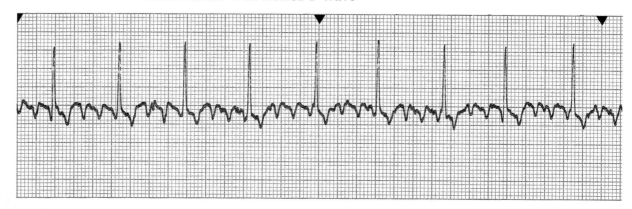

rhythmic heart blocks reviewed in Chapter 8. The physiological problem is one of conduction. The atria are firing before the junction has repolarized. The junction and ventricles are in their refractory periods and are unable to *capture or propagate* the action potentials of the atrial ectopic impulse.

The normal function of the atrioventricular node is to delay impulse conduction. In atrial flutter, it does its job well. This is very much to the advantage of the heart for a ventricular response to every F wave would result in a rapid ventricular rate with very short filling time and acutely reduced cardiac output.

The QRS complexes of atrial flutter are almost always regular. When it is irregular, the irregularity is regular and the F wave to R wave ratio varies in a regular pattern, such as two to one, then three to one, then two to one again. This is called **atrial flutter with variable block.**

Atrial Fibrillation

Atrial fibrillation is a very common dysrhythmia. It occurs in patients with healthy hearts and those with cardiac disease. Atrial fibrillation may be a paroxysmal event lasting for minutes or hours. It also may be a chronic dysrhythmia lasting for weeks or months. A few of the causes of this dysrhythmia include myocardial infarction, pulmonary embolus, hypertension, coronary artery disease, cardiac valvular stenosis, and many more.

Atrial fibrillation has fibrillatory atrial impulses called **fibrillatory waves** or f waves. The QRS complexes fall within normal limits. (Fibrillatory waves are represented by a lowercase "f" to differentiate them from flutter waves.) The f waves theoretically occur at a rate of 350 or more beats per minute. The atrial rate is not actually measurable. The atrial rate is characteristically represented as a wavy or even a flat baseline. In an atrial fibrillation rhythm some occasional f waves may resemble flutter waves. This occurs in atrial fibrillation at the slower rates around 350 atrial BPM. These occasional, flutter-like, fibrillatory waves are not well defined, regular, and repeated, as F waves are, throughout the rhythm.

The ventricular rate of atrial fibrillation is usually within a normal sinus rate range. It also may be slow or fast. The lack of an organized atrial depolarization and mechanical contraction robs the heart of its atrial kick. Ventricular filling is compromised and cardiac output is diminished. *Atrial fibrillation is generally not a life-threatening dysrhythmia and should not be confused with life-threatening ventricular fibrillation.*

Course fibrillatory (f) waves may be distinguished from flutter (F) waves because they are not regular, and are repeated throughout the rhythm.

FIGURE 6-8
Atrial Flutter with Variable Block

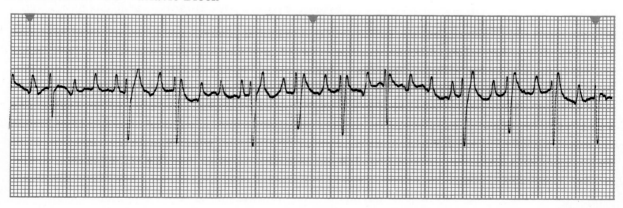

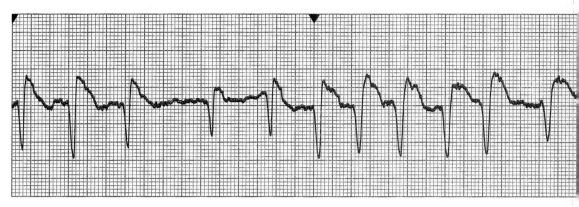

FIGURE 6-9
Atrial Fibrillation

Atrial fibrillation has irregularly irregular R to R intervals throughout the rhythm.

The patient with atrial fibrillation with a normal rate of ventricular response is usually asymptomatic (from the dysrhythmia). A fast ventricular response to atrial fibrillation compromises the filling time even more and may produce a greater reduction of cardiac output. The patient in atrial fibrillation with rapid ventricular response may present with shock symptoms. If the duration is chronic, the patient may also present with congestive heart failure.

The hallmark of atrial fibrillation is that it is the only common dysrhythmia that has irregularly irregular R to R intervals throughout the rhythm.

The baseline of an atrial fibrillation between ventricular complexes (and their T waves) is usually an irregular wavy line. It also may be flat when the atrial rate is very fast because the fibrillatory waves are very small.

Baseline artifact may be differentiated from atrial fibrillation by the regularity of the QRS complexes and by the presence of P waves under the superimposed artifact.

Baseline artifact may mimic atrial fibrillation. Baseline artifact can usually be ruled out by evaluation of the QRS complexes of the rhythm. The QRS complexes of atrial fibrillation are almost always irregularly irregular. Another indication of a normal rhythm with baseline artifact is that the artifact is usually small and may be superimposed over a visible, consistently regular P wave.

Summary

Rhythms and dysrhythmias originating from foci above the ventricles are supraventricular. Sinus rhythms and dysrhythmias originate in the sinoatrial node. Atrial dysrhythmias originate from foci in the atria.

Sinus rhythms include sinus bradycardia, sinus arrhythmia, sinus arrest, normal sinus rhythm, regular sinus rhythm, and sinus tachycardia. Sinus rhythms are identified as those rhythms with a normal cardiac complex and a rate of under 150 beats per minute.

Sinus bradycardia, normal sinus rhythm, and sinus tachycardia differ on the EKG only in rate. Sinus bradycardia is a sinus rhythm with a rate less than 60 beats per minute. Normal sinus rhythm is a sinus rhythm with no abnormalities and a rate within the range from 60 to 100 beats per minute. Regular sinus rhythm is the name given to normal sinus rhythm which has some abnormality such as ectopy superimposed on the rhythm. Sinus tachycardia is a sinus rhythm within the range of 100 to 150 beats per minute:

Sinus arrhythmia is a benign dysrhythmia with a normal rate of 60 to 100 beats per minute. It occurs in normal persons. It is distinguished by a slowing of cardiac rate in association with the vagal influence of respiratory expiration.

It is irregular, but the irregularity occurs in a cycle associated with respiration. The rhythm is considered regularly irregular. It is differentiated from the pauses associated with ectopy by the absence of premature contractions.

Sinus arrest occurs when a complete cardiac cycle is dropped from the rhythm, as a result of the sinoatrial node's failure to fire. It is differentiated from ectopic pauses by the absence of premature contractions. It is differentiated from sinus arrhythmia because its occurrence is not cyclical. It usually occurs in an underlying regular sinus rhythm of normal rate.

Atrial tachycardia is a supraventricular tachydysrhythmia with a range of rate from 150 to 250 beats per minute. It has a normal cardiac complex and arises from ectopic foci within the atria. It is sometimes called paroxysmal atrial tachycardia (PAT) because of its tendency to occur in paroxysms. Atrial tachycardia with aberrancy may be indistinguishable from ventricular tachycardia.

Atrial flutter is a supraventricular tachydysrhythmia with a range of atrial rate from 250 to 350 beats per minute. Its ventricular rate may vary from normal to tachycardic. This dysrhythmia is usually associated with myocardial pathology. The atrial waves are flutter waves and are generally rounded, regular, and slightly pointed. The ventricular response is usually regular. Ventricular response may occasionally be regularly irregular with a variable atrioventricular conduction ratio of F waves to QRS complexes.

Atrial fibrillation is a supraventricular tachydysrhythmia with an unmeasurable atrial rate of 350 or more beats per minute. The ventricular response is usually in a normal range, but may be bradydysrhythmic or tachydysrhythmic. The ventricular response is irregularly irregular. The QRS complexes are within normal limits. The baseline may be wavy or flat. Occasional f (fibrillatory) waves may mimic F (flutter) waves, but will not be regular and repeated throughout the dysrhythmia. Baseline artifact may mimic atrial fibrillation, but may be differentially evaluated by comparison of the R to R intervals for regularity.

Self-Study Questions

1. What is the single most important criterion of dysrhythmia recognition?
2. Discuss the difference between normal sinus rhythm and regular sinus rhythm.
3. List and discuss the differential characteristics of five sinus dysrhythmias.
4. Differentiate, by rate, between sinus bradycardia, normal sinus rhythm, sinus tachycardia, atrial tachycardia, atrial flutter, and atrial fibrillation.
5. Discuss the classification difference between sinus dysrhythmias and atrial dysrhythmias.
6. Discuss the differentiation between sinus arrhythmia, sinus arrest, and regular sinus rhythm with premature ectopy.
7. Discuss the major differences between atrial flutter and fibrillatory waves.
8. Discuss the term block when applied to atrial flutter.
9. Explain how atrial rate is determined when QRS complexes may be superimposed over flutter waves.
10. What is the hallmark of atrial fibrillation?
11. Discuss the physiological mechanism by which cardiac output is compromised by tachydysrhythmia and bradydysrhythmia.
12. Explain how atrial fibrillation may be differentiated from baseline artifact.
13. Explain how course f waves may be differentiated from F waves.

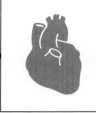

**You can go to any place
and any time you wish to go.
You must begin by knowing
you've already arrived.**

RICHARD BACH

7

Junctional Dysrhythmias

OBJECTIVES

- Identify the characteristics and clinical significance of all major junctional dysrhythmias, including junctional rhythm, accelerated junctional rhythm, and junctional tachycardia.

- Perform an electrocardiogram analysis and differentially diagnose these dysrhythmias, including all major sinus and atrial dysrhythmias.

- Identify indications for therapeutic intervention.

KEY TERMINOLOGY

accelerated junctional rhythm
junction
junctional dysrhythmia
junctional escape rhythm
junctional rhythm
junctional tachycardia
myopathy
nodal rhythm
premature junctional contractions

Junctional dysrhythmias, also known as nodal rhythms, are usually an escape mechanism. This results in the junctional dysrhythmias frequently being called junctional escape rhythms.

The foci driving the heart originate in the myocardial junction. The atria depolarize in a retrograde fashion, from the junction upward. This produces the abnormal P waves associated with premature junctional contractions. The ventricles depolarize from the junction downward in a fairly normal fashion. This produces QRS complexes of normal duration. The combination of abnormal or buried P waves with normal QRS complexes is classically junctional.

The junction has an intrinsic firing rate of 40 to 60 beats per minute. Failure of the sinoatrial node and atria to pace the heart result in less dominant pacemakers becoming dominant. The junctional firing rate is then dominant to the ventricular firing rate of 15 to 40 beats per minute. Junctional dysrhythmias are usually driven by the most automatic pacemaker of the junction in response to the failure of the sinoatrial node. This results in the dysrhythmias being regular. This regularity is an identifying characteristic used to differentiate fine atrial fibrillation with slow ventricular response from junctional dysrhythmia.

Junctional dysrhythmias are classified in three categories, as determined by rate. These are junctional rhythm, accelerated junctional rhythm, and junctional tachycardia. The apparent interchangeability of the terms "junctional rhythm" and "junctional dysrhythmia" may be confusing. The term "dysrhythmia" in this context applies to the junctional rhythms as a group because they are abnormal rhythms. The term "junctional rhythm" is the name of a junctional dysrhythmia. The terms may be used interchangeably.

Junctional rhythm is a run of three or more consecutive junctional contractions. Extended pauses in sinus and atrial conduction will normally result in junctional escape mechanisms. The dysrhythmia is usually extremely regu-

Fine atrial fibrillation with a flat baseline and slow ventricular response may be differentiated from junctional dysrhythmia by the regularity of junctional rhythm.

FIGURE 7-1
Junctional Rhythm

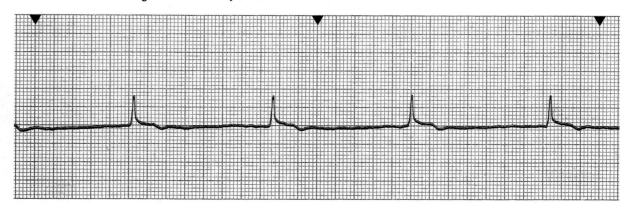

lar. P waves are either buried, inverted, retrograde and following the QRS complex, or abbreviated. The rate is within a range of 40 to 60 beats per minute and is usually around 60.

Accelerated junctional rhythm is a dysrhythmia which exceeds the intrinsic firing rate of the junctions. It is a junctional rhythm with a rate greater than 60 beats per minute but less than 100 beats. This describes a rate faster than normal for the junctional region, but not fast enough to qualify as a tachydysrhythmia. It has the other characteristics of junctional rhythm.

Tachydysrhythmia has been previously defined as a dysrhythmia with a rate greater than 100 beats per minute. Junctional tachycardia is a junctional rhythm with a rate of over 100 beats per minute. It has the other characteristics of junctional rhythm.

Junctional tachycardia may be difficult to distinguish from atrial tachycardia because of the tendency of atrial tachycardia to back up its P waves to the preceding complex's T wave. Clinically junctional tachycardia and atrial tachycardia have the same significance and are managed in the same manner. The lack of importance for differentiation between the two is indicated by the common usage of *supraventricular* as a descriptive identification.

Junctional dysrhythmias may occur in response to digitalis toxicity, myocardial infarction, ischemia, electrolyte imbalance, parasympathetic or sympathetic stimulation, and cardiac atrial **myopathy.**

FIGURE 7-2
Accelerated Junctional Rhythm

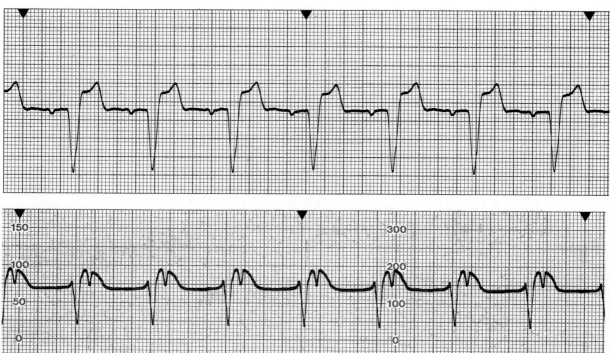

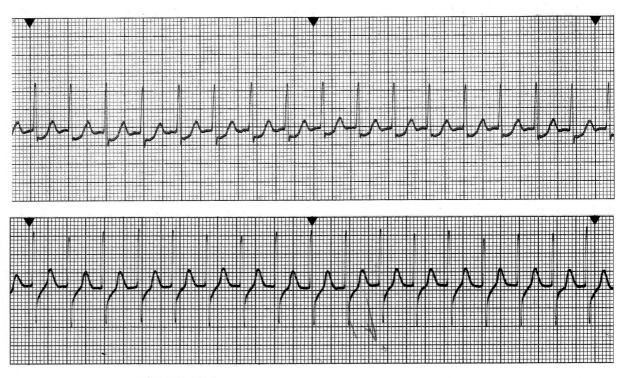

FIGURE 7-3
Junctional Tachycardia

Management is directed at elimination of the cause. The bradydysrhythmia junctional dysrhythmia that is hemodynamically symptomatic is managed initially with **parasympathetic blocking agents.** If it does not respond, it is subsequently managed with **sympathetic stimulating agents.** The use of a mechanical pacemaker is rarely necessary. The tachydysrhythmia junctional dysrhythmia is managed in the same manner as atrial tachycardia.

Summary

Junctional dysrhythmias are usually escape rhythms that are compensating for the failure of the sinoatrial node and atria to pace the heart.

Junctional dysrhythmias are categorized into three dysrhythmias, as determined by rate. Junctional rhythm has a rate of 40 to 60 beats per minute. Accelerated junctional rhythm has a rate of 60 to 100 beats per minute. Junctional tachycardia has a rate of over 100 beats per minute. Each junctional dysrhythmia has the characteristics of premature junctional contractions, regularity, and is a run of three or more consecutive junctional beats.

Clinical significance and management of slow junctional rhythms are the same as for sinus bradycardia. Junctional tachycardia is managed in the same manner as atrial tachycardia.

Self-Study Questions

1. Discuss and differentiate between the three junctional dysrhythmias. Include an evaluation of rate.
2. Explain the role of the automaticity of the junctions in determining the rate of junctional rhythm.
3. Differentiate between junctional rhythm without P waves and a slow atrial fibrillation with a flat baseline.
4. Discuss why junctional rhythms are frequently labeled *escape* rhythms. Why does the junction escape overdrive suppression before the ventricles do?
5. Discuss the indications for therapeutic management of junctional dysrhythmias.

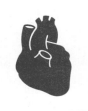

I know not how . . .
For fear of what might fall,
so to prevent
The time of life . . .
To stay the providence
of some high powers
That govern us below

If we do meet again,
why, we shall smile;
If not, why, then,
this parting was
well made. . . .

SHAKESPEARE

8

Heart Blocks

OBJECTIVES

■ Identify the characteristics and clinical significance of all major forms of dysrhythmic heart block, including first degree heart block, second degree Wenckebach (Mobitz I) heart block, second degree Mobitz II heart block, and third degree (complete) heart block.

■ Perform an electrocardiogram analysis and differentially diagnose these dysrhythmias, including sinus, atrial, and junctional dysrhythmias.

■ Identify indications for therapeutic intervention.

KEY TERMINOLOGY

atrioventricular node
automaticity
bradydysrhythmia
bundle branch block
bundle of His
cardiac output
cardiogenic shock
conductivity
heart block dysrhythmias
   complete
   first degree
   Mobitz I
   Mobitz II
   second degree
   third degree
   Wenckebach
hemodynamically symptomatic
ischemia
pacemaker (mechanical)
parasympathetic effect
sympathetic effect

Heart blocks are a common form of bradydysrhythmia and are particularly easy to recognize. The term block refers to an interruption of cardiac conduction along the normal conduction pathway, much like a road block interrupts traffic along a normal roadway. Cardiac conduction does not stop because of a heart block, no more than a road block stops traffic. A *detour* occurs. That detour is measurable on the EKG and permits the clinician to diagnose the dysrhythmia.

The conduction pathway is either impaired or completely disabled in most heart blocks. The most susceptible area of the pathway is at the atrioventricular node and in the bundle of His. The intra-atrial pathways and Purkinje fibers are so numerous that an infarct or other event affecting them, which

FIGURE 8-1
Roadblock with Detour

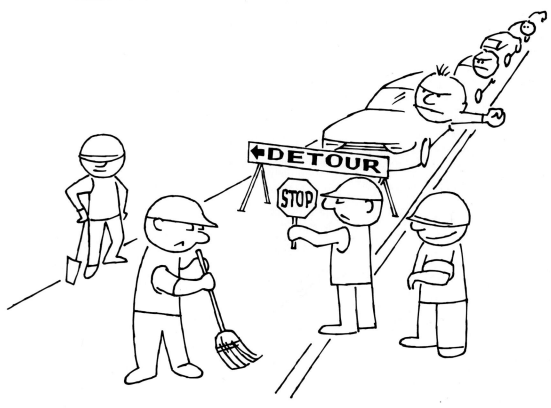

may have a dysrhythmic effect, will rarely have a substantial dysrhythmic blocking effect on the normal conduction pathway. When the pathway is affected, the most common result is either a slowing of conduction or a stoppage of conduction at the atrioventricular node or along the bundle of His. The more severe the effect, the higher is the degree of block.

Heart block may be a form of dysrhythmia or it may refer to damage along the bundles of His. A block along the bundle of His is a **bundle branch block.** Bundle branch block cannot be diagnosed from the single monitoring lead. Bundle branch block may be diagnosed from the 12-lead electrocardiogram. In the 12 leads, an extra R wave, called R prime, appearing in specific leads, indicates a bundle branch block.

Heart block dysrhythmias are categorized as **first degree heart block; second degree-Wenckebach heart block,** also known as **second degree-Mobitz I; second degree-Mobitz II heart block;** and **third degree heart block,** also known as **complete heart block.** Second degree Wenckebach (Mobitz I) will be referred to in this text as **Wenckebach block** for brevity. The designation Mobitz I is equally correct.

These heart blocks share criteria, as was mentioned in the introduction, but each one has a slightly different set of criteria that makes them easy to differentiate (see Table 8-1 on p. 91).

> **Bundle branch block cannot be diagnosed from a single monitoring lead.**

First Degree Block

First degree block has a normal to slow rate. It is regular, with a regular RR interval, regular PP interval, and regular PR interval. The QRS interval is within normal limits. The only abnormality is the PR interval, which is elongated (or prolonged). The PR interval is elongated or prolonged (greater than twenty-hundredths seconds) and regular (all PRIs are elongated and alike). It has a normal P:R ratio of 1:1.

The term regular indicates that all complexes or intervals are alike. They may be normal and alike or they may be abnormal and alike. Regularity does not necessarily imply the measured wave or interval is normal.

FIGURE 8-2
First Degree Block

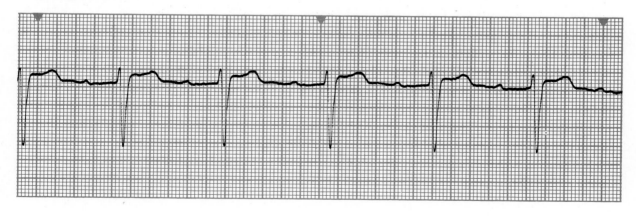

First degree block is generally considered a nonmalignant dysrhythmia, because it does not produce any symptoms or compromise cardiac output. It may be a precedent to higher degree heart block and should be watched carefully in the emergent patient.

Second Degree Wenckebach Block

Second degree Wenckebach block has a low normal to slow rate. Wenckebach has a cycle in which conduction of each atrial impulse through the atrioventricular node is increasingly difficult. Each PR interval in the cycle is longer because of the slowing, difficult conduction. The QRS complexes are within normal limits. The cycle is completed when one P wave is not conducted through the junction to be captured by the ventricles. This results in a **dropped QRS complex.** The conduction system recovers slightly during the pause resulting from the nonconducted beat. The next cycle then starts.

The overall rhythm is irregular. Its irregularity occurs in a regular cycle. This gives rise to the term *regularly irregular.*

A definitive characteristic of Wenckebach is a PR interval that gets longer with each QRS in the cycle. Eventually the last PR interval (in the cycle) gets so long that the impulse is not conducted to the ventricles. This results in a dropped QRS complex. The last P wave of a cycle has no following QRS complex.

The P to P interval is regularly irregular and gets progressively shorter through a cycle. The RR intervals also get slightly shorter between each pair of complexes in the cycle, but not as fast as the P to P interval. Therefore the progressively longer PR interval occurs.

Wenckebach is distinctively marked by clusters of cardiac complexes. Bigeminal or trigeminal ectopy with their pauses may mimic these clusters, but Wenckebach has no premature beats and has a progressively longer PR interval. Ectopic beats never have an elongated or prolonged PR interval. **Group beating,** as this is called, is the hallmark of Wenckebach and is frequently the result of digitalis toxicity. The QRS intervals are within normal limits.

Wenckebach is distinctively marked by clusters of cardiac complexes, with progressively longer PR intervals within the cluster.

FIGURE 8-3
Wenckebach Block

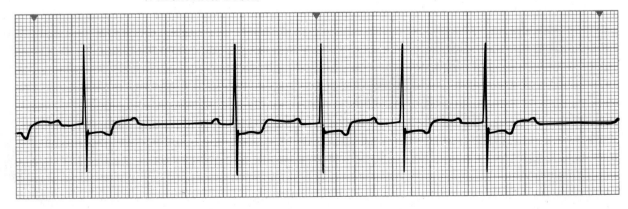

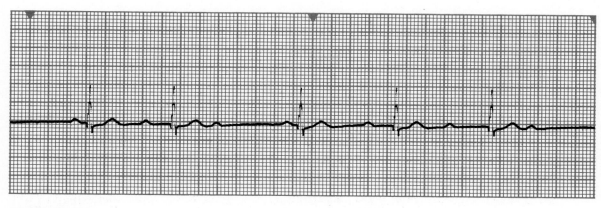

FIGURE 8-4
Wenckebach with Variable Block

   The P:R ratio of a Wenckebach rhythm is less than 2:1, but greater than 1:1, such as three P waves to two QRS complexes (3:2) or four P waves to three QRS complexes (4:3). The P:R ratio in the cycles is usually consistent throughout the rhythm. It may vary, as with three P waves to two QRS complexes (3:2), followed by four P waves to three QRS complexes (4:3), and then three P waves to two QRS complexes again (3:2).

Mobitz II

Second degree Mobitz II has a slow to low normal rate. It is regular, with regular RR interval, regular P to P interval, regular P:R ratio, and regular (remember, regular means "alike," not necessarily normal) PR interval. It has a regular P:R ratio of greater than 1:1, such as two P waves to one QRS com-

Second degree Mobitz II block has a clue to its differential characteristics in its name. The 2 of Mobitz II is a reminder of the P:R ratio being 2 or more to 1.

FIGURE 8-5
Mobitz II Heart Block

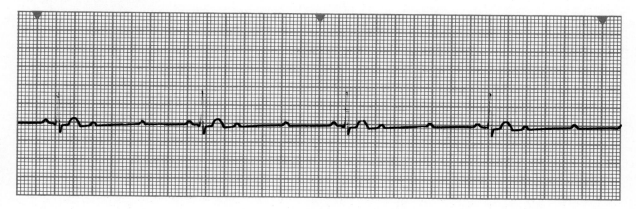

The PR intervals of third degree heart block are irregularly irregular.

plex (2:1) or three waves to one QRS complex (3:1). The PR interval may be elongated, within normal limits, or even (less frequently) abbreviated. The QRS interval is usually wide.

Mobitz II heart block does not occur normally. Any patient presenting with Mobitz II should be watched carefully for advancement to third degree heart block. It may also be a warning of impending cardiac arrest. Use of a pacemaker may be required for these patients.

Third Degree (Complete) Block

Third degree block (or complete heart block) is one of the easiest rhythms to recognize. Its ventricular rate is slow to low normal, usually around 40 beats per minute. It is a life-threatening dysrhythmia, which may acutely compromise cardiac output.

It is both regular and irregular. The ventricular activity is extremely regular and each R to R interval is identical. The atrial activity is also regular and each P to P interval is identical. The atria and the ventricles are operating completely independently of each other with a resulting irregular PR interval. While each anatomical division of the heart is regular to itself, their activities are not related in this dysrhythmia. They are irregular to each other. The conduction system is completely interrupted at the junction. The atria are firing at their own automatic intrinsic rates and the ventricles are firing at their own automatic intrinsic rates.

The characteristics of third degree (or complete) heart block include a regular R to R interval, a regular P to P interval, and an irregular PR interval.

FIGURE 8-6
Third Degree (Complete) Heart Block
Atrial rate is 70. Ventricular rate is 40.

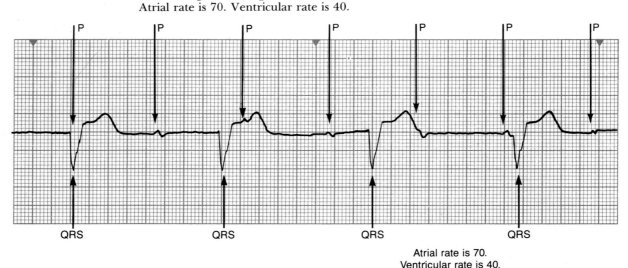

Atrial rate is 70.
Ventricular rate is 40.

TABLE 8-1   Criteria of Heart Blocks

Degree of Block	RRI	PPI	PRI	P:R
1ST	Reg	Reg	Reg & Elong	1:1
2nd Wenckebach	Reg-Irr Shortens	Reg-Irr Shortens	Reg-Irr Lengthens	>1:1 & <2:1
2nd Mobitz II	Reg	Reg	Reg & May Be Abnormal	2:1 or >2:1
3rd	Reg	Reg	Irr-Irr	>1:1

The rates are usually around 40 for ventricular activity and 60 to 80 for atrial activity. The ventricular complexes are usually paced by a junctional pacemaker and are within normal limits. However, the ventricles may be paced by an idioventricular pacemaker and have wide QRS complexes.

The only rhythm that comes close to this in rate with an irregular PR interval is Wenckebach, and it has a regularly irregular RR interval. Wenckebach also has a regularly irregular P to P interval.

AV Dissociation

AV dissociation is a minor dysrhythmia which is very similar to third degree heart block. It has a ventricular rate which is faster than complete heart block. The ventricular rate is faster than the atrial rate.

The atrial stimuli and ventricular stimuli are independent of each other. An atrial stimulus may be conducted to the ventricles if it happens to occur when the ventricles are repolarized from their last ectopic contraction. This may give the appearance of a third degree heart block with a fast ventricular response and occasional normally conducted beats. This is a minor dysrhythmia and is mentioned here to prevent confusion, hopefully. Some clinicians choose to not distinguish between AV dissociation and third degree heart block.

Indications for Management

Blocks are significant to the patient because as bradydysrhythmias they present the threat of impaired cardiac output with a resulting cardiogenic shock, and possibly death. It is common for a patient in block, especially a lower (first or second) degree, to be perfusing adequately.

Patients with block should be managed in the emergency situation symptomatically. Blocks usually result in a bradydysrhythmia or less frequently a slow normal rate. Therapeutic management of block will result in an increase in rate. The increase in cardiac rate will directly increase myocardial oxygen demand. It is probable, if the patient is suffering myocardial infarction, the increased oxygen demand will contribute to myocardial ischemia. The increase in ischemia may directly increase the infarction. Heart blocks, in the emergency setting, are managed only if the patient is **hemodynamically symptomatic.**

Hemodynamic symptoms are shock symptoms that indicate a lack of adequate cardiovascular perfusion. These symptoms include a diminished level of consciousness, diaphoresis, fatigue, dyspnea, mucosa and nail bed blanching, and other general signs of shock.

First degree block generally requires no therapeutic intervention, although the condition causing the block may require intervention.

Second and third degree blocks may require management. Initial management usually addresses parasympathetic and sympathetic influences on the heart to increase conductivity and rate (automaticity). Permanent definitive therapy for advanced block will require the surgical implantation of a **mechanical pacemaker.**

> **Heart blocks, in the emergency setting, are therapeutically managed only if the patient is hemodynamically symptomatic, because of the risk of increasing an infarction.**

Summary

Damage to the conduction system of the heart results in abnormal conduction patterns causing dysrhythmias known as heart blocks. There are four forms of heart block: first degree, second degree Wenckebach (or Mobitz I), second degree Mobitz II, and third degree (or complete) heart block.

First degree heart block is a regular sinus rhythm with a prolonged PR interval. It is generally an asymptomatic dysrhythmia.

Wenckebach block is a dysrhythmia occurring in cycles with groups of normal QRS complexes. Within each cycle there is one more P wave than QRS complexes. Each PR interval is progressively longer until one has no subsequent QRS complex. The cycle then starts anew.

Mobitz II block is marked by the presence of two or more P waves to each QRS complex. Each PR interval is regular. The QRS complexes are usually widened.

Third degree (or complete) heart block has regular atrial activity and regular ventricular activity. Atrial activity and ventricular activity, while regular, are not coordinated with each other. The atrial rate is usually 60 to 80 complexes per minute while the ventricular rate is usually around 40 complexes per minute. The PR interval is irregularly irregular.

Therapeutic management of heart block is performed on an as-needed basis. Lower forms of block, especially first degree, require no management other than observation. Higher forms of block are initially managed with parasympathetic antagonism or sympathetic stimulation. Definitive therapy for higher forms of block requires the surgical implantation of a mechanical pacemaker.

Self-Study Questions

1. List and differentiate between the four types of heart block dysrhythmia.
2. Discuss a form of block which is not a dysrhythmia.

3. What dysrhythmia other than heart block may have more than one atrial complex per ventricular complex?

4. Discuss how the rhythm in question 3 above is differentiated from second or third degree heart blocks.

5. Discuss the indications for therapeutic intervention in heart block patients.

6. What dysrhythmia (from an earlier chapter) other than Wenckebach was regularly irregular?

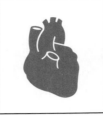

**All bodies are subject to change;
so it comes to pass
that each body is mortal.**

CICERO

9

Ventricular Dysrhythmias

OBJECTIVES

■ Identify the characteristics and clinical significance of all ventricular dysrhythmias, including asystole, ventricular tachycardia, ventricular fibrillation, idioventricular rhythm, and ventricular ectopy with clinical significance.

■ Perform an electrocardiogram analysis and differentially diagnose these dysrhythmias, including sinus dysrhythmias, atrial dysrhythmias, junctional dysrhythmias, and heart blocks.

■ Identify indications for therapeutic intervention.

KEY TERMINOLOGY

aberrancy
advanced life support
agonal rhythm
apnea
apneic
asystole
atrioventricular block
basic life support
cardiac arrest
cardiorespiratory arrest
chemotherapeutic measures
dysfunctional
electromechanical dissociation
  (EMD)
hemodynamic compromise
hemodynamic decompensation
hypokalemia
hypotension

hypotensive
idioventricular
idioventricular rhythm
  accelerated
pericardial tamponade
pericardiocentesis
torsade de pointes (TDP)
ventricular asystole
ventricular dysrhythmia
ventricular fibrillation
  coarse
  fine
ventricular tachycardia
  pulseless

Ventricular dysrhythmia is of particular importance in the dysrhythmic patient. It is the ventricles that produce cardiac output. Without effective atria, ventricular output may be compromised, but without effective ventricles there is no cardiac output. **Ventricular dysrhythmia** is often a precedent to life-threatening **cardiorespiratory arrest.** Dysrhythmias, in general, are frequently categorized as ventricular or supraventricular, indicating the dysrhythmia's origin in or above the ventricles (junctional or atrial). This indicates the importance of recognizing ventricular dysrhythmia. Supraventricular tachydysrhythmias include sinus tachycardia, atrial tachycardia, atrial flutter, atrial fibrillation, and junctional tachycardia.

Ventricular Tachycardia

Ventricular dysrhythmia is often a precedent to life-threatening cardiorespiratory arrest.

Ventricular tachycardia is a run of three or more consecutive PVCs. Ventricular tachycardia may occur in an isolated run, but commonly persists for an extended period of time, and is life threatening. Clinically, it may occur with or without pulses.

The patient who has a pulse is usually **hypotensive** because the fast rate of the tachycardia compromises ventricular filling time and reduces cardiac output. Ventricular tachycardia with a pulse is also ominous because of its tendency to degenerate to ventricular fibrillation without a pulse.

The pulseless **cardiac arrest** patient is **apneic** and/or pulseless and will require **basic life support** initially and **advanced life support** therapies to survive.

Ventricular tachycardia usually has a rate range of 100 to 220 beats per minute. Sinus P waves may exist between ventricular complexes if there is **atrioventricular block.** Such P waves will have no regular relationship to the QRS complexes. The rhythm is usually regular. The cardiac complexes meet the criteria for PVCs and have QRS complexes that are wide.

Supraventricular tachycardia with **aberrancy** or bundle branch block may mimic ventricular tachycardia. Differentiation may not be possible. A diagnosis of atrial fibrillation with aberrancy may be made based on the irregularity of atrial fibrillation as contrasted to the regularity of ventricular tachycardia. The presence of QRS duration of fourteen-hundredths (0.14) seconds (or greater) suggests the origin is ventricular. Ultimately the clinical presentation of the patient may indicate the presence or absence of **hemodynamic decompensation** associated with ventricular tachycardia. The clinician would be wise, when in doubt, to conservatively manage the dysrhythmia as if it were the more serious ventricular dysrhythmia until it can be ruled out. Hemodynamic decompensation is the rapid onset of shock symptoms due to the sudden failure of the cardiovascular system's compensating mechanisms.

The causes of ventricular tachycardia are the same as those for PVCs, listed in Chapter 5. Major causes include myocardial infarction complicated with ischemia, acidosis, and electrolyte imbalance.

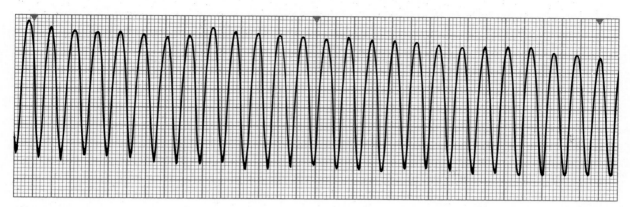

FIGURE 9-1
Ventricular Tachycardia

Torsade de Pointes

Torsade de pointes (TDP) is a relatively rare form of ventricular tachycardia. It is mentioned here because recognition of it is important to clinical management (see Figure 9-2 on p. 98). Torsade de pointes may be aggravated by conventional ventricular tachycardia management protocols.

The term **torsade de pointes** literally translated from the French means *twisting of the points.* The QRS complexes of the ventricular tachycardia tend to rotate from a negative deflection to a positive deflection in a period of 5 to 20 beats. During the rotation the points of the QRS complexes when upright or down (for a series of beats) may show a clockwise or counterclockwise rotation (of the R wave) from complex to complex. Torsade usually has a rate of 200 to 250 beats per minute. The amplitude of the complexes may continually change from complex to complex.

Warning signs of the development of torsade de pointes in the EKG of the high-risk patient include a prolongation of the QT (or QTU) interval, prominent U waves, very large T waves, and ventricular bigeminy with close coupling (R on T).

Common causes include hypokalemia and quinidine therapy. Quinidine blood levels in the normally therapeutic range (nontoxic levels) may be associated with torsade. Severe bradycardia is a major predisposing factor.

Management of torsade de pointes is directed at eliminating the cause, which is usually drug toxicities or electrolyte imbalance. Suspect intoxications include primarily quinidine, and, less frequently, phenothiazines and tricyclic antidepressants. Vagal stimulation, intravenous lidocaine, overdrive pacing with mechanical pacemakers, and even cautiously administered intravenous isoproterenol may be effective in terminating torsade de pointes.

> **Recognition of torsade de pointes is important because management is different from other forms of ventricular tachycardia.**

> **Any patient presenting with severe bradycardia, who is also taking quinidine or who has prolonged QT intervals, should be considered at risk of torsade de pointes.**

Ventricular Fibrillation

Ventricular fibrillation is one of the four forms of cardiac arrest. The other three forms are **asystole, pulseless ventricular tachycardia,** and **electromechanical dissociation.** Ventricular fibrillation is the most disorganized of all

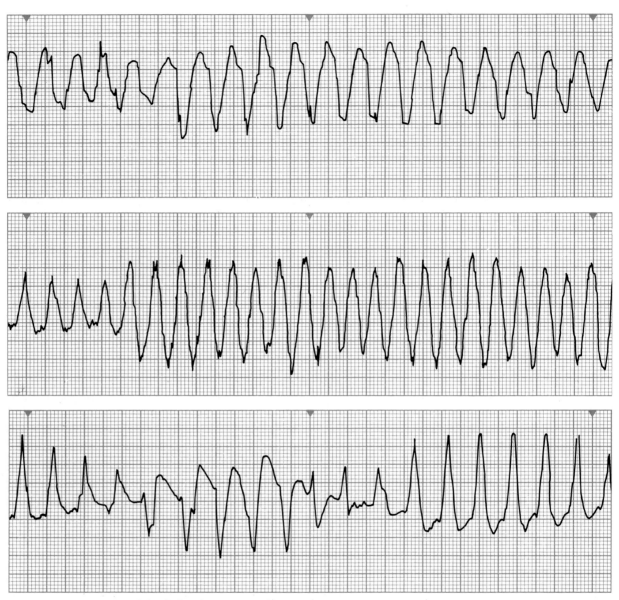

(Torsade de pointes courtesy of Dr. Fahrid Ullah.)

FIGURE 9-2
Torsade de Pointes

possible cardiac rhythms. Areas of cardiac cells depolarize independently. The myocardium lacks an effective muscular contraction. There is no cardiac output. The myocardium has a quivering muscular activity.

The EKG of ventricular fibrillation reveals an irregular wavy baseline that has no organized, repeated wave patterns. Fibrillatory waves that are easily visible are described as **coarse ventricular fibrillation.** Waves that are small (low amplitude) and almost flat line are described as **fine ventricular fibrillation.** Coarse ventricular fibrillation is successfully defibrillated more frequently than fine fibrillation. The distinction between coarse and fine fibrillation is somewhat subjective.

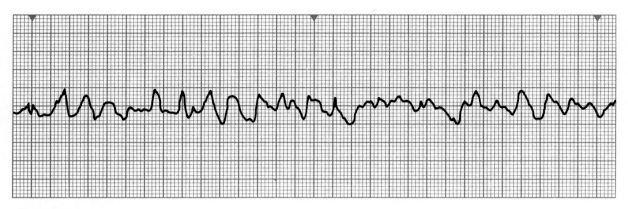

FIGURE 9-3
Coarse Ventricular Fibrillation

Warning dysrhythmias, such as ventricular tachycardia or the five types of warning ventricular ectopy listed in Chapter 5, may precede ventricular fibrillation. Ventricular fibrillation shares the common causes of ventricular tachycardia and PVCs. It also may occur spontaneously.

The definitive therapy for ventricular fibrillation is defibrillation. Defibrillation produces a stimulus much stronger than the normal cardiac stimuli. That stimulus depolarizes all cells that are in a repolarized or relative refractory period. This depolarization places all the cells of the heart at a uniform stage of polarization. The intent of defibrillation is to produce a uniform state of polarization to enable the natural pacemakers of the heart to reassert their influence on cardiac conduction and return to a normal (or at least a perfusing) rhythm. Clinical studies have demonstrated defibrillation is more successful when performed shortly after the onset of the dysrhythmia.

Defibrillation in ventricular fibrillation should be attempted at the earliest possible opportunity. Defibrillation should not delay the initiation of basic life support unnecessarily. If the initial attempts to defibrillate are unsuccessful, drug therapies, especially oxygenation, may make the myocardium receptive to a successful attempt.

FIGURE 9-4
Fine Ventricular Fibrillation

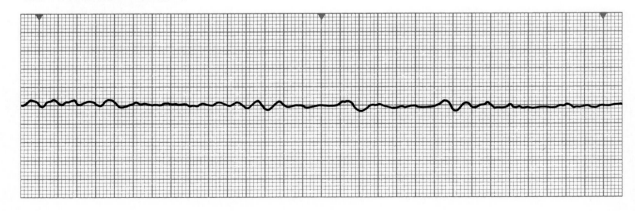

Idioventricular Rhythm

Any rhythm originating in the ventricles is considered **idioventricular.** Some rhythms, such as ventricular tachycardia or fibrillation, have additional criteria that provide a more specific identification.

Idioventricular rhythm is a regular, slow rhythm with wide ventricular complexes without P waves. The intrinsic firing rate of the ventricles is 15 to 40 beats per minute. The rate for idioventricular rhythm is 40 beats per minute or less.

A rhythm with idioventricular characteristics, that is faster than 40 beats per minute but not fast enough to be considered tachycardia (100 beats per minute), is called **accelerated idioventricular rhythm.**

Ventricular Asystole

Asystole is literally translated as *without contractions.* More accurately, the arrhythmia is completely without electrical activity. There are no waves and no complexes. The rhythm is a flat line on the EKG. The patient is clinically in cardiac arrest, both pulseless and apneic. **Ventricular asystole** is also known as **ventricular standstill.**

FIGURE 9-5
Idioventricular Rhythm

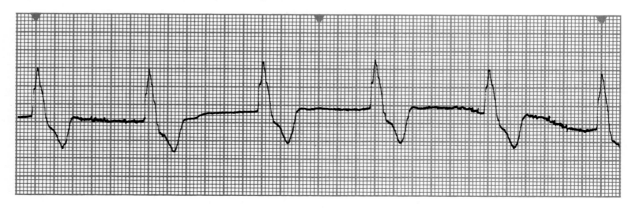

FIGURE 9-6
Accelerated Idioventricular Rhythm

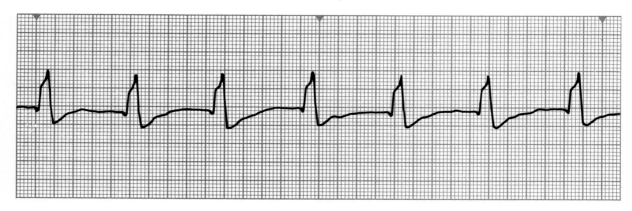

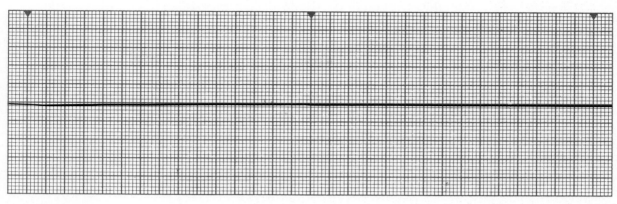

FIGURE 9-7
Asystole

Ventricular fibrillation, that is refractory to defibrillation, will degenerate to asystole. Asystole may also result from myocardial infarction, ischemia, hyperkalemia, digitalis toxicity, prolonged sinus arrest, and complete heart block without escape ectopy.

Management includes basic life support and **chemotherapeutic measures** designed to produce cardiac irritability and convert the asystole to ventricular fibrillation. Ventricular fibrillation may respond to defibrillation. Asystole may also respond to pacemaker therapy. Defibrillation is not a definitive therapeutic technique for asystole. It may, however, be employed as a last resort without harming the patient. Many clinicians feel that asystole may actually be a fine ventricular fibrillation in some cases.

Agonal Rhythm

Agonal rhythm is a dying heart rhythm (see Figure 9-8 on p. 102). It is usually ventricular, but may also be sinus or junctional in origin. It is marked by being extremely slow and irregularly becoming slower to the point of asystole. A rate of less than ten beats per minute is common. This dysrhythmia usually precedes ventricular asystole. Agonal rhythm usually occurs as a result of (failing) escape ectopy occurring in an underlying asystole. Agonal rhythm is managed as asystole.

Electromechanical Dissociation

Electrical activity as measured on the EKG is normally associated with mechanical muscular contraction. The failure of the myocardium to mechanically respond to the normal electrical depolarization is **electromechanical dissociation (EMD).** Electromechanical dissociation is not genuinely a dysrhythmia; rather, it is a *condition.* The electrical rhythm is frequently a normal sinus rhythm. Any rhythm having QRS complexes without associated pulses is technically an electromechanical dissociation. Many clinicians consider pulseless ventricular tachycardia a form of electromechanical dissociation because it has QRS complexes without mechanical contractions. Pulseless ventricular tachycardia has specific treatment indications and is usually more precisely identified.

Electromechanical dissociation may occur when the ventricular myocardium has sustained such damage as to be **dysfunctional.** Another theory suggests electrolyte imbalance may precipitate a neuromuscular dysfunction.

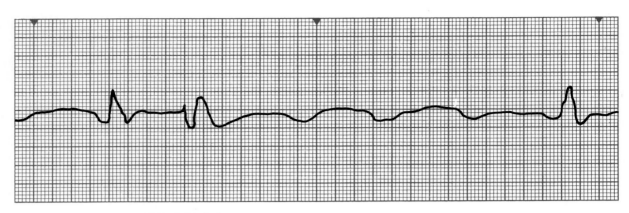

FIGURE 9-8
Agonal Rhythm

It is essential to clinically assess the patient to confirm cardiac complexes are associated with mechanical activity.

Pericardial tamponade must be suspected in any patient presenting with electromechanical dissociation.

Management of electromechanical dissociation cardiac arrest includes immediate basic life support and subsequent advanced life support drug therapy to restore mechanical activity.

Pericardial tamponade may mimic electromechanical dissociation. Pericardial tamponade occurs when the heart chambers or vessels bleed into the pericardial sac. Rupture of a ventricular aneurysm may occur with myocardial infarction and precipitate a pericardial tamponade. The blood accumulates within the sac eventually compressing (or tamponing) the heart. It is marked by a progressive diminishment of cardiac output, a narrowing pulse pressure, distended neck veins, and shock symptoms. A pulseless tamponade may be distinguished from electromechanical dissociation by the presence of diminished heart sounds. A pulseless tamponade will quickly degenerate into a less viable dysrhythmia such as ventricular fibrillation.

Management of pericardial tamponade, also known as *cardiac tamponade,* requires removal of the blood in the pericardial sac. A needle may be inserted and excess blood drained out. This **pericardiocentesis,** when performed on a viable patient usually results in a dramatic improvement. Diagnosis of tamponade must be considered in any patient presenting with electromechanical dissociation.

Summary

Ventricular dysrhythmias are categorically the most serious of all dysrhythmias, because they may be hemodynamically life threatening and because they frequently precede or cause cardiac arrest.

Ventricular tachycardia is differentiated from the other five forms of tachycardia by their designation as supraventricular tachycardias. Ventricular tachycardia with a pulse may be life threatening because of hemodynamic compromise. It may also present without pulses in the clinically cardiac-arrested patient. This dysrhythmia is marked as a run of three or more consecutive PVCs, wide QRS complexes, and a regular rate of between 100 and 220 beats per minute.

Differentiation of ventricular tachycardia from supraventricular tachycardia with aberrancy may be most difficult or impossible. Some diagnostic clues include the regularity of the rhythm, the duration of the QRS complexes, and the rate. A conservative approach to tachydysrhythmia of uncertain origin is to manage it as ventricular tachycardia until definitive diagnosis is established.

Torsade de pointes is a rare form of ventricular tachycardia which results from drug toxicity. It may be aggravated by conventional antidysrhythmic therapies normally used for ventricular tachycardia. It is marked by a rotation of the QRS complexes.

Ventricular fibrillation is a disorganized rhythm without meaningful muscular activity. It has no cardiac output. The victim is in cardiac arrest. Defibrillation is the definitive therapy and should be attempted as soon as possible after the onset of the dysrhythmia and initiation of basic life support.

Idioventricular rhythm is any rhythm that originates in the ventricles. The term specifically applies to ventricular rhythms that are not fast enough to qualify as ventricular tachycardia and too regular to qualify as fibrillation. A rate of 40 beats per minute or less is normal for this dysrhythmia. A rate greater than 40 but less than 100 is considered accelerated idioventricular rhythm.

Asystole is the absence of electrical activity. Electrocardiographic representation is a flat uninterrupted baseline. Management is directed at converting it to ventricular fibrillation so defibrillation may be attempted.

Agonal rhythm is a dying heart rhythm. It is marked by very slow complexes that are irregularly becoming slower. It usually represents escape ectopy superimposed on an asystolic rhythm.

Electromechanical dissociation is a syndrome in which the EKG may be normal or dysrhythmic, but has no associated mechanical muscular contractions of the heart. It may be imitated by pericardial tamponade. It is essential to clinically evaluate the cardiac patient because of the possibility of electromechanical dissociation. Pericardial tamponade may be effectively managed with pericardiocentesis.

Self-Study Questions

1. Discuss the clinical significance of the categorization of ventricular and supraventricular dysrhythmia.
2. Discuss identifying characteristics of all six major forms of tachydysrhythmia.
3. Discuss identifying characteristics that may assist in distinguishing ventricular tachycardia from supraventricular tachycardia with aberrancy.
4. Discuss identifying characteristics of torsade de pointes and differences in clinical approach.
5. Discuss the differentiation between and significance of fine and coarse ventricular fibrillation.
6. Discuss idioventricular rhythm and list the four major dysrhythmias that may be classified as idioventricular.
7. Discuss the four major forms of cardiac arrest. Identify the initial management approach to cardiac arrest.
8. Explain why each cardiographic patient needs to be clinically assessed.
9. Differentiate between the clinical presentations of the electromechanical dissociation patient and the pericardial tamponade patient.
10. Explain the role of defibrillation in managing ventricular dysrhythmias and when it should be performed.

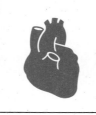

**What if a man does not keep pace
with his companions?
Perhaps it is because he hears
a different drummer.
Let him step to that music he hears,
however measured or far away.**

HENRY DAVID THOREAU

10

Pacemaker Rhythms

OBJECTIVES

■ Identify the characteristics of pacemaker rhythms, including pacemaker rhythm, synchronous pacemaker rhythm, pacer rhythm with failure to capture, and pacer rhythm with failure to fire.

■ Differentiate between demand, fixed rate, and activity related pacemakers.

■ Perform an electrocardiogram analysis and differentially diagnose these dysrhythmias, including sinus, atrial, junctional, ventricular, and heart block dysrhythmias.

■ Identify indications for therapeutic management.

KEY TERMINOLOGY

atrioventricular synchronous
   pacing
automatic implantable cardioverter
   defibrillators
bradydysrhythmia
cardiac output
catheterization
demand rate
failure to capture
failure to fire
failure to pace
hemodynamically symptomatic
pacemaker
   activity related
   demand
   external
   fixed rate
   temporary
pacemaker pulse generator
pacemaker rhythm
parasympathetic stimulation
spike
telemetry
vagal tone
vein
   pulmonary
   subclavian
wire electrode

A mechanical **pacemaker** is an electronic device used to generate an **artificial action potential** in the heart. A pacemaker is used in bradydysrhythmia, in which the patient's heart is not producing an effective cardiac output.

Pacemakers may be used on a temporary basis for transient bradydysrhythmia or on a permanent basis for serious, permanent bradydysrhythmia. Third or second degree heart blocks are commonly managed with **permanent pacemaker** therapy. Pacemakers are indicated for bradydysrhythmias that are hemodynamically symptomatic, with signs and symptoms such as lightheadedness, fainting, confusion, or weakness.

Temporary pacemakers are commonly used for bradydysrhythmias occurring during myocardial infarction and for those resulting from increased **vagal tone** (parasympathetic stimulation).

Pacemakers used on a permanent basis are surgically implanted under the skin, usually in the area just below the right clavicle and occasionally in the abdominal area. The pacemaker is palpable and clearly visible because of its

FIGURE 10-1
Pacemaker: Pulse Generator, Electrode, and Programmer

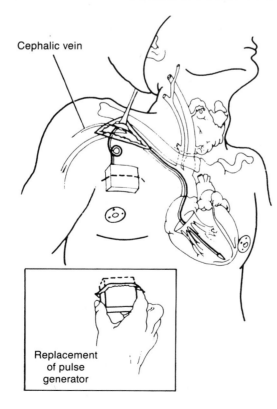

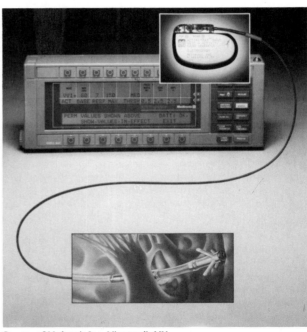

Courtesy of Medtronic Inc., Minneapolis MN.

Left: Cephalic vein insertion and pulse generator placement. (From Furman, S.: Heart Lung 7[5]:813, 1978.)

distention under the skin. Temporary pacemakers are external with an electrode catheterized through a central vein.

Pacemakers have two major parts. The **pacemaker pulse generator** is the sterile sealed circular frame which contains the adjustment, timing, and discharge components and the battery. The **wire electrode** is a wire coming from the casing, threaded through the systemic venous system (either the **subclavian vein** or, less frequently, other large veins) into the right ventricle.

Most pacemakers are adjustable by electronic signals, called **telemetry.** A computerized programming unit is used to set the pacemaker (see Figure 10-1). Settings are made for rate, duration, and strength of the pacemaker impulse. Adjustments may be made without requiring a surgical procedure. One brand of pacemaker was, in the past, tuned to a microwave frequency for its telemetric adjustments. While this is no longer a problem, it accounts for warnings to pacemaker users to avoid microwave ovens. Theoretically if the microwave is defective and leaking radiation, it could cause an undesired adjustment in the pacemaker.

Pacemaker Catheterization

Venous catheterization is usually used for the insertion of the pacemaker. It produces less complications in long-term therapy and less bleeding than **arterial catheterization, pulmonary vein catheterization,** or **transmyocardial** (through the myocardial wall) **catheterization.** Some complications of pacemaker therapy include infection, hemorrhage, chest muscle response to the pacer impulse, embolism, perforation of the myocardial wall by the electrode, battery failure, and even dysrhythmia.

The right ventricle is targeted for the pacer electrode because the left ventricle is inaccessible through the deep pulmonary vein or arteries. Impulses in the right ventricle are conducted through the ventricular septum into the left ventricle and produce an effective bilateral contraction of the heart.

External Pacing

External pacemakers are occasionally employed in emergency situations when expediency is essential. They are more easily applied and do not require venous catheterization. External pacemakers discharge their electrical stimulus through electrodes that are applied to the anterior and posterior chest wall. The electrodes are very similar to the electrodes used for cardiac monitoring. The electrodes are then connected to an external pacing mechanism. External pacing has a higher incidence of undesired pacing of chest wall and body muscles.

Pacemaker Rhythm

The impulse occurring when a pacemaker fires is a vertical deflection known as a **spike.** The spike is usually short, very fast and only rarely shows a return to baseline. It may be negative, positive, or biphasic. The pacemaker spike is usually set without width (showing no return to baseline) because a small rapid charge is effective for pacing. An impulse of longer duration would cause more rapid battery depletion.

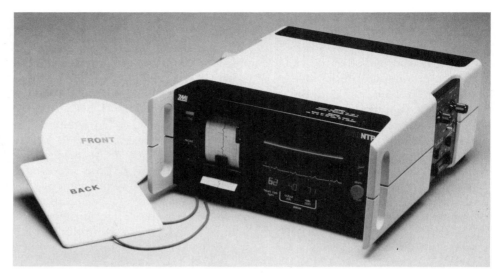

Photo courtesy of ZMI Corporation

FIGURE 10-2
External Pacemaker

The spike is normally followed by a QRS complex. The QRS complex frequently shows an RR′ wave, indicating the left ventricle is depolarizing shortly after the right ventricle. The QRS complex may originate in the junction or in the ventricle, depending on the anatomical shape of the heart and the physical location of the pacemaker. The QRS complex may be normal in duration (if the origin is in the junction) or wide (if the origin is in the ventricle). A wide (greater than 0.10 seconds) QRS complex in response to a pacemaker spike is very common.

An EKG with a pacemaker spike in it is called simply **pacemaker rhythm.** A spike without a following QRS complex occurs when the heart fails to capture the impulse and respond with a propagated action potential/depolarization wave. This is a **failure to capture.** Failure to capture may occur as a result of increased cardiac disease, myocardial infarction of a critical mass of the myo-

FIGURE 10-3
Pacemaker Rhythm

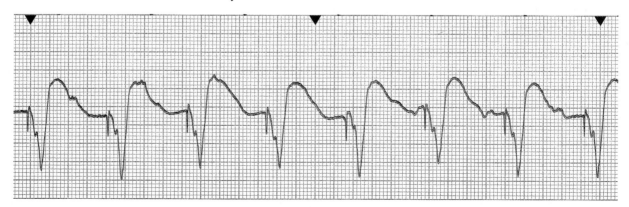

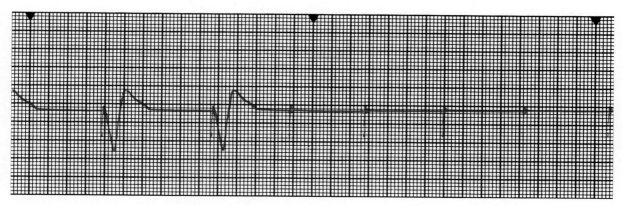

FIGURE 10-4
Pacemaker Rhythm with Failure to Capture

cardium, shifting of the tip of the electrode, perforation of the ventricular wall by the electrode, or even an increase in the threshold action potential of the myocardium.

Pacemaker Types

Most pacemakers are designed to fire only when needed. The need is determined by cardiac rate. These pacemakers fire when the rate drops below a specified setting, such as 70 beats per minute. To do this, the pacemaker has a sensing mechanism in the pulse generator to sense the cardiac rate. These pacemakers *fire on demand* from the heart rate and are known as **demand pacemakers.** A demand pacemaker will only show pacer spikes on an EKG when the intrinsic rate of the heart is slower than the intrinsic setting of the pacemaker. A pacemaker rhythm may show a mixture of regular rhythm, borderline bradydysrhythmia, and pacer beats.

Another type of pacemaker operation is a fixed rate mode. The pacemaker is set to fire at a fixed rate regardless of any underlying natural cardiac activity. **Fixed rate pacemakers** are very rarely used. The EKG appearance of a fixed rate pacemaker would be regular pacer beats superimposed over any existing natural complexes. There may be no natural complexes if the fixed rate is fast enough to overdrive the innate automaticity of the heart. Routinely, demand pacemakers are switched temporarily to a fixed rate mode when the pacemaker rate is being checked during a patient examination. It is remotely possible that this switch could occur accidentally in response to environmental factors.

Activity Related Pacing

Many patients become weak and dizzy with physical exertion because their mechanical pacemakers do not increase cardiac rate in response to exercise as their natural cardiac pacemaker did. An **activity related pacemaker** has an additional capacity to be set to vary cardiac rate in response to physical activity. The pacemaker has a built-in sensor which detects musculoskeletal vibrations

Holter monitor of normal cardiac response vs. Activitrax

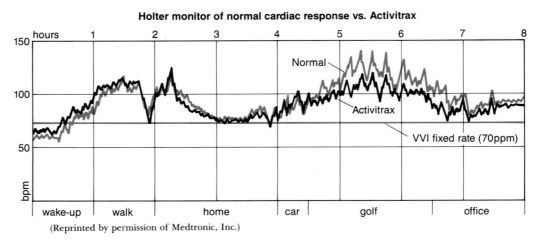

(Reprinted by permission of Medtronic, Inc.)

FIGURE 10-5
Activitrax and Normal Cardiac Comparison

associated with exercise and increases the pacing rate in response to the vibrations. It also has a minimum **demand rate** setting for pacing at rest. The pacemaker also has a maximum setting. Sensitivity may be adjusted to eliminate unwanted responses to vibration in patients who may have an unusually active environment. This type of pacemaker is frequently used to replace the older demand rate type pacemaker merely by changing pulse generators and leaving the original electrode in place.

The obvious advantage of the device is that it removes many of the activity related restrictions on the pacemaker patient. In one study by Medtronic, Incorporated, a continuous monitor was applied to a patient with a normal, healthy heart. An activity related pacemaker was externally applied to the pectoral muscle and a comparative analysis was performed. Figure 10-5 illustrates a response of the pacemaker which is almost identical to the natural cardiac response.

Atrioventricular Synchronous Pacing

Occasionally a pacemaker rhythm will be seen in which two pacemaker spikes are evident in each cardiac complex. The first pacer spike paces the atrium and the second paces the ventricles, very soon after the first. This type of pacing is used when the patient requires atrial kick to maintain adequate cardiac output. Single chamber (ventricular) pacing is not adequate for these patients. The first spike is usually smaller than the second.

A mild variation of this occurs when a pacemaker has a sensing device which receives a stimulus from the natural atrial contraction and the stimulus from the atrium triggers the pacemaker impulse. The pacemaker impulse then stimulates a ventricular response very soon after the normal atrial contraction. **Atrioventricular synchronous pacing** is most useful in atrioventricular block

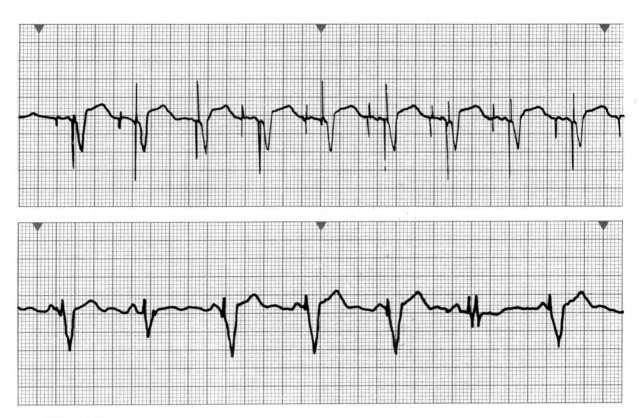

FIGURE 10-6
Atrioventricular Synchronous Pacing
Each complex in the top EKG has two pacer spikes. The first (and smaller) paces the
atria. The second paces the ventricles. The rhythm in the bottom EKG results from a
pacer spike which is in response to an effective natural atrial rate. The pacemaker
senses atrial activity and paces ventricular activity.

which has a good natural atrial activity. The advantage is the sinoatrial node
continues to indirectly pace the entire heart, allowing it to respond normally to
vagal, sympathetic, and exercise influences. It also allows the heart to improve
stroke volume by taking advantage of the atrial kick. The rhythm is marked by
a normal P wave followed by a pacemaker spike and a pacemaker-type ventricular QRS complex.

Failure to Pace

A pacemaker may malfunction for a number of reasons. The most common
causes are battery failure and wire electrode failure. Failure of the pacemaker
is recognized on the EKG by the absence of pacemaker spikes and a return of
the underlying bradydysrhythmia, for which the pacemaker was implanted.
The total absence of pacemaker spikes is a **failure to pace** or **failure to fire** (see
Figure 10-7 on next page). This assumes pacer spikes are absent from a slow
dysrhythmia. If the cardiac rate is not slow, the pacemaker may be functioning
normally in a demand mode.

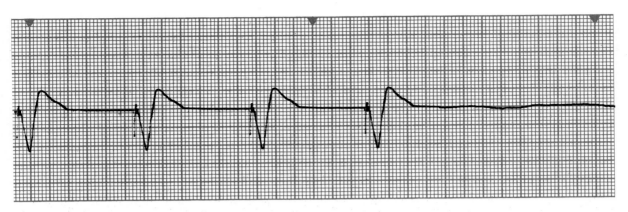

FIGURE 10-7
Pacemaker Rhythm with Failure to Pace

Defibrillation with Pacemakers

Defibrillation in the pacemaker patient should never be withheld because of potential damage to the pacemaker. Ventricular fibrillation is immediately life threatening. Defibrillation in which the electrical current passes through the pulse generator may burn out the pacemaker circuits. However pulse generators are always more replaceable than is the patient. **Automatic Implantable Cardioverter Defibrillators** may one day be incorporated into pacemaker devices.

Summary

Mechanical pacemakers are used to pace the heart in patients with significant bradycardia. They may be used temporarily for transient bradydysrhythmia or permanently for chronic dysrhythmia, such as second or third degree heart block.

Mechanical pacemakers consist of two parts, the casing containing the electronic components, and the wire electrode. They have adjustable settings for rate and mode. Those adjustments are made by telemetric signal.

Pacemakers are inserted, either into the right atrium or through the atrium into the right ventricle, by a catheter in a central vein such as the right subclavian.

Pacemaker rhythms show a spike. Pacemakers occasionally make use of the atrial conduction in association with ventricular pacing. This atrioventricular synchronous pacing senses atrial activity and triggers a ventricular response in time to take advantage of atrial stroke volume. A pacemaker may also use two electrodes to pace both the atrium and ventricles in sequence to produce an atrial stroke volume.

A pacemaker rhythm may have natural heartbeats between pacemaker beats if the pacemaker is operating in the demand mode. The pacemaker in the demand mode functions only when the heart rate drops below the established setting for the pacemaker. Pacemakers have a fixed rate mode, which is rarely used except to check the settings of the pacemaker. A third type of mode is the activity related mode, in which the pacemaker responds to physical exercise with an increase in rate.

Two problems with pacemakers include failure to capture and failure to pace. Failure to capture is a failure of the heart to respond to the pacemaker stimulus and is represented by an absence of cardiac complexes after a spike on the EKG. Failure to pace is a mechanical failure of the pacemaker to generate an impulse and is represented by an absence of spikes on the EKG.

Pacemakers are the definitive therapy for bradydysrhythmia that is hemodynamically symptomatic.

Self-Study Questions

1. List and discuss the indications for pacemaker therapy.
2. Discuss recognition of pacemaker rhythm and EKG patterns that may be present, including an RR' wave. Describe the characteristics of the pacemaker spike.
3. Differentiate between the fixed rate mode and the demand mode of pacemakers.
4. Discuss the uses and EKG recognition of demand mode pacemakers and fixed rate mode pacemakers.
5. Discuss and differentiate between failure to pace and failure to capture.
6. List at least three possible complications of pacemaker therapy.
7. Discuss the physical identification of the patient with a pacemaker.
8. Explain why pacemaker wearers are often warned about the presence of microwave ovens.

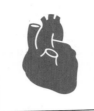

And an old man,
only a few hours before he died,
told me that he had lived
for one hundred years
without experiencing any
physical failure other than weakness;
and sitting on the bed in the hospital
of Santa Maria Nova in Florence,
he passed from this life,
giving no sign of any accident.
And I dissected his body,
in order to understand the cause
of so easy a death.
I discovered that it came to him
through a lack of blood
in the arteries that fed the heart
and the lower parts,
which were used up and dried out.

LEONARDO DA VINCI

11

Limitations of the Monitoring Lead

OBJECTIVES

- Identify and define criteria of an electrocardiogram that relate to electrocardiograms in general rather than to individual dysrhythmias or ectopy.

- Discuss P mitrale, ST segment changes, generation of a myocardial infarction, false positives or false negatives, digitalis toxicity and its role in dysrhythmia, and ectopy generation.

- Identify limited aspects of management such as oxygenation, synchronized cardioversion, carotid massage, and the Valsalva maneuver.

KEY TERMINOLOGY

analog
aneurysm
cardiotonic medication
carotid massage
catecholamine
chronic obstructive pulmonary disease
collateral circulation
concomitant
coronary artery disease
denial
dextrocardia
diaphoresis
digitalis toxicity
digitalized
dyspnea
fight or flight response
hypoxia
J point depression

Levine sign
mammalian diving reflex
myocardial infarction
    acute (AMI)
    electrocardiographic silent
    silent
necrosis
occlusion
P mitrale
pericarditis
prophylactic
pulmonary embolism
ST segment changes
ST segment depression
ST segment elevation
Stokes-Adams attack
synchronized cardioversion
Valsalva maneuver

Electrocardiography is a useful tool in conducting an examination of the patient. Twelve-lead analysis is capable of supporting the diagnosis of a variety of medical conditions, including myocardial infarction, previous myocardial infarction, pulmonary embolism, pericarditis, valvular disease, coronary artery disease, pericardial tamponade, dextrocardia, hyperthyroidism, chronic obstructive pulmonary disease, ventricular and aortic **aneurysm,** and—the list goes on.

The Monitoring Lead

The monitoring lead is useful only for diagnosing major dysrhythmia and ectopy.

Confusion arises when the clinician sees something on the monitoring lead that relates to a diagnosis on the full 12 lead. The objective of the monitoring lead is to provide ongoing current information about the patient's heart rhythm and its degree of irritability.

A number of phenomena occur in the EKG which are commonly associated with complications, such as ST segment changes. **ST segment changes** may be diagnostic of pathology in the 12 lead but only suggest it in the monitoring lead. The monitoring electrocardiogram usually has electronic devices which alter the represented electrical activity and may cause ST segment depression or elevation. The axis in the monitoring lead is slightly altered from the normal axis of the 12 lead, and allows some changes from the expected shape of the cardiac complex in the normal limb leads. Any ST segment change of one millimeter or less is not diagnostic, even in the 12-lead EKG and is identified as nonspecific.

P Mitrale

One abnormality that can be diagnosed from the monitoring lead is the notched P wave. A P wave notched in the middle to have the appearance of a camel-back shape is **P mitrale.** P mitrale is suggestive of left atrial hypertrophy.

ST and J Point Depression

ST segment depression is a depression of the ST segment below the normal baseline of the EKG. It is suggestive of myocardial ischemia. It is commonly associated with tachydysrhythmia because of the increase in oxygen demand associated with fast heart rates. ST depression is commonly confused with **J point depression.** J point depression has a J point below the baseline, but the ST segment slopes steadily upward toward baseline (see Figure 11-2). To be considered depressed, the ST segment must level out and form a segment of baseline below normal before returning to the normal baseline.

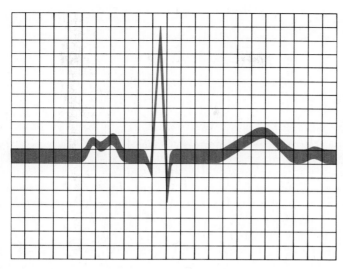

FIGURE 11-1
P Mitrale

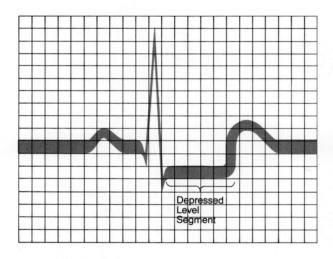

ST depression shows a
Level ST Segment which
is below baseline.

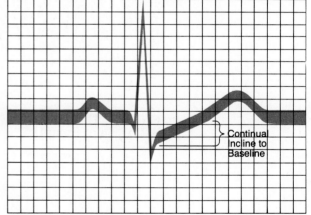

J point depression
shows a low J point
with a **continual incline**
to baseline.

FIGURE 11-2
ST Depression and J Point Depression

ST Elevation

The ST segment may also be elevated. An elevation is considered a pattern of injury and suggests myocardial infarction in the 12-lead EKG. **ST segment elevation,** like ST segment depression, must level out before returning to the baseline. The ST segment may be difficult to evaluate in the presence of T wave changes which are associated with some of the same causes as ST depression.

T Wave Changes

T waves may change to be tall, positive waves known as **hyperacute T waves** or flatten out into what is termed a **depressed T wave.** The T wave may also be inverted. *T wave changes are not diagnostic on the monitoring lead.*

Hyperacute T waves may be an early sign of acute myocardial infarction in the first few minutes of the event. It may also indicate hyperkalemia, or even a P wave buried on top of the T wave (especially with tachydysrhythmia). Hypokalemia with resulting PVCs are common in cardiac patients taking diuretics and in alcoholics who are malnourished.

The T wave, which is hyperacute with **AMI,** may become inverted in a time frame of hours to days as the infarction progresses.

Digitalis toxicity tends to fuse the T wave with the ST segment. Digitalis and a number of other medications tend to cause depressed T waves when **toxicity** develops.

R-R Prime (RR′)

The presence of an R prime (R′) wave indicates the left and right ventricles are not contracting simultaneously. This may, in the complete 12-lead EKG, indicate a form of bundle (of His) branch block. *It is not diagnostic in the monitoring lead.* An R wave that precedes the R′ prime wave may not show a complete return to baseline, but may take on an overall appearance of a notch in the QRS complex's RR′ waves.

FIGURE 11-3
RR′ (Prime) Complex

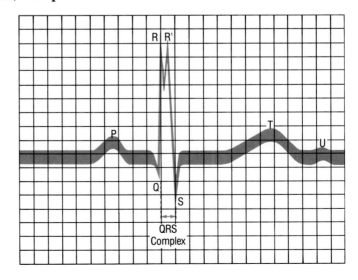

Myocardial Infarction

Myocardial infarction is almost always a concern in the patient who has cause to be electrocardiographically monitored. Thorough discussion of myocardial infarction is beyond the scope of this text, but it deserves brief attention here.

Infarction occurs when tissue is *ischemic* for a period of time resulting in **necrosis** (or tissue death). **Ischemia** is a deficiency of blood in a localized area of tissue. Infarction may occur anywhere in the body. Pulmonary infarction is common in **pulmonary embolism.** Myocardial infarction is of concern to the health care professional because it may be life threatening.

The most common complication of myocardial infarction is the development of dysrhythmia which potentially may be life threatening.

Myocardial infarction sets into motion a vicious cycle. The infarction is thought to occur as a result of reduction or occlusion of blood flow in the coronary artery to the myocardium. Other theories suggest the infarction may be secondary to the development of dysrhythmia which causes the reduction in blood flow, or it may even be secondary to spasms of the coronary artery.

Whatever the cause, the infarction impairs normal function of the heart. This, in turn, may cause a reduction in cardiac output and, in 80 percent of all cases, chest pain. The chest pain is most alarming to the patient.

An infarction without pain is a **silent myocardial infarction.** The most common symptom of the **silent MI** is severe weakness and fatigue, often accompanied by **diaphoresis.**

Other signs and symptoms include **dyspnea,** radiating pain, a feeling of constriction in the chest, and a feeling of impending doom. Pain from a heart attack may radiate anywhere in the body. The left arm, jaw, head, and groin are the most common areas of radiation. A **Levine sign** is also common. The

Chest pain is totally absent in about 20 percent of all myocardial infarctions and should not be relied upon as a warning sign of heart attack.

FIGURE 11-4
Levine Sign

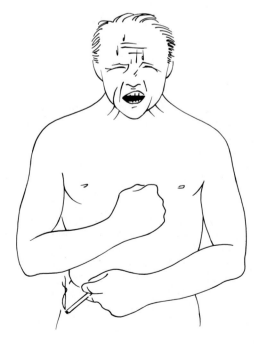

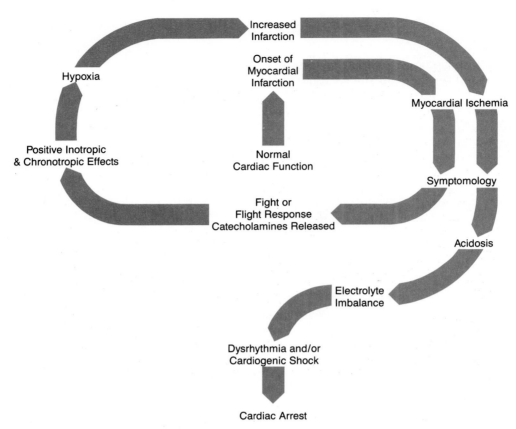

FIGURE 11-5
The Cycle of Myocardial Infarction

Levine sign is a clenched fist, usually the right, held closely over the sternum by the patient.

The most common symptom of myocardial infarction is not chest pain as one might suspect, but **denial** and a state of high anxiety. This emotional state results in stimulation of the sympathetic nervous system with the secretion of **catecholamines.**

The catecholamines secreted by the **fight or flight response** of the sympathetic nervous system stimulate the heart to work harder and faster. The additional workload increases oxygen demand and relative ischemia. The myocardial ischemia is increased, with an increase in the infarction and symptoms. As the condition worsens, pump failure or reduced cardiac output may contribute to **hypoxia,** anxiety, acidosis, electrolyte imbalance, and cardiogenic shock. All of these contribute to the infarction and generation of dysrhythmia.

The pathophysiology of the myocardial infarction indicates basic concepts of management. Initial management should include psychological aid to interrupt the anxiety-catecholamine cycle that is aggravating the myocardial infarction. There is an immediate need for supplemental oxygenation to increase the oxygen content of the blood supply to the myocardium.

Oxygen demand is reduced by restricting patient activity, and addressing afterload and preload problems. Another objective of management is to in-

Oxygen is the most essential medication in the management of myocardial infarction and should be administered even in patients who deny shortness of breath.

crease the blood supply to the myocardium by addressing the **occlusion** and increasing **collateral circulation.**

Dysrhythmia management is directed at eliminating or preventing life-threatening dysrhythmia and at reducing excessive oxygen demand.

Tachydysrhythmia

Tachydysrhythmia is generally undesirable because of its effect on oxygen demand of the myocardium. Chemotherapeutic agents or synchronized cardioversion may be used to eliminate tachydysrhythmia. Sinus and atrial tachycardias are frequently managed by treating the cause. Common causes are anxiety and caffeine use.

Synchronized Cardioversion

Synchronized cardioversion is similar to defibrillation. It uses a less powerful charge and is electronically synchronized within the defibrillator unit to discharge through the paddles to the patient on the R wave of the patient's QRS complex. The purpose of discharging on the R wave is to avoid a possible R on T phenomenon that could coincidentally occur by an untimed discharge. The R wave is the easiest portion of the cardiac complex for an electrocardiograph to automatically sense.

Carotid Massage

Carotid massage stimulates the parasympathetic nervous system by increasing aortic pressure. Carotid massage involves placing the clinician's fingers on either one of the patient's carotid arteries in the region of the sixth cervical vertebra and pressing two or three fingers on the artery. The artery should be pressed hard enough to retard normal arterial flow for 10 to 20 seconds. Massage should be stopped at the first sign of cardiac slowing. Theoretically this increases pressure in the aorta and stimulates blood pressure receptors called **baroreceptors** to produce a parasympathetic vagal response. This parasympathetic vagal response slows the heart. The right artery should be massaged first and, if there is no relief, the left may be massaged four or five minutes later.

Carotid massage may, on rare occasion, result in a conversion from tachydysrhythmia to asystole or ventricular fibrillation. The clinician is well advised, when attempting it in the emergent patient, to monitor the patient, establish a **prophylactic** intravenous line, and have resuscitative equipment and medications available.

Simultaneous bilateral carotid massage should *never* be performed.

Valsalva Maneuver

The **Valsalva maneuver** is a procedure which momentarily increases the intrathoracic pressures and results in a vagal response. It is performed by the patient who breathes in and bears down, while holding his breath, as if to strain with a difficult bowel movement. The same effect may be obtained by instructing the patient to blow up an elastic balloon, especially those that are difficult to inflate. The Valsalva maneuver is dramatic in its conversion of tachydysrhythmia to normal rhythm in the patient with anxiety induced tachydysrhythmia. The Valsalva maneuver has the same rare possibility of inducing ventricular fibrillation in the myocardial infarction patient as carotid massage. The same precautions should be taken.

Many patients found after cardiac arrest in their homes are found in the bathroom on the commode. One theory suggests these patients, usually elderly, confuse myocardial pain with constipation pain and retire to the bathroom. They strain to have a bowel movement and vagally stimulate their sick heart and arrest. Unfortunately these are circumstances in which privacy tends to delay discovery of the emergency situation.

Mammalian Diving Reflex

The **mammalian diving reflex** is a reflex found in aquatic mammals, such as whales, seals, and so on, that induces a vagolytic response to immersion in cold water or water under pressure. This enables those animals to slow their cardiac and respiratory metabolism while diving. Man has a remainder of his ancient mammalian reflex. Immersion of the head and chest in very cold water for 30 to 40 seconds will stimulate a vagal response and accomplish the same objective as carotid massage and the Valsalva maneuver. It has been clinically effective when used, but telling a patient to go soak his head in cold water is usually poor public relations.

Bradydysrhythmia

Bradydysrhythmia, such as heart block, is dealt with delicately to avoid increasing heart rate beyond what is necessary for adequate perfusion. Any increase in rate increases oxygen demand with a resulting undesired effect on myocardial ischemia. Hemodynamic symptoms include any decline in level of consciousness, diaphoresis, cyanosis, pallor, and escape ectopy. Fainting resulting from cardiac compromise is referred to as **Stokes-Adams attack.** Hemodynamically symptomatic bradydysrhythmias are first addressed by parasympathetic blocking agents to reduce possible parasympathetic induced causes of the dysrhythmias without causing beta stimulatory effects on the heart. If this avenue is ineffective, cautious efforts at sympathetic stimulation are the last chemotherapeutic avenue prior to pacemaker insertion. Pacemaker insertion is considered the definitive therapy for bradydysrhythmia.

Any pulseless dysrhythmia is initially managed with basic life-support resuscitative measures, including external chest compression and artificial respiration. Dysrhythmias are addressed secondarily.

The American Heart Association has been recognized by the National Academy of Sciences as the most appropriate organization to develop and maintain standards of care for management resuscitation of the cardiac patient.

Please refer to the *Textbook of Advanced Cardiac Life Support* of the American Heart Association for definitive standards of care.

The EKG, like any test, is subject to false positives and false negatives. A **false positive** occurs when the EKG indicates an abnormal reading that has no associated pathology. An example of a false positive would be ST depression in the monitoring lead, because it may not be true ST depression.

A **false negative** is common in the EKG and indicates a normal EKG when there is actually a medical pathology existing. It is fairly common for an acute myocardial infarction to be occurring without EKG changes. This particular false negative is called an **electrocardiographic silent MI.** This is similar to the silent MI, which is a myocardial infarction without pain.

Digitalis

Digitalis and digitalis preparations or analogs, such as Digoxin or Lanoxin, are commonly prescribed medications for cardiac patients. *The dosage range between therapeutic blood levels and toxic blood levels is small.* Digitalis is a potent **cardiotonic medication** that can rapidly make that small increase to toxic blood levels. **Digitalis toxicity** is a common cause of dysrhythmia and ectopy and may be fatal. Early recognition of digitalis toxicity is essential for appropriate management of the cardiac patient. Digitalis toxicity also needs to be recognized because it compromises the **concomitant** use of many antidysrhythmic medications and defibrillation or cardioversion. A patient taking digitalis without demonstrating toxic symptoms is said to be **digitalized.**

Noncardiac indications of digitalis intoxication are uncommon, but include loss of appetite (anorexia), vomiting, diarrhea, and visual field deficits, especially a yellow clouding of vision. Cardiac-related indications include frequent ectopy and group beating, as with the Wenckebach phenomenon.[1] Digitalis intoxication may precipitate a broad range of dysrhythmia including, but not limited to, bradydysrhythmia, such as heart block, and tachydysrhythmia, such as ventricular tachycardia, atrial tachycardia, atrial flutter, and atrial fibrillation.

> **Digitalis toxicity should be suspected in any digitalized patient presenting with dysrhythmia.**

Summary

The monitoring lead EKG is not a diagnostic tool. Its objective is to provide ongoing information about the patient's cardiac rhythm, major dysrhythmia, and an indication of cardiac irritability. The complete 12-lead electrocardiogram may be diagnostic of a variety of medical emergencies including myocardial infarction.

False positives are readings which indicate pathology when no pathology actually exists. False negatives are normal readings that fail to indicate pathology when it actually does exist. Both may exist in the EKG.

---

[1]Kevin M. McIntyre and A. James Lewis, eds., *Textbook of Advanced Cardiac Life Support* (Dallas, Texas: American Heart Association, 1983), p. 128.

Diagnostic information, which may be obtained from the complete 12-lead EKG, includes ST segment depression, which indicates myocardial ischemia; ST segment elevation, which indicates a myocardial pattern of injury; depressed J point, which is not diagnostic; T wave changes, which may indicate digitalis toxicity or electrolyte imbalance; and abnormal QRS complexes, which may indicate bundle (of His) branch block.

Myocardial infarction is a major concern of the EKG technician and patient. A variety of signs and symptoms include anxiety, denial, pain, diaphoresis, weakness, fatigue, decreased level of consciousness, and a Levine sign. Acute MI is a vicious cycle that perpetuates itself and is aggravated by the patient's autonomic nervous system fight or flight response to anxiety and pain. The pathophysiology of the cycle emphasizes the need for supplemental oxygenation and psychological aid for the victim of suspected myocardial infarction. Silent MI occurs in about 20 percent of all cases and is marked by a total absence of pain.

Tachydysrhythmia is managed clinically with sympathetic blocking agents and parasympathetic stimulating agents or therapies. Parasympathetic stimulating therapies include carotid massage and the Valsalva maneuver. Tachydysrhythmia may also respond to synchronized cardioversion.

Bradydysrhythmia is managed on an "if needed" basis in suspected AMI patients due to the risk of increasing the infarction. Any therapy that increases heart rate will increase oxygen demand and relative myocardial ischemia and risks increasing the infarction.

Digitalis and digitalis preparations are commonly prescribed cardiotonics which are extremely potent. Digitalis toxicity is a dangerous and common occurrence. It should be suspected in any digitalized patient presenting with dysrhythmia or AMI. Digitalis toxicity may precipitate any major dysrhythmia and complicates concomitant electrical and drug therapies because of drug interactions and potentiations.

Self-Study Questions

1. Discuss the major use of the monitoring lead and its limitations in diagnosis.
2. Differentiate between P mitrale and the abnormal P waves associated with premature junctional contractions.
3. Differentiate between ST segment depression and J point depression.
4. Discuss what ST segment depression or elevation represents on the monitoring lead and the full 12-lead EKG.
5. Discuss general concepts of management of acute myocardial infarction (AMI) and relate the concepts to the pathophysiology of the event. What is the most essential medication in the management of AMI?
6. Discuss general management for bradydysrhythmia in the possible AMI patient.
7. Discuss the effect of, and the general management concepts for, tachydysrhythmia in the potential AMI patient.
8. What is the definitive therapy for hemodynamically symptomatic bradydysrhythmia?

9. Discuss the initial general management of the pulseless dysrhythmic patient.
10. Discuss the precautions that should be taken prior to attempting carotid massage, Valsalva maneuver, or synchronized cardioversion.
11. Differentiate between false positive and false negative EKG readings.
12. Discuss the indications of digitalis toxicity in the digitalized patient and how that toxicity influences patient management.
13. Discuss the role of the American Heart Association in cardiac health care.

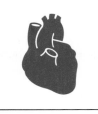

**It should be perfectly clear,
under the surface of the mud,
there's more mud there.**

CROSBY, STILLS & NASH

12

Recognition and Interpretation

OBJECTIVES

■ Identify all significant criteria for each major dysrhythmia.

■ List an organizational approach to the dysrhythmias. This approach should identify the criteria for each dysrhythmia.

■ Identify categorically, by each criterion, all dysrhythmias that criterion may apply to.

■ Perform an electrocardiogram analysis and identify any major dysrhythmia or ectopy.

■ State the clinical significance of each dysrhythmia or ectopy and the indications for therapeutic intervention.

KEY TERMINOLOGY

acardic rhythm
algorithm
bradycardic rhythm
criteria
    primary differential
    secondary differential
electromechanical dissociation
fibrillation
    atrial
    ventricular
normocardic rhythm
P on T phenomena
P:R ratio
R on T phenomena
regularity
tachycardic rhythms
unifocal
Wiederhold Algorithm

Dysrhythmia recognition will be facilitated by the knowledge that, while several **criteria** apply to a given dysrhythmia, some are more important than others. These important criteria are primary differential criteria. Primary differential criteria are rarely, if ever, absent from the dysrhythmia. Secondary differential criteria are usually present, but their absence does not rule out the dysrhythmia.

Primary and Secondary Criteria

Primary differential criteria are important diagnostic characteristics that differentiate one dysrhythmia from others. Primary criteria are rarely, if ever, absent from a dysrythmia.

Each criterion forms a piece of the puzzle. Some puzzle pieces, such as the outside borders, are the first to fall into place. These are the **primary differential criteria,** with which the secondary pieces fit. Some criteria will fit more than one puzzle, but each puzzle has only one *set of criteria.*

Secondary differential criteria include characteristics such as compensatory or non-compensatory pauses in evaluating premature contractions, the ventricular rate and saw-toothed pattern of atrial flutter, the wavy baseline of atrial fibrillation, P mitrale, T wave, ST segment, or J point changes, the relation of sinus arrhythmia to respiration, **P on T phenomena** associated with tachydysrhythmia, **R on T phenomena,** and in general, any criteria other than the primary six listed in this chapter.

Secondary differential criteria are diagnostic characteristics that differentiate one dysrhythmia from others. Secondary characteristics are usually present but their absence does not rule out the dysrhythmia.

Comparison Between Complexes

Regular sinus rhythms are characteristically **unifocal.** Unifocal cardiac complexes are all shaped alike. This facilitates the recognition of abnormal beats by comparing the abnormal beat to the rest of the beats in the rhythm. A PAC, for example, may be so premature that the P wave will fall on the T wave of the preceding complex. The P will not be obviously visible. The preceding complex, if a regular complex, should have a T wave exactly like the T waves of other regular beats in the rhythm. If the T wave is changed and taller, the clinician may safely determine the change represents a P on T phenomena (do not confuse this with the life-threatening R on T phenomena).

This criterion may also apply to dysrhythmia, such as atrial fibrillation. Fibrillatory (f) waves in a slow fibrillation (350 impulses per minute is relatively slow for atrial fibrillation) may be coarse enough to occasionally resemble flutter (F) waves. Comparison of the apparent flutter (F) wave to the rest of the rhythm will show it is not "regular" throughout the rhythm and thereby rule out the possibility of atrial flutter.

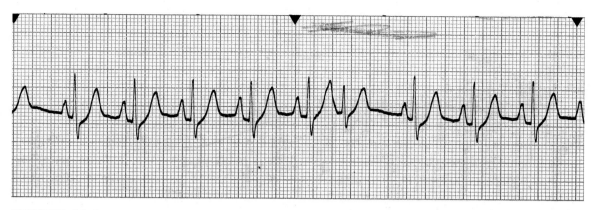

FIGURE 12-1
PAC with P on T
The elevated T wave of the normal beat preceding the PAC indicates a P wave
on the T.

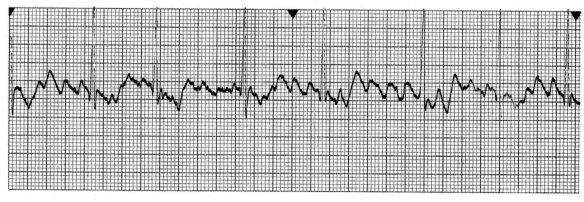

FIGURE 12-2
Atrial Fibrillation with Coarse Waves

Comparison Within Complexes

It may be difficult, sometimes, to distinguish the end of the QRS complex from
the start of the ST segment. The measurement of the QRS duration is an
essential primary differential criterion and this distinction must be made. The
QRS complex represents rapid electrical conduction. The stylus is moving rapidly over the graph paper. The paper is heat sensitive and is marked by the
stylus heat. When the stylus travels slowly, it exposes the graph paper to more
heat and the line it produces is a thick black line. When the stylus moves rapidly, it exposes the graph paper to less heat and the line it produces is a thin
black line. The thickness of the line may help make the determination of the **J
point.** The J point is the point at which the QRS complex ends and the ST
segment begins. This technique is only effective if the stylus heat is properly
adjusted. An overly hot stylus will eliminate any such distinctions.

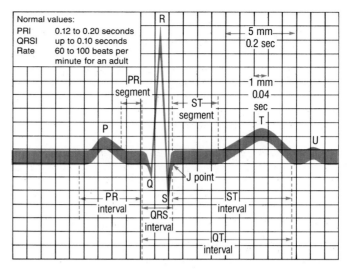

FIGURE 12-3
The Normal Electrocardiographic Cycle

Dysrhythmia Differentiation

Knowledge of the criteria of each dysrhythmia is essential to recognition. A cliché in the profession states, "One only sees what one looks for and only recognizes what one knows." This knowledge is most effectively used for dysrhythmia recognition when the dysrhythmia is approached via the criteria, rather than approaching the criteria through the dysrhythmia. This is a form of cross-indexing the dysrhythmias by their criteria. Rather than list each dysrhythmia's criteria, the clinician should be able to take one criterion and list all dysrhythmias that may share that criterion. Primary criteria are evaluated first, followed by secondary criteria, which help complete the evaluation.

For example, there are only four major dysrhythmias that have more than one P wave per QRS complex. The clinician may, after recognizing the presence of a **P:R ratio** that is greater than 1:1, concentrate on differential characteristics between only these four. An additional primary differential criterion that applies to these dysrhythmias is **rate.** Of the four dysrhythmias with more than one P wave per QRS complex, only one is tachycardic. The dysrhythmias are atrial flutter, Wenckebach, Mobitz II, and third degree block. Atrial flutter is the tachycardic dysrhythmia. Additional primary criteria and secondary criteria may be evaluated to determine the dysrhythmia if it is not tachycardic.

The single most important primary differential criterion is rate. Dysrhythmias group themselves by rate.

The single most important primary differential criterion is rate.

Acardic Rhythms

An **acardic rhythm** is one that has no waves or organized electrical activity. Rhythms that have no electrical activity have no electrocardiographic rate. There are only two dysrhythmias that have no rate. The absence of cardiac

TABLE 12-1   Bradycardic Dysrhythmias

Heart Block	Sinoatrial Rhythms	Junctional Rhythms	Ventricular Rhythms
First Degree	Sinus Bradycardia	Junctional Rhythm	Idioventricular
Wenckebach (Mobitz I)	Agonal		*Agonal
Mobitz II	Atrial Fibrillation		
Third Degree			

*May be sinus or ventricular in origin

complexes is associated with only **asystole** and **ventricular fibrillation.** An additional condition that has an electrocardiographic rate, but no pulse rate, is **electromechanical dissociation.**

Acardic Dysrhythmia

Flat Line = Asystole
Wavy Line = Ventricular Fibrillation

Bradycardic Rhythms

Bradycardic rhythms are those with rates less than 60 beats per minute. They include the following nine major dysrhythmias; first degree heart block, Wenckebach heart block, Mobitz II heart block, third degree heart block, sinus bradycardia, junctional rhythm, idioventricular rhythm, agonal rhythm, and atrial fibrillation with slow ventricular response. The heart blocks can cross the 60 beats per minute border slightly and are occasionally on the slow side of normal rate. Atrial fibrillation may also cross the rate border from bradydysrhythmia to normal rate and even tachydysrhythmia. However, only these nine major dysrhythmias need be considered with a bradydysrhythmia.

Normocardic Rhythms

Normocardic rhythms may include any rhythm with a rate between 60 and 100 beats per minute. These include the following nine dysrhythmias or rhythms: normal, or "regular sinus" with ectopy, sinus rhythm (NSR is listed

TABLE 12-2   Normocardic Rhythm and Dysrhythmias

Heart Block	Sinoatrial Rhythms	Junctional Rhythms	Ventricular Rhythms
First Degree	Normal Sinus Rhythm	Accelerated Junctional Rhythm	Accelerated Idioventricular Rhythm
Wenckebach (Mobitz I)	Sinus Arrhythmia		
Mobitz II	Sinus Arrest		
Third Degree	Atrial Fibrillation		

TABLE 12-3   Tachycardic Dysrhythmias

Sinoatrial	Junctional	Ventricular
Sinus Tachycardia Atrial Tachycardia Atrial Flutter Atrial Fibrillation	Junctional Tachycardia	Ventricular Tachycardia

although it is not dysrhythmic); sinus arrhythmia; sinus arrest; accelerated junctional rhythm; first degree heart block; Wenckebach block; Mobitz II block; complete heart block; and atrial fibrillation.

Tachycardic Rhythms

Tachycardic rhythms are dysrhythmias with rates faster than 100 beats per minute. There are six major dysrhythmias that may be tachycardic. These include sinus tachycardia, atrial tachycardia, atrial flutter, atrial fibrillation, junctional tachycardia, and ventricular tachycardia.

The first primary differential criterion limits the possibilities of dysrhythmia to no more than nine. This simplifies identification.

TABLE 12-4   Dysrhythmias Listed by Rate

Acardia	Bradycardia	Normocardia	Tachycardia
Asystole Ventricular Fibrillation	First Degree Wenckebach	*First Degree *Wenckebach	Sinus Tachycardia Atrial Tachycardia
	Mobitz II Third Degree Sinus Bradycardia	*Mobitz II Third Degree Normal Sinus Rhythm	Atrial Flutter *Atrial Fibrillation Junctional Tachycardia
	Agonal	Sinus Arrhythmia	Ventricular Tachycardia
	Atrial Fibrillation Junctional Rhythm	Sinus Arrest Atrial Fibrillation Accelerated Junctional Rhythm	

*May occur in more than one rate category

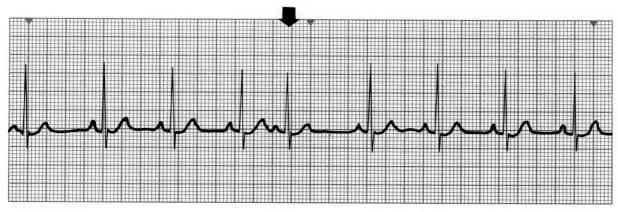

FIGURE 12-4
Regular Sinus Rhythm with PAC

Regularity

The **regularity** of a rhythm is the second primary differential criterion. It is second only to rate in importance. The regularity is determined by measuring the RR intervals. An artificial distinction must be made between determining irregularity caused by ectopic contractions and irregularity caused by dysrhythmia.

Irregularity caused by ectopy is marked by a shortened R to R interval prior to the premature contraction and an immediate elongated R to R interval following the premature contraction. This sequence of short-long intervals distinguishes irregularity caused by ectopy.

TABLE 12-5   Dysrhythmias Listed by Regularity

Regular	Irregular
Asystole	Agonal Rhythm
Idioventricular	Ventricular Fibrillation
Junctional	Wenckebach Block
Complete Heart Block	Atrial Fibrillation
Mobitz II	Sinus Arrhythmia
Sinus Bradycardia	Sinus Arrest
First Degree Block	
Normal Sinus Rhythm	
Accelerated Junctional Rhythm	
Sinus Tachycardia	
Atrial Tachycardia	
Ventricular Tachycardia	
Junctional Tachycardia	
Atrial Flutter	

TABLE 12-6   Dysrhythmias Listed by P:R Ratios

P:R = 0:1	P:R = 1:1	P:R > 1:1
Agonal Rhythm	Agonal Rhythm	Wenckebach Block
Idioventricular Rhythm	First Degree Block	Mobitz II Block
Junctional Rhythm	Sinus Bradycardia	Third Degree Block
Atrial Fibrillation	Normal Sinus Rhythm	Atrial Flutter
Accelerated Junctional Rhythm	Junctional Rhythm	
Ventricular Tachycardia	Accelerated Junctional Rhythm	
Junctional Tachycardia	Sinus Arrhythmia	
	Sinus Arrest	
	Sinus Tachycardia	
	Atrial Tachycardia	

Dysrhythmia recognition concentrates on the underlying rhythm. To evaluate the underlying rhythm, irregularity caused by ectopy (unless it is a run of three or more beats) should be temporarily disregarded.

P to R (P:R) Ratio

A third primary criterion that is related to rate is the **P to R ratio.** The ratio of P waves to QRS complexes is the P:R ratio and is normally 1:1. A ratio greater than or less than 1:1 will cause a difference of atrial rate from ventricular rate. The ventricular rate is of primary concern, but the atrial rate must be evaluated to determine dysrhythmias such as atrial flutter, atrial fibrillation, and heart block.

PR Intervals

The fourth primary criterion is the measurement of the **PR interval.** The PR interval is measured for duration and regularity. Only junctional rhythm has an abbreviated or retrograde PR interval. Only Wenckebach and third degree block have irregular PR intervals.

TABLE 12-7   Dysrhythmias Listed by PR Interval

Normal PRI	Elongated PRI	Irregular PRI
Sinus Bradycardia	First Degree Block	Wenckebach Block
Normal Sinus Rhythm	*Mobitz II Block	Third Degree Block
Mobitz II Block		
Sinus Tachycardia		
Atrial Tachycardia		
Sinus Arrhythmia		

*May be normal or elongated

QRS Interval

The last (fifth) general primary criterion is the **QRS interval.** Only third degree heart block, Mobitz II, and ventricular rhythms may have wide QRS intervals.

Dysrhythmia Identification

A methodical approach to rhythm analysis using these five primary criteria will enable the clinician to distinguish all major dysrhythmia and differentiate between them. The only exception is differentiation between asystole and ventricular fibrillation in which a sixth primary criterion is applied. That criterion is the **absence** of electrical activity, which distinguishes asystole.

The clinician should identify the dysrhythmia and confirm that identification by applying the secondary criteria which were listed earlier in the text.

The Wiederhold Algorithm

A step-by-step approach to the decision-making process in which alternative pathways are determined by circumstances is an **algorithm.** The **Wiederhold Algorithm** incorporates these primary criteria of rhythm analysis (see Figure 12-5). It provides a step-by-step approach which will make dysrhythmia identification simple to learn. Use of the algorithm and practice at recognition of waves, intervals, segments, and complexes will enable the clinician to recognize all major dysrhythmia. This will provide a foundation for additional learning in 12-lead electrocardiography.

TABLE 12-8   Dysrhythmias Listed by QRS Intervals

Wide QRS	Normal QRS	Absent QRS
Idioventricular Rhythm	*Agonal Rhythm	Ventricular Fibrillation
Ventricular Tachycardia	Wenckebach Block	Asystole
*Agonal Rhythm	Mobitz II Block	
*Third Degree Block	*Third Degree Block	
	First Degree Block	
	Junctional Rhythm	
	Accelerated Junctional Rhythm	
	Normal Sinus Rhythm	
	Sinus Arrhythmia	
	Sinus Arrest	
	Sinus Tachycardia	
	Atrial Tachycardia	
	Atrial Flutter	
	Atrial Fibrillation	
	Junctional Tachycardia	

*May be wide or normal

The Wiederhold Algorithm

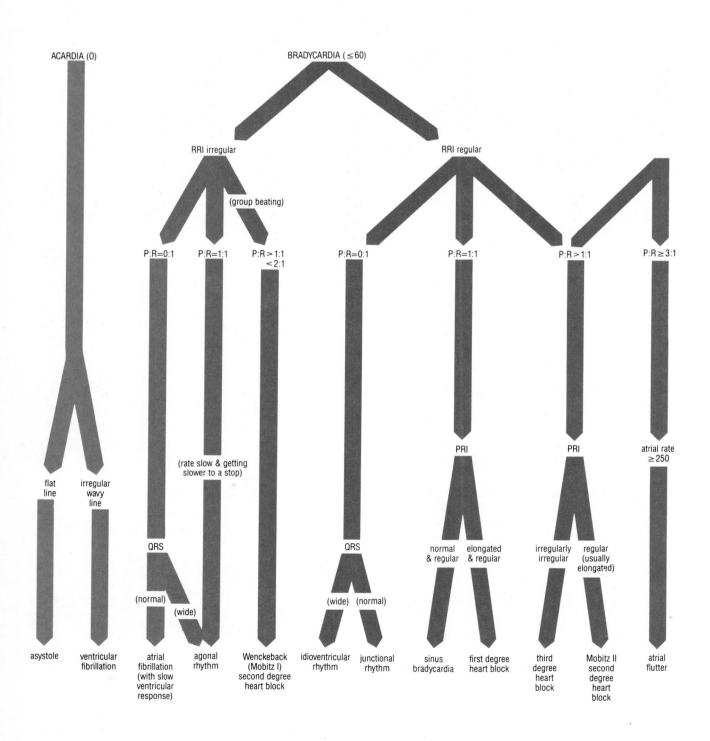

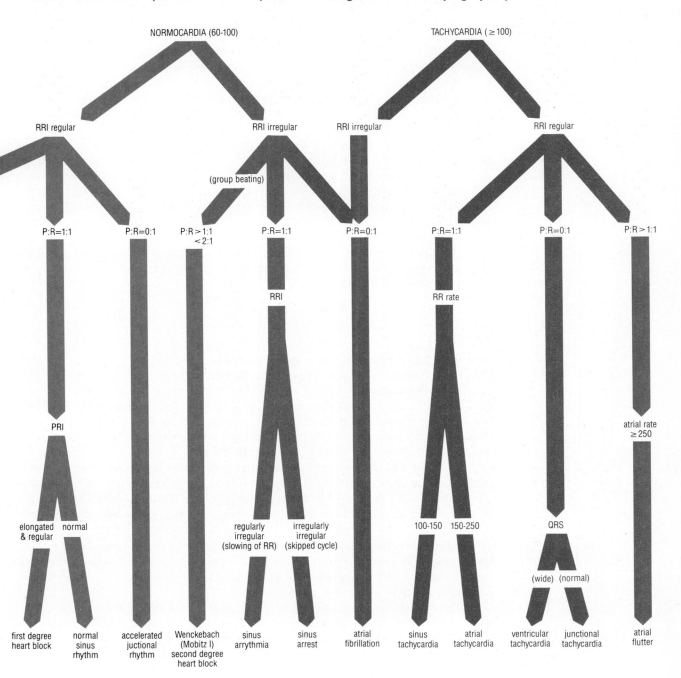

LEGEND
RRI—R to R interval
P:R—P to R ratio (normal 1 to 1)
(only upright, unabbreviated P
waves are indicated)
PRI—PR interval (normal .12 to .20 sec.)
QRS—QRS interval (normal to .12 sec.)

This algorithm is designed to facilitate recognition of major dysrhythmias. Many dysrhythmias are marked by premature or escape ectopy. This ectopy and its associated pauses should be temporarily disregarded to utilize the algorithm to recognize the underlying dysrhythmia.

NORMOCARDIA (60-100)

TACHYCARDIA (≥ 100)

RRI regular

RRI irregular

RRI irregular

RRI regular

(group beating)

P:R=1:1

P:R=0:1

P:R > 1:1
< 2:1

P:R=1:1

P:R=0:1

P:R=1:1

P:R=0:1

P:R > 1:1

RRI

RR rate

PRI

atrial rate
≥ 250

elongated
& regular

normal

regularly
irregular
(slowing of RR)

irregularly
irregular
(skipped cycle)

100-150

150-250

QRS

(wide)

(normal)

first degree
heart block

normal
sinus
rhythm

accelerated
juctional
rhythm

Wenckebach
(Mobitz I)
second degree
heart block

sinus
arrythmia

sinus
arrest

atrial
fibrillation

sinus
tachycardia

atrial
tachycardia

ventricular
tachycardia

junctional
tachycardia

atrial
flutter

It should be noted that electromechanical dissociation is a condition requiring clinical evaluation for recognition. It is not a true dysrhythmia. It is therefore not recognizable by dysrhythmia interpretation techniques, including this algorithm.

The first step in the algorithm is to identify the ventricular (and atrial, if they are not the same) rate.

After identifying the rate, as a second step, determine if the underlying rhythm (excluding ectopy) is regular or irregular.

In the third step the P:R ratio is evaluated and a differentiation is made between 0:1 (no P waves), 1:1 (one P wave to each QRS complex), or greater than 1:1 (more than one atrial complex per QRS complex).

The fourth and fifth steps may not be necessary. A majority of the major dysrhythmias are identified at this point. Additional evaluation may require evaluation of either the PR interval (fourth step) or the QRS interval (if no P wave exists).

All major dysrhythmias, except agonal rhythm, asystole, and ventricular fibrillation, have been identified at this point. The absence of electrical activity differentiates asystole from ventricular fibrillation. Agonal rhythm may have a normal or wide QRS complex but it is irregular, very slow, and getting slower until it becomes asystolic. There are only two major rhythms with totally irregularly irregular ventricular complexes. These are atrial fibrillation and agonal rhythm.

Pacemaker rhythm is defined as a *rhythm* and is not a dysrhythmia. It is therefore not included in the Wiederhold Algorithm. It is easily recognizable by the presence of spikes.

Summary

Dysrhythmia recognition will require an approach to the dysrhythmia through the criteria, rather than an approach to criteria from the dysrhythmia. This is a form of cross-indexing the dysrhythmias by their criteria. Primary differential criteria are criteria that are major identification tools in differentiating between dysrhythmias. Secondary differential criteria are identification tools that assist or confirm identification of major dysrhythmia. The secondary criteria are not always present in each dysrhythmia.

Comparison between complexes in a rhythm and between waves in a complex is essential to identifying dysrhythmia. Complexes in a normal rhythm should look alike. The QRS complex should have a thinner black line than the P wave, T wave, or any segments. This change in line helps identify the QRS complex.

There are five major primary differential criteria. These include rate, regularity, P:R ratio, PR interval, and QRS interval. One additional (sixth) primary criterion that is unique to asystole is the total absence of electrocardiographic activity.

Dysrhythmia interpretation is made easier by a methodical approach to the primary criteria. The Wiederhold Algorithm is a systematic approach to the primary criteria that differentiates between all major forms of dysrhythmia. To identify dysrhythmia, the algorithm systematically evaluates rate, regularity, P:R ratio, and either PR interval, or if there is no P wave, QRS interval. The sixth additional primary criterion is applied to acardic rhythms to differentiate between asystole and ventricular fibrillation. Electromechanical dissociation is not a dysrhythmia; rather, it is a condition which must be recognized from clinical findings. Electromechanical dissociation is not identified by the algorithm.

Self-Study Questions

1. Discuss and define primary differential criteria and secondary differential criteria. Identify the single most important differential criterion.
2. List all major dysrhythmias by classification of rate.
3. List all major dysrhythmias by classification of rate and regularity.
4. List and differentiate between two major dysrhythmias that are regularly irregular.
5. List and differentiate between the three major dysrhythmias that are irregularly irregular.
6. List and differentiate between four major dysrhythmias that have more than one definable atrial wave.
7. List and differentiate between eight major dysrhythmias that have no P waves.
8. List the single dysrhythmia that has no electrical activity.
9. Identify the major rhythm that has spikes.
10. Identify the associated rates for six tachydysrhythmias.
11. Discuss and differentiate between four forms of heart block and include an evaluation of PR intervals, PR ratios, RR regularity, PP regularity, and PR regularity. Include an evaluation of rate.
12. Discuss and differentiate between all major dysrhythmias that have an elongated or prolonged PR interval.
13. Identify the single dysrhythmia that may cross all rate lines from bradydysrhythmic to tachydysrhythmic.
14. Discuss why an ectopic beat causes irregularity preceding it and following it.

> *And further, by these, my son, be admonished:*
> *of making many books there is no end;*
> *and much study is a weariness of the flesh.*
> *Let us hear the conclusion of the whole matter. . . .*
>
> ***ECCLESIASTES 12:11–12***

Glossary

This glossary is intended as a convenient reference to electrocardiographic terms and includes a pronunciation guide for hard-to-pronounce words. The definitions in many cases are limited in scope for the purpose of brevity. You are encouraged to refer to a medical dictionary or a more comprehensive electrocardiography or cardiology text for additional clarification.

abbreviation   a shortened form

aberrant (a-'ber-ənt)   a deviation from normal

absolute refractory period   *see* refractory period

acardia (a-'kärd-ē-ə)   absence of the heart or heartbeat

acardic rhythm   having no cardiac rhythm—asystole or ventricular fibrillation

accelerated junctional rhythm   a junctional rhythm with a rate faster than the normal automatic rate of the junctions (40 to 60 beats per minute) but not fast enough to be considered tachycardic (over 100 beats per minute)

action potential   the electrical energy developed in a specialized cardiac conduction cell or muscle cell which causes a response from the cell

adrenergic (ad-rə-'nər-jik) **hormonal influence**   sympathetic nervous system influence on the body via the group of drugs, known as catecholamines, secreted by the kidneys

adrenergic receptor site   a cellular chemoreceptor site that combines with an adrenergic drug or hormone to alter the function of the cell; predominant classifications are alpha, beta, and dopaminergic

afterload   the arterial resistance against which the ventricle of the heart must pump

agonal ('ag-ən-ᵊl)   pertaining to death or dying

agonal rhythm   a cardiac rhythm associated with patient death; also known as "dying heart rhythm"

algorithm ('al-gə-rith-əm)   a special method of solving a problem or making conclusions using a repetitive decision-making process

alpha receptor site   a cellular chemoreceptor site; *see* adrenergic receptor site

amplitude ('am-plə-t(y)üd)   referring to size, extent of movement, or strength; the height of a wave on the EKG

analog ('an-ᵊl-òg)   a chemical compound having a similar structure to another; may have a similar or opposite action to the other drug.

anastomosis (ə-nas-tə'mō-səs)   an articulation or communication between two vessels

aneurysm ('an-yə-riz-əm)   a bulge or sac formed by an abnormal dilatation of the wall of an artery or chamber of the heart

anion ('an-ī-ən)   a negatively charged ion; an ion which has accepted an electron.

anode ('an-ōd)   the positive electrode of an EKG lead

aorta (ā-'òrt-ə)   the main trunk of the arterial system; arises from the left ventricle of the heart; carries blood from the heart into the systemic circulatory circuit

aortic valve   the organic valve between the left ventricle and the aorta

apex ('ā-peks)   the point of a cone or conical structure; the distal point of the left ventricle of the heart

apnea ('ap-nē-ə)   without breathing; respiratory arrest

arrhythmia (ā-'rith-mē-ə)   absence of rhythm, especially pertaining to the heartbeat; irregular heartbeat

artifact ('ärt-i-fakt)   a changed appearance produced artificially; interference in an electrocardiogram

asystole (a-'sis-tə-lē)   cardiac standstill; absence of cardiac conduction and contraction

atrial (ā-trē-əl) **flutter**   a cardiac dysrhythmia characterized by an atrial rate between 250 and 350 beats per minute; ventricular rate is usually less than the atrial rate

atrial kick   referring to the distension of the ventricles which results from contraction of the atria, forcing blood into the partially filled ventricles

atrial systole   contraction of the atria

atrial tachycardia   a cardiac dysrhythmia characterized by an atrial rate between 150 and 250 beats per minute

atrioventricular (ā-trē-ō-ven-'trik-yə-lər) **block**   referring to a difference in atrial and ventricular rates

atrioventricular node   a node of specialized cardiac muscle fibers at the base of the inter-atrial septum which transmits the cardiac impulse generated by the sinoatrial node; *aka* node of Aschoff & Tawara

atrioventricular synchronous pacing   a pacemaker rhythm in which the ventricles are stimulated shortly after the atrial contraction; this pacing maximizes stroke volume by using atrial kick and may allow the heart to respond to natural atrial pacing

atrium ('a-tre-əm)   the upper chamber of each half of the heart; *pl* atria

auricula (ò-'rik-yə-lə)   a small conical tissue mass on the upper anterior portion of each atrium; an obsolete term for atrium

automaticity (ȯt-ə-mə-'tis-ət-ē) referring to the unique ability of cardiac muscle tissue to spontaneously generate an impulse which can result in muscular contraction

AV dissociation (general) a term applied to any dysrhythmia in which the atrial stimuli are not conducted in a normal manner to the ventricles; (specific) a term applied to a dysrhythmia very similar to third degree heart block, but which has a ventricular rate equal to or faster than the atrial rate

aVF (augmented voltage left foot) referring to a unipolar electrocardiographic lead in which the positive electrode is attached to the patient in the area of an extremity, in this case the left foot; the voltage of the EKG is augmented 50% electronically inside the electrocardiograph

aVL (augmented voltage left arm) refer to aVF

aVR (augmented voltage right arm) refer to aVF

axis a line of measurement between two points; the standard locations for EKG leads; *pl* axes

baroreceptor (bar-ō-ri-'sep-tər) a nerve ending which senses changes in blood pressure

baseline on the electrocardiogram, the isoelectric line from which waves and deflections are measured

benign (bi-'nīn) having no negative effect on the body

beta receptor site a cellular chemoreceptor site; *see* adrenergic receptor site

bicuspid (bī-'kəs-pəd) **valve** valve between the left atrium and left ventricle of the heart; having two cusps to the value; *see* mitral valve

bifurcate ('bī-fər-kāt) to separate into two divisions

bigeminal (bī-'jem-ən-ᵊl) occurring in pairs; every other heartbeat

biphasic a wave with both negative and positive portions

bipolar limb lead referring to an EKG lead in which there is both a negative and positive electrode used to create the axis

blind defibrillation defibrillation of a pulseless victim of cardiac arrest without interpretation of the EKG by qualified personnel

brachiocephalic (brā-kē-ō-sə-fal-ik) **trunk** pertaining to the artery which arises from the aorta and provides the initial pathway for the circulation of blood to the right head and arm areas; obsolete term is innominate artery

bradycardia (brād-i-'kärd-ē-ə) referring to a heart rate slower than normal (usually slower than 60 beats per minute); a synonym is bradydysrhythmia

bradycardic rhythm an abnormally slow (rate less than 60 beats per minute) cardiac rhythm

bradydysrhythmia *see* bradycardia

bundle branch one of the divisions of the bundle of His

bundle branch block an interruption of normal cardiac conduction through the bundle of His or one of its branches; bundle branch block should not be confused with the block dysrhythmias (first, Wenckebach, Mobitz II, and third degree)

bundle of His a small band of specialized cardiac muscle fibers that originates in the AV node, passes through the junction, divides into the left and right bundles which distribute to the left and right ventricles, terminating in Purkinje fibers; propagates the cardiac impulse to the ventricles

calibration (kal-ə-'brā-shən) the standardization of the EKG machine; the sensitivity of the stylus is set to read 10 millimeters in height in response to a one millivolt charge

cardiac ('kärd-ē-ak) **arrest** the cessation of pulses, followed shortly by cessation of respiration and absence of blood pressure; clinical death

cardiac contraction a contraction of the heart

cardiac cycle the period from the beginning of one heartbeat to the beginning of the next heartbeat; electrocardiographically one complete cycle of waves and complexes including the PQRST and possibly U waves

cardiac irritability an increase of automaticity to an undesired level at which ectopic contractions or cardiac dysrhythmias occur

cardiac output the amount of blood pumped by each ventricle in one minute; usually 5 liters in the average adult at rest, or 3.0 liters per square meter of body surface per minute

cardiac oxygen need the amount of oxygen required by the heart; varies in response to muscular activities, including cardiac rate and contractility

cardiac reserve the potential capacity of the heart to function well beyond its resting state, in response to physiological or psychological demands

cardiac standstill cardiac arrest; *see* asystole and ventricular fibrillation

cardiogenic ('kärd-ē-ō-'jen-ik) **shock** shock resulting from abnormal function of the heart

cardiorespiratory arrest a stoppage of cardiac contractions and spontaneous respirations

cardiotonic (kärd-ē-ō-'tän-ik) **medication** one of a group of medications which produces or restores normal muscle tone of the heart

carotid (kə-'rät-əd) **bodies** located in the carotid arteries; structures, which respond to changes in arterial oxygen and/or pressure levels

carotid massage a technique of stimulating a vagal response by occluding carotid artery blood flow

catecholamine (kat-ə-'kō-lə-mēn) any one of a group of natural hormones secreted by the adrenal glands or cortex of the kidneys; agents which have sympathetic actions and include epinephrine, norepinephrine, dopamine, and others

cathode ('kath-ōd)   the negative electrode of an EKG lead

cation ('kat-ī-ən)   a positively charged ion; an ion which has donated an electron

cholinergic (kō-lə-'nər-jik) **effect**   a parasympathetic response to acetylcholine or acetylcholine-like agents

chordae tendineae ('kȯr-dē 'tən-də-nē-ē)   small tendinous cords which connect the leaves of cardiac valves to the papillary muscles of the ventricular endocardium

chronic obstructive pulmonary disease   a group of chronic diseases marked by increasing obstruction to pulmonary function, increasing limitation on physical activity, and erosion of respiratory reserve volume; major forms of COPD include emphysema, bronchitis, and asthma

chronotropic ('krä-nə-träp-ik) **effect**   having an effect on timing, a positive chronotropic effect increases the cardiac rate; a negative chronotropic effect decreases the cardiac rate

chronotropy   having an effect on the rate of contraction of the heart

circumflex artery   a division of the left coronary artery

close coupled beats   a pair of cardiac contractions in which the second of the pair follows the first very closely; the second beat is located (or threatens to locate) on the T wave of the first beat

collateral circulation   circulation provided by anastomosing vessels or adjacent vessels

compensation   one physiological system or portion of a system making up for a defect in another system or portion of a system (for example, initial hypovolemia will be compensated for by an increase in cardiac rate to maintain cardiac output)

compensatory ('kəm-pen(t)-sə-tōr-ē) **pause**   a pause in cardiac rhythm following a premature contraction; the pause is of sufficient duration to allow the cardiac rhythm to resume (with the following complex) the normal cycle, as if the timing had been uninterrupted

complex   referring to the QRS waves of the cardiac cycle; it is immaterial whether all three waves are actually present (for example, an R and an S wave without a Q wave in a cardiac cycle is still considered a QRS complex)

concomitant (kən-'käm-ət-ənt)   occurring at the same time; to take two medications at the same time

conduction   the transmission of the cardiac impulse through the myocardium

conduction system   a system of specialized cardiac cells which have greater automaticity and conductivity than other cardiac cells. Its major components include the SA node, the intra-atrial pathways, AV node, bundle of His and its divisions, and the Purkinje fibers

conductivity   a measure of the ability of a cardiac cell or group of cells to capture and conduct an external stimulus

contractility (kän-trak-'til-ət-ē)   referring to the ability to contract; strength of contraction

contraction   a shortening or tightening of a muscle

coronary ('kȯr-ə-ner-ē) **artery**   one of two primary arteries that perfuse the heart; they arise from the right and left aortic sinuses at the base of the aorta

coronary artery disease   arteriosclerosis or atherosclerosis affecting the coronary arteries; may be symptomatic with angina, myocardial infarction, or sudden death syndrome, or may be asymptomatic

coronary sinus   the cavity which is the terminal of coronary circulation; it empties its venous blood into the right atrium

coronary sulcus ('səl-kəs)   a fissure on the surface of the heart in which the coronary vessels lie

coronary veins   pertaining to the venous return of coronary circulation; they empty into the coronary sinus

couplet (kəp-lət)   a pair of two abnormal contractions occurring consecutively

coupling interval   the interval between a premature complex and the preceding normal beat

cusp ('kəsp)   one of the leaf-like divisions of a cardiac valve

defibrillation (dē-fib-rə-'lā-shən)   stopping fibrillation of the heart, usually by universal depolarization with external electrical energy; the intent is to permit the heart to resume its natural routine electrical activity on its own after defibrillation

defibrillator   an electrical device used to deliver an electrical defibrillation to the heart; one who defibrillates

deflection (di-'flek-shən)   a movement away from baseline on an electrocardiogram

denial   a negative answer to inquiry about symptoms; it may occur as a psychological defense mechanism in which the patient is subconsciously refusing to accept intolerable ideas; a common occurrence with myocardial infarction, even in highly educated medical personnel

depolarization (dē-pō-lə-rə-'zā-shən)   reversal of polarization of cardiac cells' resting membrane potentials, associated with conduction of an impulse and normally associated with muscular contraction

depressed wave   a wave which is flatter (has less amplitude) than normal

dextrocardia ('dek-strō-,kärd-ē-ə)   a congenital abnormality in which the heart is located in the right side of the thorax with the apex pointing toward the right side

diaphoresis (dī-ə-fə-'rē-səs)   profuse perspiration, usually seen as a thin layer of perspiration over the whole body rather than in concentrated areas of heat, such as under the arms

digitalized   referring to a patient who is taking digitalis or a digitalis preparation

dysfunction (dis-'fənk-shən)   an impairment in the function of an organ or system

dyspnea ('dis(p)-nē-ə)   having difficulty breathing

dysrhythmia (dis-'rith-mē-ə)   abnormal cardiac rhythm

ECG   *see* EKG

ectopic (ek-'täp-ik)   a cardiac impulse originating at a site other than the node

ectopic focus   a site of origin of a cardiac complex other than the normal SA node; *pl* foci

ectopy ('ek-tə-pē)   conducted premature or escape complexes from a site other than normal

Einthoven's (īn-'tō-vənz) **triangle**   a triangle that is the mathematical model of the three standard EKG limb leads; named after Willem Einthoven, Dutch physiologist, in honor of his discovery of the mechanism of the electrocardiogram

EKG   abbreviation; *see* electrocardiogram

electrocardiogram (i-lek-trō-'kärd-ē-ə-gram)   a record of the electrical activity of the heart

electrocardiograph (i-lek-trō-'kärd-ē-ə-graf)   a device for recording electrical activity of the heart

electrode (i-'lek-trōd)   a conductive device through which an electric current is applied to an object or person; may be positive (anode) or negative (cathode)

electrolyte (i-'lek-trə-līt)   a substance which in solution dissolves to form ions that will conduct an electrical charge

electromechanical dissociation (i-lek-trō-mə-kan-i-kəl dis-ō-sē-ā-shən)   a condition in which the EKG reveals electrical cardiac activity that is not matched with muscular, mechanical activity

electrophysiology (i-lek-trō-fiz-ē-'äl-ə-jē)   the study of the electrical properties of living cells

elongation (ē-lȯn-'gā-shən)   lengthening of an interval

embolism ('em-bə-liz-əm)   a traveling particle which causes an occlusion of circulation

endocardium (en-dō-'kärd-ē-əm)   the serous membrane lining the inner surface of the cavities of the heart; it is continuous with the intima of the arteries

epicardium (ep-ə-'kärd-ē-əm)   the serous, visceral layer of the pericardium; the innermost layer of the pericardium and the outermost layer of the myocardium

escape beat   a contraction from an ectopic pacemaker, occurring due to failure or impairment of normal (faster) pacemakers; ectopic response to failure of overdrive suppression

extra systole ('ek-strə 'sis-tə-lē)   a premature contraction of the heart, usually originating from a site other than the SA node

failure to capture   failure of the myocardium to respond to the stimulus of a pacemaker

failure to fire   failure of a pacemaker to function

false negative   a test result that wrongly rules out a diagnostic category

false positive   a test result that wrongly indicates a diagnostic category

fibrillation (fib-rə-'lā-shən)   uncoordinated action by individual muscle cells and may be atrial or ventricular in origin; ventricular fibrillation generates no cardiac output or pulses and is immediately life threatening; atrial fibrillation is the most common dysrhythmia and is clinically less significant than ventricular fibrillation

fibrillatory (fib-rə-'lə-tō-rē) **wave**   the atrial wave associated with the dysrhythmia atrial fibrillation; occasional f waves may be coarse enough to resemble P waves, but they are not regular or unifocal in shape

fight or flight response   the response of the sympathetic division of the autonomic nervous system to stress, anxiety, or pain; catecholamines are secreted with a detrimental effect upon myocardial infarction

flutter wave   the atrial wave associated with the dysrhythmia atrial flutter; flutter waves are more pointed than the normal P wave and are very regular at a rate of 250 to 350 beats per minute

focus ('fō-kəs)   a site or place of origin; the normal focus for cardiac activity is the SA node; *pl* foci

Frank-Starling effect   refers to the effect that the greater a muscle is stretched, the more forceful its subsequent contraction will be; a primary determinant of cardiac output; *aka* Starling's law

fusion ('fyü-zhən) **beat**   a cardiac contraction incorporating characteristics from two foci

f wave   *see* fibrillation wave

F wave   *see* flutter wave

heart block   a condition in which normal cardiac conduction is impaired; there are several forms usually with the higher degree being more clinically significant; complete heart block (*aka* third degree heart block) is usually the most clinically significant, frequently requiring insertion of a pacemaking device

hemodynamic (hē-mō-dī-'nam-ik) **compromise** a weakening of the cardiovascular system; the cardiovascular system fails to maintain adequate perfusion pressures; signs and symptoms are those of shock

hemodynamic decompensation the sudden failure of the body's compensating mechanisms; the process includes an initial onset of disability, secondary body mechanisms begin to compensate for the disability, and finally the compensating mechanisms fail

hemodynamically symptomatic (sim-tə-'mat-ik) having the signs or symptoms of shock

hyperacute ('hī-pər-ə-'kyüt) extremely acute

hypertrophy (hī-'pər-trə-fē) enlargement or overgrowth of a muscle; *athletic H* strengthening and thickening of the myocardium as a result of exercise; *pathologic H* diseased enlargement of the myocardium as a result of enlargement of the ventricle chambers and stretching of the myocardial muscle walls (this is due to chronic illness such as congestive heart failure or hypertension)

hypokalemia (hī-pō-kə-lē-mē-ə) abnormally low body levels of the electrolyte potassium

hypotension ('hī-pō-ten-chən) abnormally low blood pressure

hypoxia (hip-'äk-sē-ə) generalized reduction of oxygen supply to body tissues; *syn* hypoxemia

idiojunctional (id-ē-ə-'jən(k)-shən-ᵊl) having a site of origin in the junction of the heart

idioventricular (id-ē-ə-ven-'trik-yə-lər) having a site of origin in one of the ventricles of the heart

infarction (in-'färk-shən) formation of an area of tissue necrosis, resulting from inadequate perfusion; usually associated with myocardial infarction but applies as well to any potentially infarcted area of the body such as pulmonary or intestinal, etc

innervation (in-ər-'vā-shən) the supply of nerves and their influence to a part

inotropic (ē-nə-'trō-pik) **effect** any change in the force of muscular contraction; *negative i* denotes decreasing contraction; *positive i* denotes increasing contraction

inotropy ('ē-nə-trə-pē) denotes a measure of muscular contractility

internodal (int-ər-'nōd-ᵊl) **pathways** the paths of the conduction system and the cardiac impulses between the SA node and the AV node

interpolated (in-'tər-pə-lāt-əd) **beat** the occurrence of an ectopic beat, which is not significantly premature and occurs between two normal beats

interval a horizontal measurement on a electrocardiogram from one point of a complex, wave, or baseline to another point; a finite period of time

intra-atrial (in-trə-'ā-trē-əl) **pathways** the paths the conduction system and cardiac impulses take within the atria of the heart

inversion an electrocardiographic presentation opposite of what is normal for a given lead; *note* students frequently confuse this with negative deflection—inversion may be, but does not have to be negatively deflected

irritability the ability of the cardiac cells to respond to an impulse; a condition in which the heart responds excessively to a stimulus

ischemia (is-'kē-mē-ə) a reduction of oxygenated blood to a localized area of tissue

isoelectric (ī-sō-i-'lek-trik) having no electrical charge; the baseline of the EKG divides an area of positive from an area of negative measurements and is isoelectric

J point the point in the EKG at which the QRS complex ends and the ST segment begins

J point depression the J point is below baseline and the ST segment slopes continuously up to baseline

junction ('jən(k)-shən) the area of cardiac tissue which separates the atria from the ventricles

junctional ('jən(k)-shən-ᵊl) **dysrhythmia** any one of the three junctional dysrhythmias: junctional rhythm, accelerated junctional rhythm, and junctional tachycardia

junctional escape rhythm a junctional rhythm of three or more consecutive beats occurring as a result of depressed automaticity of the atria

junctional rhythm a cardiac dysrhythmia in which the primary pacemaker is within the junction

junctional tachycardia a junctional rhythm of three or more consecutive beats with a rate greater than 100 beats per minute

Kent fibers accessory conduction fibers which travel from the atria to the ventricles; *aka* as bundles of Kent

Levine sign the physical sign of holding the fist, usually the right, clenched in the mid-sternum area; it is associated with acute myocardial infarction

LGL *see* Lown-Ganong-Levine syndrome

limb leads referring to one of the six EKG leads in which an axis uses an electrode attached to one or more of the body's limbs

Lown-Ganong-Levine syndrome a supraventricular tachycardia associated with short PR intervals (usually less than twelve-hundredths seconds) and a normal QRS interval; usually referred to as LGL syndrome

mammalian (mə-'mā-lē-ən) **diving reflex**   a parasympathetic response to increased thoracic or atmospheric pressure or cold water; slowing of cardiac rate, respiration, and other body functions

MCL₁   a monitoring EKG lead, known as modified chest lead I, and also as Marriott's chest lead

mediastinum (mēd-ē-ə-'stī-nəm)   the thoracic cavity between the two lungs in which the heart and great vessels lie

mitral ('mī-trəl) **valve**   the bicuspid valve located between the left atrium and left ventricle

multifocal (məl-ti-'fō-kəl)   having multiple areas of origin (foci); cardiac complexes which are shaped unalike; *syn* multiformed

multiformed   *see* multifocal

myocardial (mi-ə'kärd-ē-əl) **infarction**   an infarction affecting the myocardium; *see* infarction

myocardium (mī-ə-'kärd-ē-əm)   the (middle) muscle layer of the wall of the heart; referring to the heart in general

myopathy (mī-'äp-ə-thē)   disease of the heart (myocardium) muscle

necrosis (nə-'krō-səs)   cellular or tissue death

net deflection   a measurement of both the negative and positive size of the QRS complex of the EKG; it is determined to be either negative or positive by subtracting the smaller deflection from the larger, if the QRS is biphasic

nodal ('nōd-ᵊl) **contraction**   a second name for junctional contraction

nodal rhythm   a synonym for junctional rhythm

node ('nōd)   a tissue mass, refers to the sinoatrial (SA node) or the atrioventricular (AV) node

non-compensatory pause   a pause following an ectopic contraction; the pause is not long enough to allow the cardiac rhythm to resume its original rhythm as if it had been uninterrupted; associated with PACs and sometimes with PJCs

normal sinus rhythm (NSR)   the most desirable cardiac rhythm; it is a regular sinus rhythm with a rate of 60 to 100, which contains no ectopic beats

normocardia (nȯr-mō-'kärd-ē-ə)   referring to having a heart rate within normal ranges of 60 to 100 beats per minute

normocardic (nȯr-mō-'kärd-ık) **rhythm**   having a cardiac rate of 60 to 100 beats per minute

occlusion (ə-'klü-zhən)   an obstruction or closing of a vessel or container

overdrive suppression   referring to the suppression of cardiac pacemakers by a superior pacemaker with a faster intrinsic firing rate; the faster pacer propagates an impulse through the myocardium before other pacemakers can fire

PAC   premature atrial contraction; a contraction which originates in the atrium and occurs early in the cardiac rhythm

pacemaker   a cardiac cell or group of cells which automatically initiates a cardiac impulse that propagates to other regions of the heart; a mechanical device which is therapeutically implanted in patients requiring external pacing such as with chronic symptomatic, complete heart block

pacemaker pulse generator   the electronic components of a pacemaker

pacemaker rhythm   any cardiac rhythm which includes cardiac contractions occurring in response to pacemaker impulses

pacer   a pacemaker

papillary ('pap-ə-ler-ē) **body**   a muscular tissue in the ventricles of the heart to which the chordae tendineae attach; *aka* papillary muscle

parasympathetic (par-ə-sim-pə-'thet-ik)   pertaining to the craniosacral division of the autonomic nervous system

parasympathetic influence   the effect of the parasympathetic nervous system on the cardiovascular system

parasympathetic stimulation   stimulation of the parasympathetic nervous system; it may be accomplished by vagal maneuvers such as the Valsalva maneuver, immersion in cold water, or chemotherapeutic means

parasystole (par-ə-'sis-tə-lē)   an abnormally prolonged period of time between systole and diastole; a cardiac dysrhythmia attributed to the interaction of two foci independently initiating cardiac impulses at different rates (not to be confused with heart block)

paroxysm ('par-ək-siz-əm)   a sudden episode of signs or symptoms of a disease or dysrhythmia

paroxysmal (par-ək-'siz-məl)   occurring in paroxysms

paroxysmal atrial tachycardia   an atrial tachycardia which starts and stops suddenly; atrial tachycardia is a cardiac dysrhythmia marked by a rate between 150 and 250 beats per minute

PAT   *see* paroxysmal atrial tachycardia

pericardial tamponade (per-ə-'kärd-ē-əl 'tam-pə-nād)   progressive compression of the heart by the accumulation of blood or other fluid within the pericardial sac

pericardiocentesis (per-ə-kärd-ē-ō-sen-'tē-səs)   to surgically remove fluid from the pericardial cavity

pericarditis (per-ə-kär-'dīt-əs)   inflammation of the pericardium

pericardium (per-ə-'kärd-ē-əm)   the fibroserous sac enclosing the heart and the roots of the great vessels

PJC   (premature junctional contraction) a contraction which originates in the junction or at the AV node and occurs early in the cardiac rhythm; *aka* premature nodal contraction

P mitrale ('mi-trəl)   an abnormality of the P wave where there appears to be an indentation or "notch" in the middle of the P wave

PNC   premature nodal contraction, a contraction which originates in the junction or at the AV node and occurs early in the cardiac rhythm

polarized ('pō-lə-rīzd)   the condition of a cardiac cell being either positively or negatively charged, depending on the separation of charged ions by the cellular membrane and cellular ion "gates" or "channels" through the membrane

P on T phenomena   the P wave of a cardiac complex is falling on the T wave of the preceding cardiac complex; common in tachycardias and in some forms of blocks

precordial (prē-kȯr-jəl) **lead**   referring to one of the standard six chest leads of the complete 12-lead EKG

preload (prē-'lōd)   the pressure of venous blood entering the left (systemic) or right (pulmonic) atrium of the heart; a significant determinant of cardiac workload

premature   to occur before scheduled; early

premature junctional contractions   ectopic cardiac beats originating in the junction or atrioventricular node

prognosis (präg-'nō-səs)   a prediction of a patient's condition

prolapsed valve   displacement of a cardiac valve, usually resulting in its reversal of position due to pressures exerted by the ventricle

propagated ('präp-ə-gāt-id) **action potential**   an action potential of a cardiac cell, which is perceived by an adjacent cell, that in turn depolarizes in response to the action potential and propagates it to other adjacent cardiac cells

prophylactic (prō-fə-'lak-tik)   an action intended to prevent disease or dysrhythmia

pulmonary ('pu̇l-mə-ner-ē) **artery**   referring to the artery which carries unoxygenated blood from the right ventricle to the lungs

pulmonary embolism   an embolism occurring in the lungs

pulmonary vein ('vān)   referring to one of the veins which carries oxygenated blood from the lungs to the left atrium of the heart

Purkinje (per-kin-jē) **fiber**   atypical cardiac muscle fibers which form part of the conduction system of the heart

PVC   premature ventricular contraction; a contraction which originates in the ventricle and occurs early in the cardiac rhythm

QRS complex   the portion of an electrocardiogram composed of any combination of one or more of the Q, R, or S waves and/or primes of those waves

receptor (ri-'sep-tər) **site**   a cellular chemoreceptor site that combines with an adrenergic drug or hormone to alter the function of the cell; predominant classifications are alpha, beta, and dopaminergic

reentry (rē-'en-trē)   referring to a phenomenon in which the cardiac impulse, instead of following a normal conduction pathway, follows a circuitous path allowing the impulse to repropagate a cell or group of cells it just passed through; an hypothesized cause of tachycardia

refractory (ri-'frak-tə-rē) **period**   a period in which the cardiac cell is either resistant (relative refractory) or impervious (absolute refractory) to stimulation

regular sinus rhythm   a sinus rhythm that is regular but has an abnormality of some kind, such as ectopic beats in the otherwise regular rhythm; a normal sinus rhythm with an isolated abnormality

relative refractory period   *see* refractory period

repolarization (rē-pō-lə-rə-'zā-shən)   the recovery of a depolarized cardiac cell to its resting state (and charge)

resting membrane potential   the electrical potential difference that exists across a cellular membrane between the inside and the outside of a resting, "polarized" cell

retrograde ('re-trə-grād)   occurring backward; a P wave that is inverted or follows the QRS complex

rhythm ('rith-əm)   the regular occurrence of an impulse and cardiac cycle

R on T phenomena   the QRS complex of a premature contraction falls on the T wave of the preceding cardiac complex; also refers to defibrillation in which the energy may be discharged during the T wave

run   three or more ectopic beats in a row

SA node   *see* sinoatrial node

segment   a portion of the baseline in an electrocardiogram

septum ('sep-təm)   a wall dividing two cavities; the division between the two atria and between the two ventricles

silent MI   a myocardial infarction without pain; a myocardial infarction without the normally associated electrocardiographic changes in the 12-lead electrocardiogram

sinoatrial (sī-nō-'ā-trē-əl) **node**   a group of specialized cardiac cells located at the articulation of the superior vena cava and the right atrium; normally the dominant pacemaker of the heart

sinus ('sī-nəs)   referring to a cardiac complex or rhythm originating at the SA node; a physiological cavity having a relatively narrow opening; *see* coronary sinus

sinus arrest a dysrhythmia in which one (or more) complete cardiac complex is omitted from the rhythm; *syn* sinus pause

sinus arrhythmia a benign dysrhythmia in which the heart beat and electrocardiogram slow during or just after respiratory expiration and prior to inspiration

sinus bradycardia (brād-i-'kärd-ē-ə) a sinus rhythm slower than 60 beats per minute

sinus rhythm a cardiac rhythm originating in the SA node

sinus tachycardia (tak-i-'kärd-ē-ə) a sinus rhythm with a regular rate greater than 100 beats per minute and less than 150 beats per minute

sodium-potassium pump an active transport mechanism of the cell in which sodium is pumped out of the cell and potassium is pumped into the cell; requires the expenditure of cellular energy

spike a deflection away from baseline in the EKG; it usually does not show a return to baseline, and may be a form of artifact or represent a pacemaker rhythm

Stokes-Adams attack a fainting spell of cardiac origin

strip chart recorder the part of the EKG machine that imprints the EKG paper with the line representing the patient's EKG

stroke volume the amount of blood pumped with each ventricular contraction of the heart (approximately 70 ml in the average adult at rest)

ST segment depression a depression of the ST segment of the EKG below normal baseline

ST segment elevation an elevation of the ST segment of the EKG above normal baseline

stylus ('stī-ləs) the heated probe of the electrocardiograph that inscribes the electrocardiograph paper

supraventricular ('sü-prə-ven-'trik-yə-lər) referring to a location above the ventricles

supraventricular dysrhythmia any cardiac dysrhythmia not originating in the ventricles

sympathetic (sim-pə-'thet-ik) referring to the sympathetic nervous system, which is the thoracolumbar division of the autonomic nervous system; affects the system through direct innervation and via chemical transmitters which are classified as alpha, beta, or dopaminergic stimulating (or blocking) adrenergic drugs

synchronized cardioversion ('sin-krə-nīzd 'kärd-ē-ō-'vər-zhən) electrical discharge through a defibrillating device; discharge is timed to occur during the QRS complex and avoid the T wave of any existing EKG complexes; if no QRS complex can be monitored the cardioverter will not discharge

systole ('sis-tə-lē) the contraction of the heart, especially the ventricles

tachycardia (tak-i-kärd-ē-ə) having a heart rate faster than normal (usually a rate of over 100 beats per minute); *syn* tachydysrhythmia

tachycardic (tak-i-kär-dik) **rhythms** any rhythm with a rate greater than 100 beats per minute, including ventricular tachycardia, junctional tachycardia, sinus tachycardia, atrial tachycardia, atrial flutter, and atrial fibrillation

tachydysrhythmia (tak-i-dis-'rith-mē-ə) *see* tachycardia

telemetry (tə-'lem-ə-trē) making of measurements (such as an EKG) and the transmission of them by radio

threshold potential a measure of the electrical charge on the cell, at the point in time when depolarization will begin

tricuspid (trī-'kəs-pəd) **valve** the three cusped valve which separates the right atrium from the right ventricle

trigeminal (trī-'jem-ən-°l) occurring in every third heartbeat

unifocal (yü-nē-'fō-kəl) having only one origin; cardiac complexes which are shaped alike

unipolar (yü-ni-'pō-lər) **limb lead** referring to an EKG lead in which there is no single negative electrode; the EKG axis runs from a point, posterior to the heart, created electronically as a combination of three physical leads to a positive lead on an extremity

vagal ('vā-gəl) **tone** pertaining to the degree of stimulation or blockade of the vagus nerve

Valsalva ('val-sal-və) **maneuver** a vagal stimulating procedure accomplished by forcing exhalation against a closed glottis; the resulting increase in intrathoracic pressure causes vagal stimulation and may slow the heart rate (it also occurs when straining to defecate, cough, gag, or vomit)

valve ('valv) a membranous structure in a canal or passage which prevents backward flow of material flowing through it

vascular ('vas-kyə-lər) **compartment** the volume of the cardiovascular system, including the veins, capillaries, arteries, and chambers of the heart; it varies with changes in the size of the blood vessels (vasomotor tone)

vasoconstriction (vā-zō-ken-'strik-shən) referring to a decrease in the lumen of vessels of the circulatory system

vasomotor tone (vā-zə-'mōt-ər) a reference to the degree of constriction or relaxation of the blood vessels; a decrease in vasomotor tone allows relaxation and dilation of the blood vessels and increases the size of the vascular compartment;

an increase causes constriction of the blood vessels and results in a decrease of the vascular compartment

ventricle ('ven-tri-kəl)   either of the two lower chambers of the heart; the right ventricle pumps blood into the pulmonary circulatory system; the left ventricle pumps blood into the systemic circulatory system

ventricular (ven-'trik-yə-lər) **fibrillation**   a life-threatening dysrhythmia in which the patient is pulseless and apneic; the myocardium is depolarizing in a totally random manner without effective muscular activity

ventricular flutter   a form of ventricular tachycardia in which the ventricular complexes cannot be distinguished from the T waves and the ST segments; the rate is usually one hundred eighty (180) to two hundred sixty (260) beats per minute, but may be faster

ventricular systole   contraction of the ventricles

VPB   (ventricular premature beat) a contraction which originates in the ventricle and occurs early in the cardiac rhythm; *aka* PVC

wandering atrial ('ā-trē-əl) **pacemaker**   a dysrhythmia in which the atrial focus shifts from focus to focus with each cardiac cycle; the P waves are differently formed

wave ('wāv)   a double oscillation (a deflection away from and a return to) from the baseline in an EKG.; a progressive contraction spreading rhythmically in a muscle

Wiederhold (wē-dər-hōld) **algorithm**   an algorithmic, step-by-step procedure using five steps of primary differential criteria to identify all major cardiac dysrhythmias

wire electrode   the electrode portion of a pacemaker; it is inserted into the right ventricle, usually through venous access pathways; less commonly, it is also inserted through the wall of the ventricle

Wolff-Parkinson-White   the association of supraventricular rhythms with pre-excitation, marked by a short PR interval that frequently slurs upward into the QRS complex, which is usually wide; *aka* anomalous atrioventricular excitation

Index

A

Practice EKG Rhythms

Practice at interpretation is essential in order to become a skilled clinician, proficient at dysrhythmia recognition. Practice is most effective if mistakes and correct evaluations can be confirmed.

These practice EKGs have been carefully selected to provide a representative sampling of dysrhythmias. Because these EKGs are **accurate reproductions** of genuine clinical cases, some may appear light. The primary criteria can still be derived, indicating one of the strengths of an analytical approach to dysrhythmia recognition.

An index to the EKGs is supplied with the interpretations of the author as well as additional consultants. Your interpretation or the interpretation of your instructor may vary occasionally. This is to be expected and confirms that medicine is truly an art. It is important that your interpretations be based on consistent, definable evaluative tools. Good luck and good learning.

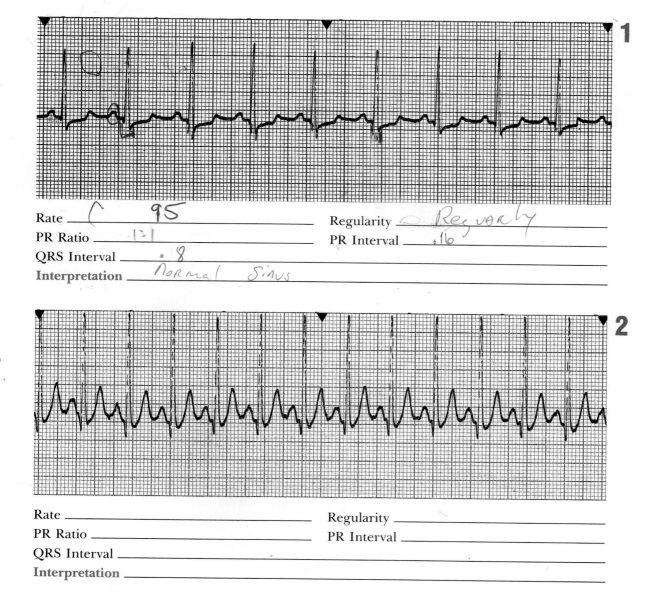

1

Rate _____ 95 _____ Regularity ___ Regularly ___

PR Ratio ___ 1:1 ___ PR Interval ___ .16 ___

QRS Interval ___ .8 ___

Interpretation ___ Normal Sinus ___

2

Rate _____ Regularity _____

PR Ratio _____ PR Interval _____

QRS Interval _____

Interpretation _____

3

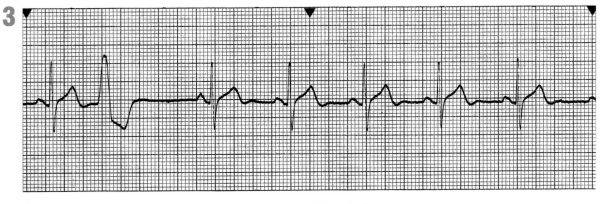

Rate _____   Regularity _____

PR Ratio _____   PR Interval _____

QRS Interval _____

Interpretation _____

4

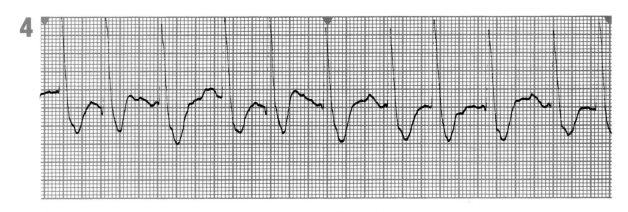

Rate _____   Regularity _____

PR Ratio _____   PR Interval _____

QRS Interval _____

Interpretation _____

5

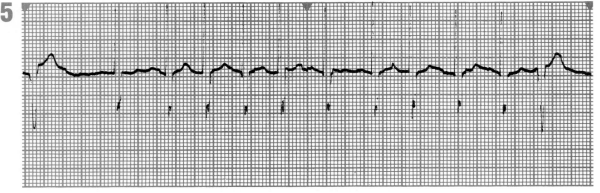

Rate _____   Regularity _____

PR Ratio _____   PR Interval _____

QRS Interval _____

Interpretation _____

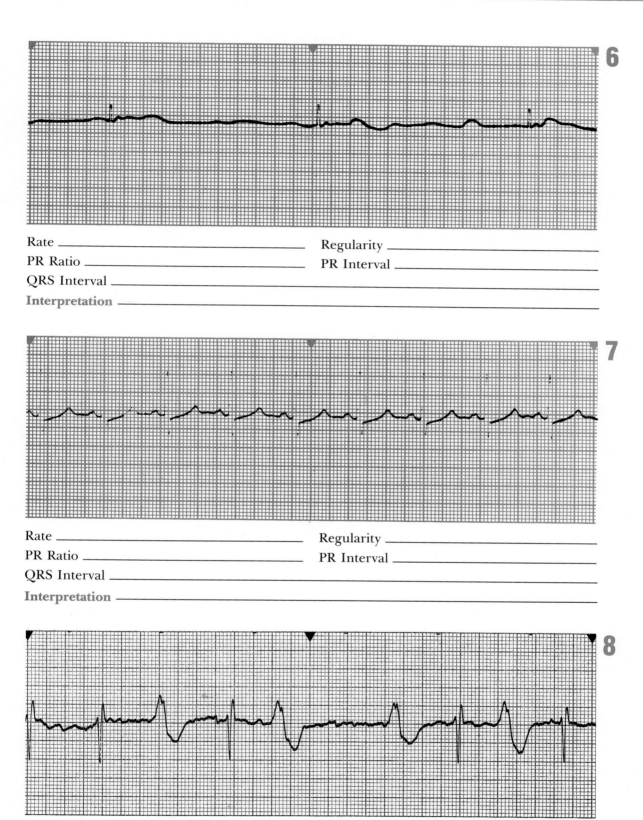

6

Rate _____ Regularity _____

PR Ratio _____ PR Interval _____

QRS Interval _____

Interpretation _____

7

Rate _____ Regularity _____

PR Ratio _____ PR Interval _____

QRS Interval _____

Interpretation _____

8

Rate _____ Regularity _____

PR Ratio _____ PR Interval _____

QRS Interval _____

Interpretation _____

9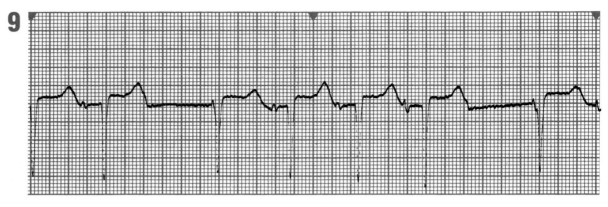

Rate _____   Regularity _____

PR Ratio _____   PR Interval _____

QRS Interval _____

Interpretation _____

10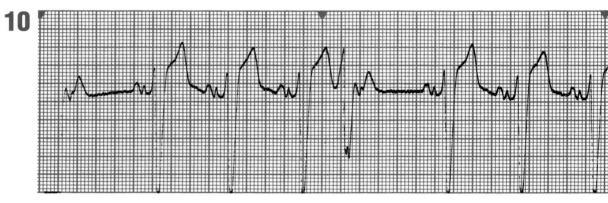

Rate _____   Regularity _____

PR Ratio _____   PR Interval _____

QRS Interval _____

Interpretation _____

11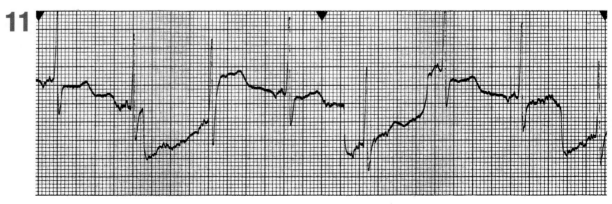

Rate _____   Regularity _____

PR Ratio _____   PR Interval _____

QRS Interval _____

Interpretation _____

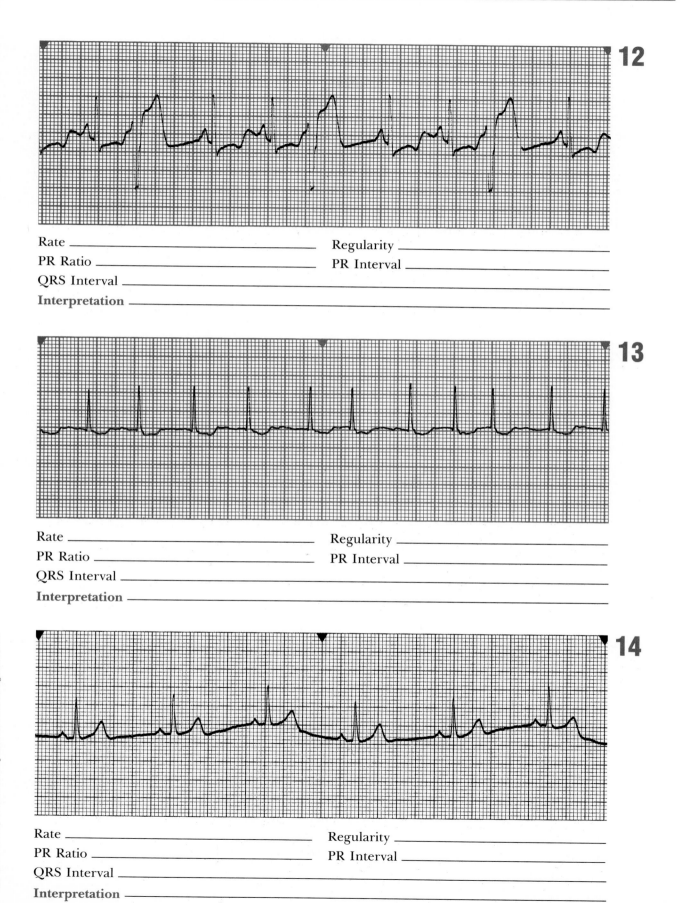

12

Rate _____   Regularity _____

PR Ratio _____   PR Interval _____

QRS Interval _____

Interpretation _____

13

Rate _____   Regularity _____

PR Ratio _____   PR Interval _____

QRS Interval _____

Interpretation _____

14

Rate _____   Regularity _____

PR Ratio _____   PR Interval _____

QRS Interval _____

Interpretation _____

15

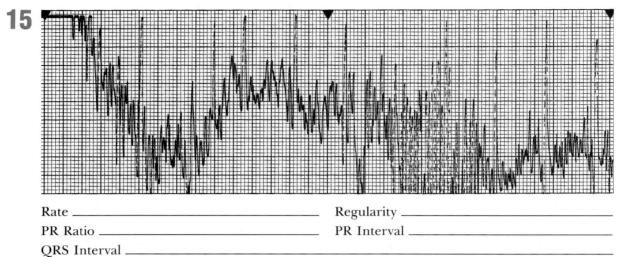

Rate _____ Regularity _____

PR Ratio _____ PR Interval _____

QRS Interval _____

Interpretation _____

16

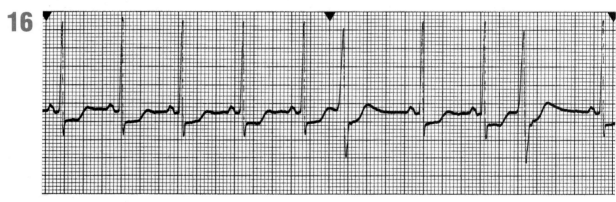

Rate _____ Regularity _____

PR Ratio _____ PR Interval _____

QRS Interval _____

Interpretation _____

17

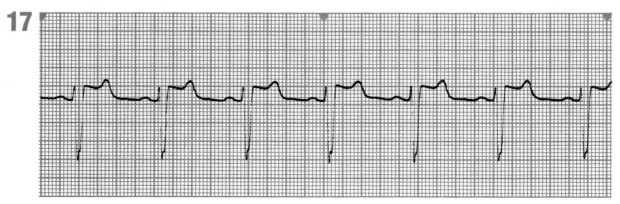

Rate _____ Regularity _____

PR Ratio _____ PR Interval _____

QRS Interval _____

Interpretation _____

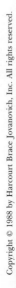

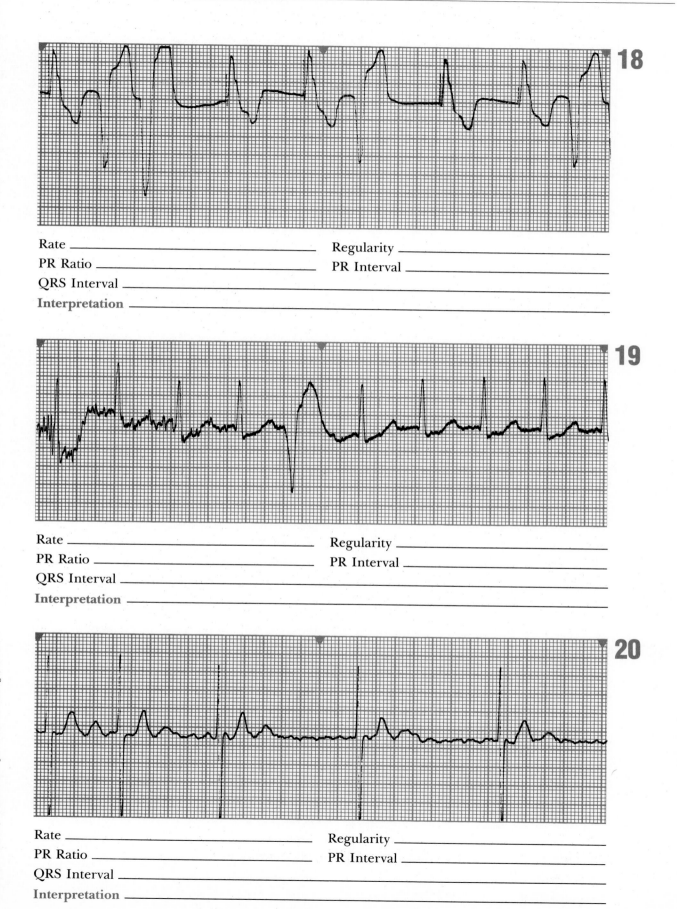

18

Rate _____ Regularity _____

PR Ratio _____ PR Interval _____

QRS Interval _____

Interpretation _____

19

Rate _____ Regularity _____

PR Ratio _____ PR Interval _____

QRS Interval _____

Interpretation _____

20

Rate _____ Regularity _____

PR Ratio _____ PR Interval _____

QRS Interval _____

Interpretation _____

21

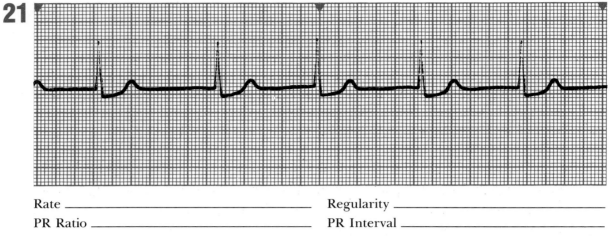

Rate _____   Regularity _____

PR Ratio _____   PR Interval _____

QRS Interval _____

Interpretation _____

22

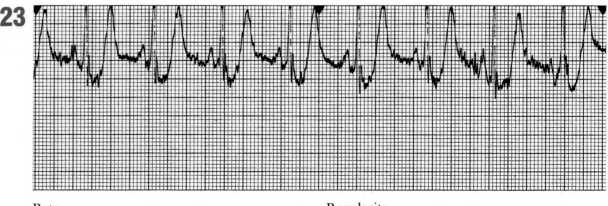

Rate _____   Regularity _____

PR Ratio _____   PR Interval _____

QRS Interval _____

Interpretation _____

23

Rate _____   Regularity _____

PR Ratio _____   PR Interval _____

QRS Interval _____

Interpretation _____

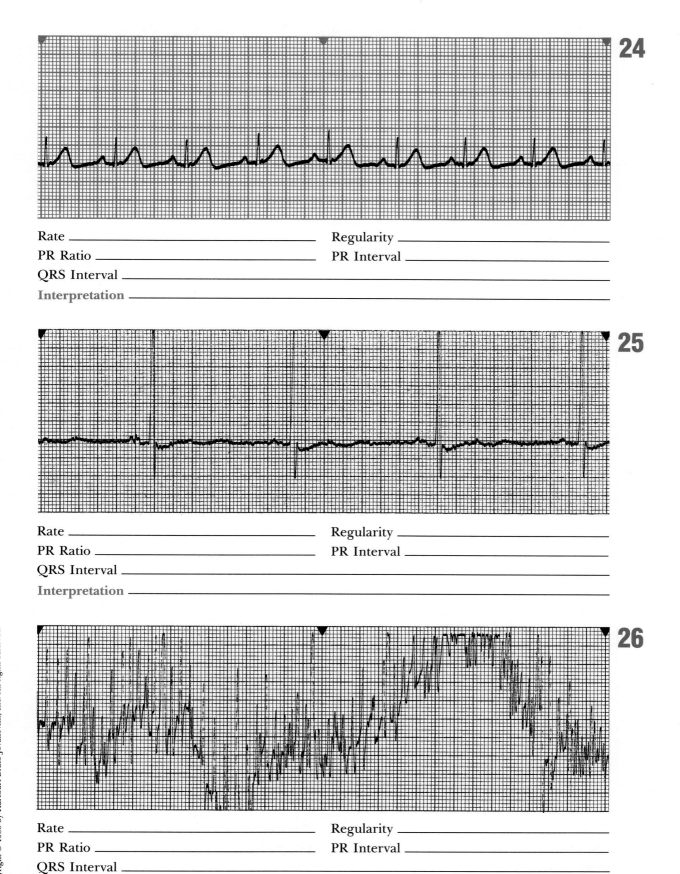

24

Rate _____   Regularity _____

PR Ratio _____   PR Interval _____

QRS Interval _____

Interpretation _____

25

Rate _____   Regularity _____

PR Ratio _____   PR Interval _____

QRS Interval _____

Interpretation _____

26

Rate _____   Regularity _____

PR Ratio _____   PR Interval _____

QRS Interval _____

Interpretation _____

27

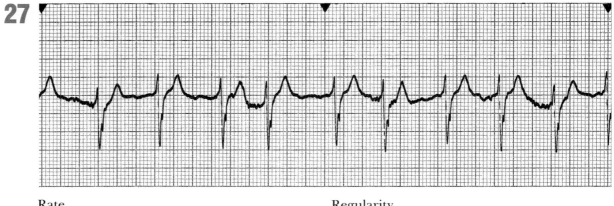

Rate _____   Regularity _____

PR Ratio _____   PR Interval _____

QRS Interval _____

Interpretation _____

28

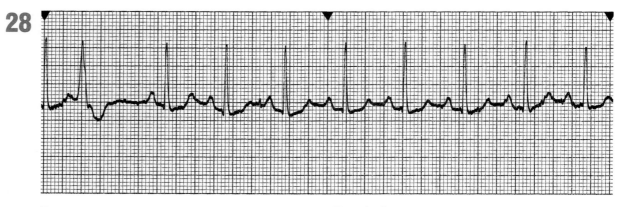

Rate _____   Regularity _____

PR Ratio _____   PR Interval _____

QRS Interval _____

Interpretation _____

29

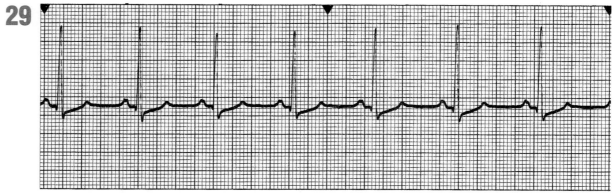

Rate _____   Regularity _____

PR Ratio _____   PR Interval _____

QRS Interval _____

Interpretation _____

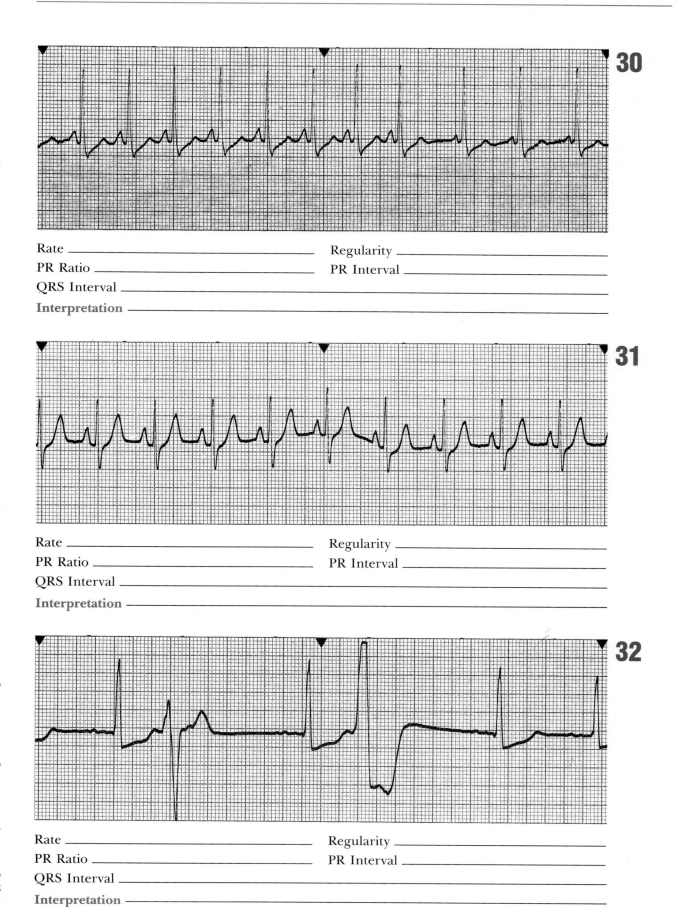

30

Rate _____ Regularity _____

PR Ratio _____ PR Interval _____

QRS Interval _____

Interpretation _____

31

Rate _____ Regularity _____

PR Ratio _____ PR Interval _____

QRS Interval _____

Interpretation _____

32

Rate _____ Regularity _____

PR Ratio _____ PR Interval _____

QRS Interval _____

Interpretation _____

33

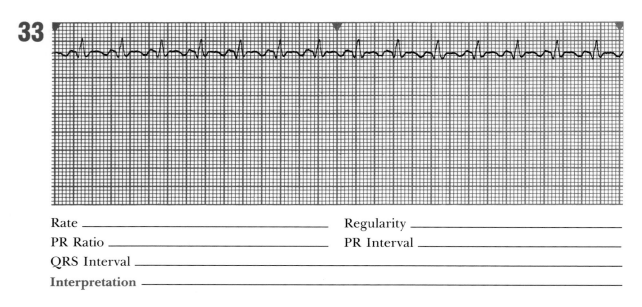

Rate _____ Regularity _____

PR Ratio _____ PR Interval _____

QRS Interval _____

Interpretation _____

34

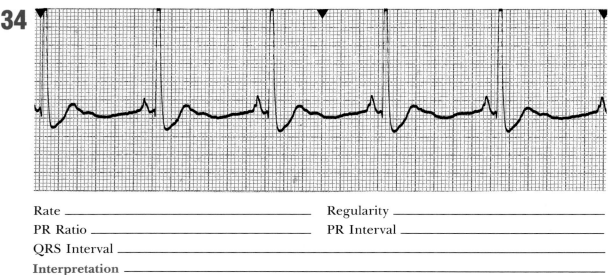

Rate _____ Regularity _____

PR Ratio _____ PR Interval _____

QRS Interval _____

Interpretation _____

35

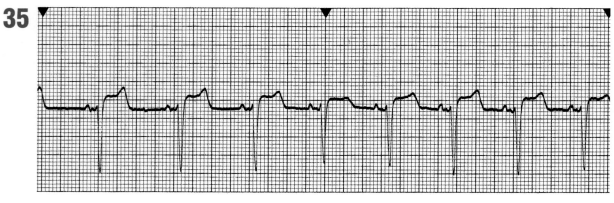

Rate _____ Regularity _____

PR Ratio _____ PR Interval _____

QRS Interval _____

Interpretation _____

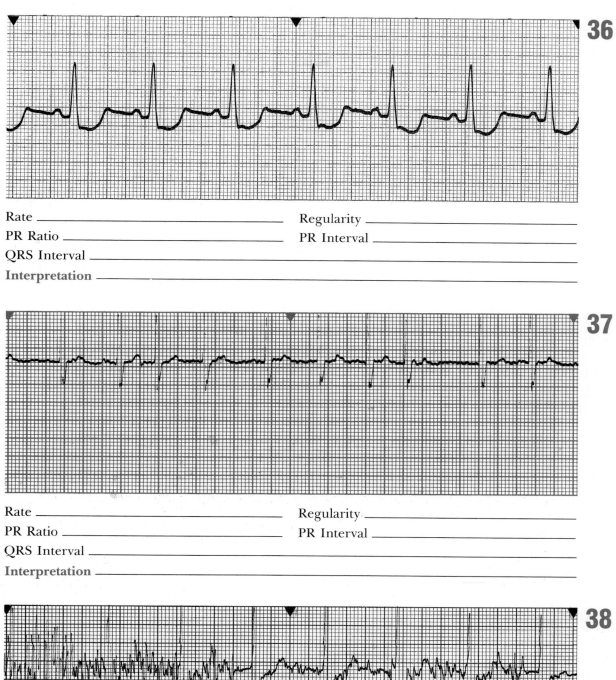

36

Rate _____ Regularity _____

PR Ratio _____ PR Interval _____

QRS Interval _____

Interpretation _____

37

Rate _____ Regularity _____

PR Ratio _____ PR Interval _____

QRS Interval _____

Interpretation _____

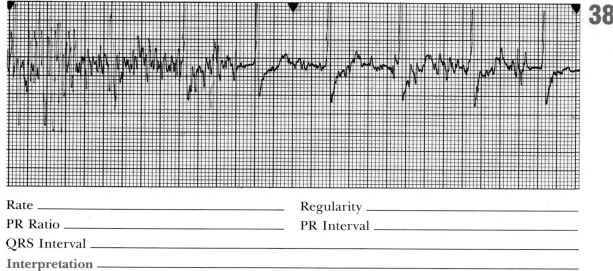

38

Rate _____ Regularity _____

PR Ratio _____ PR Interval _____

QRS Interval _____

Interpretation _____

39

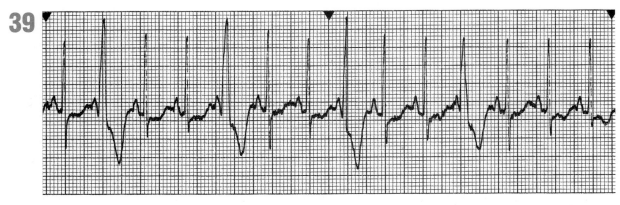

Rate _____ Regularity _____

PR Ratio _____ PR Interval _____

QRS Interval _____

Interpretation _____

40

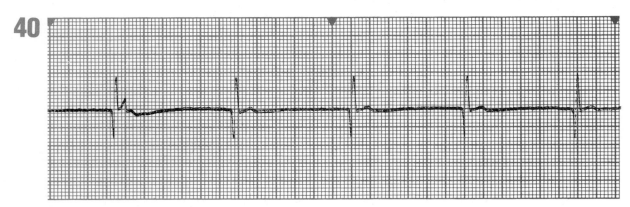

Rate _____ Regularity _____

PR Ratio _____ PR Interval _____

QRS Interval _____

Interpretation _____

41

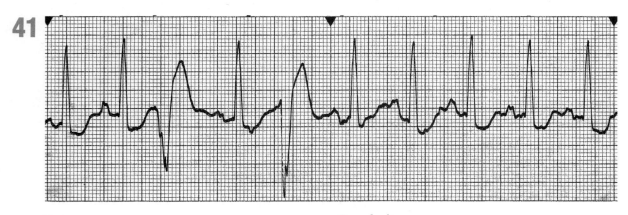

Rate _____ Regularity _____

PR Ratio _____ PR Interval _____

QRS Interval _____

Interpretation _____

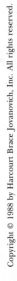

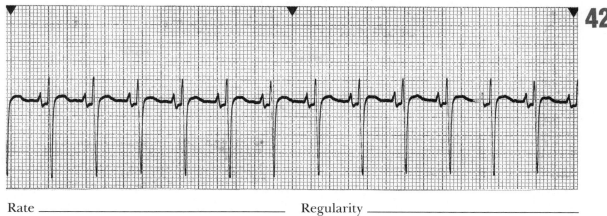

Rate _____ Regularity _____

PR Ratio _____ PR Interval _____

QRS Interval _____

Interpretation _____

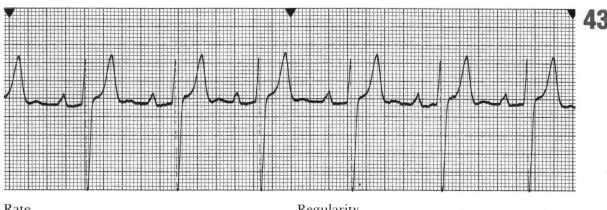

Rate _____ Regularity _____

PR Ratio _____ PR Interval _____

QRS Interval _____

Interpretation _____

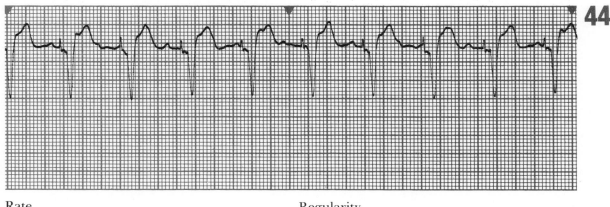

Rate _____ Regularity _____

PR Ratio _____ PR Interval _____

QRS Interval _____

Interpretation _____

45

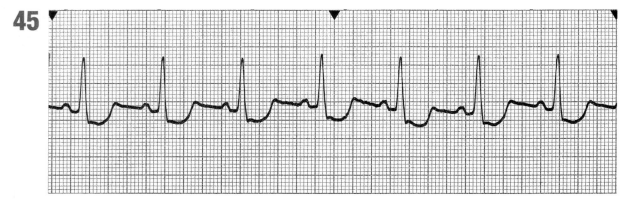

Rate _____ Regularity _____

PR Ratio _____ PR Interval _____

QRS Interval _____

Interpretation _____

46

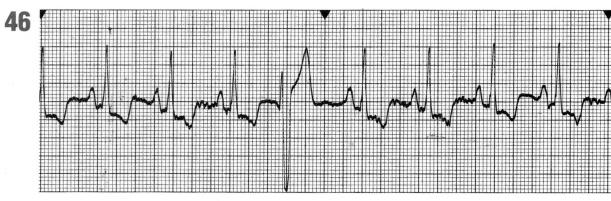

Rate _____ Regularity _____

PR Ratio _____ PR Interval _____

QRS Interval _____

Interpretation _____

47

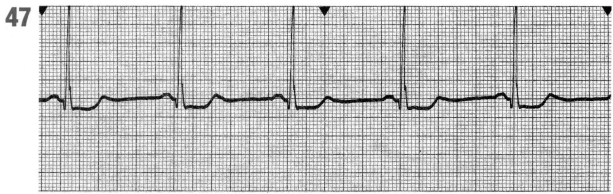

Rate _____ Regularity _____

PR Ratio _____ PR Interval _____

QRS Interval _____

Interpretation _____

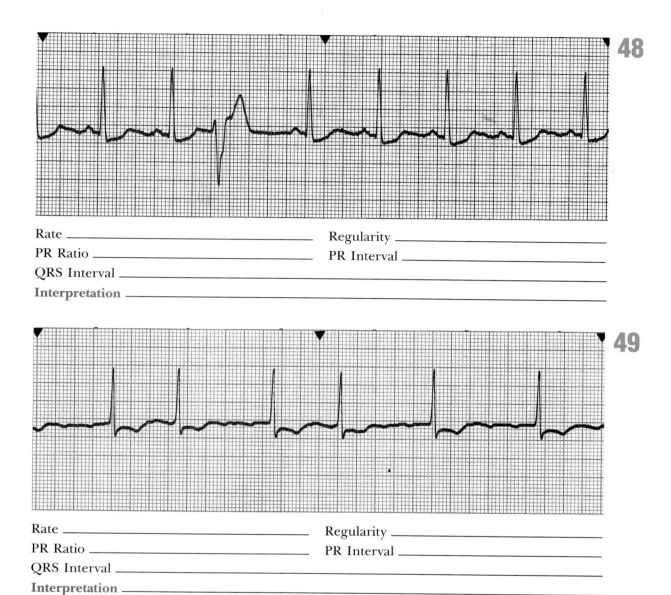

48

Rate _____ Regularity _____

PR Ratio _____ PR Interval _____

QRS Interval _____

Interpretation _____

49

Rate _____ Regularity _____

PR Ratio _____ PR Interval _____

QRS Interval _____

Interpretation _____

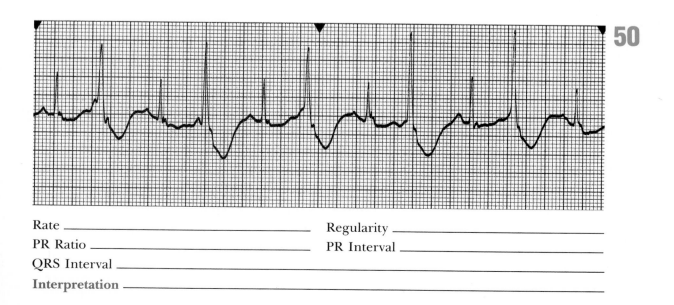

50

Rate _____ Regularity _____

PR Ratio _____ PR Interval _____

QRS Interval _____

Interpretation _____

51

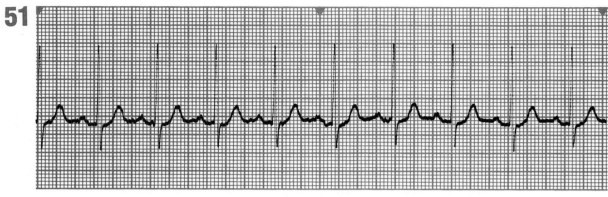

Rate _____   Regularity _____

PR Ratio _____   PR Interval _____

QRS Interval _____

Interpretation _____

52

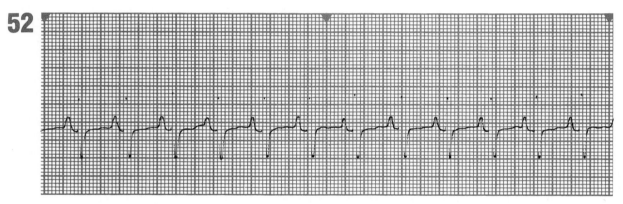

Rate _____   Regularity _____

PR Ratio _____   PR Interval _____

QRS Interval _____

Interpretation _____

53

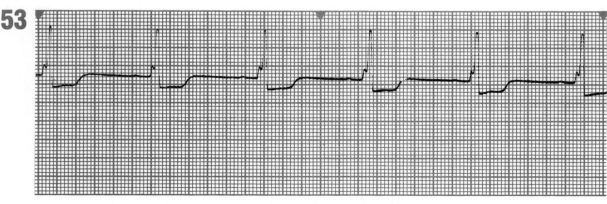

Rate _____   Regularity _____

PR Ratio _____   PR Interval _____

QRS Interval _____

Interpretation _____

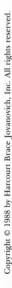

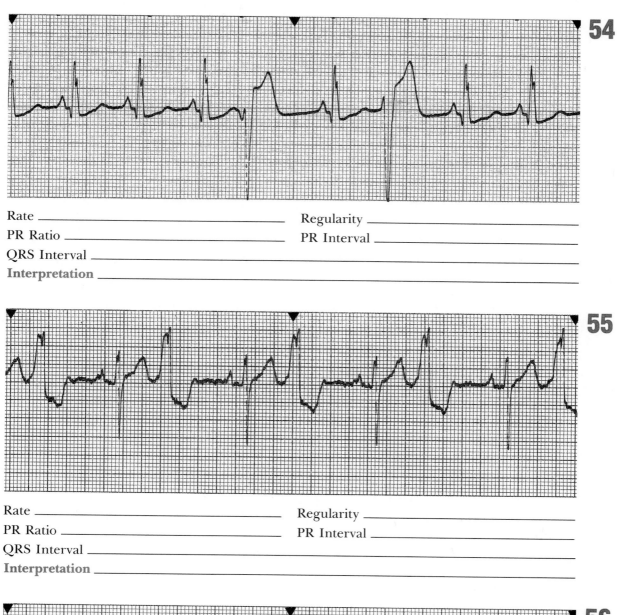

54

Rate _____   Regularity _____

PR Ratio _____   PR Interval _____

QRS Interval _____

Interpretation _____

55

Rate _____   Regularity _____

PR Ratio _____   PR Interval _____

QRS Interval _____

Interpretation _____

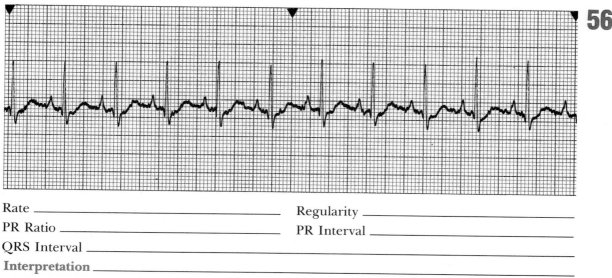

56

Rate _____   Regularity _____

PR Ratio _____   PR Interval _____

QRS Interval _____

Interpretation _____

57

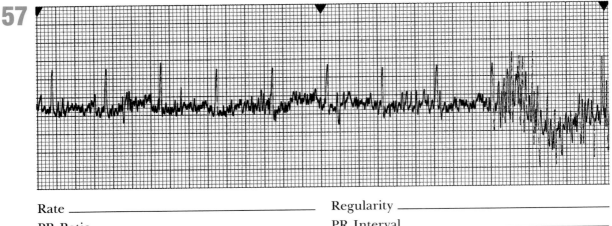

Rate _____   Regularity _____

PR Ratio _____   PR Interval _____

QRS Interval _____

Interpretation _____

58

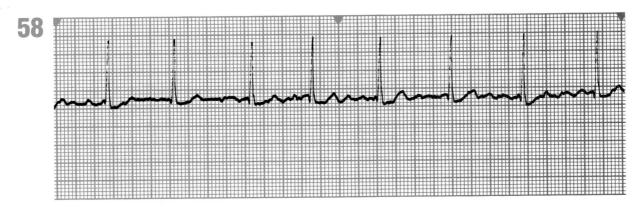

Rate _____   Regularity _____

PR Ratio _____   PR Interval _____

QRS Interval _____

Interpretation _____

59

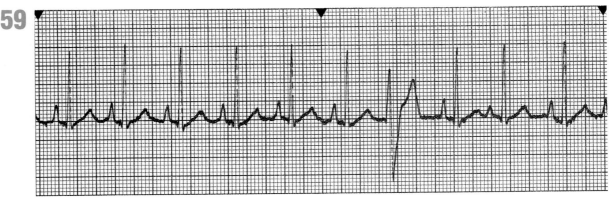

Rate _____   Regularity _____

PR Ratio _____   PR Interval _____

QRS Interval _____

Interpretation _____

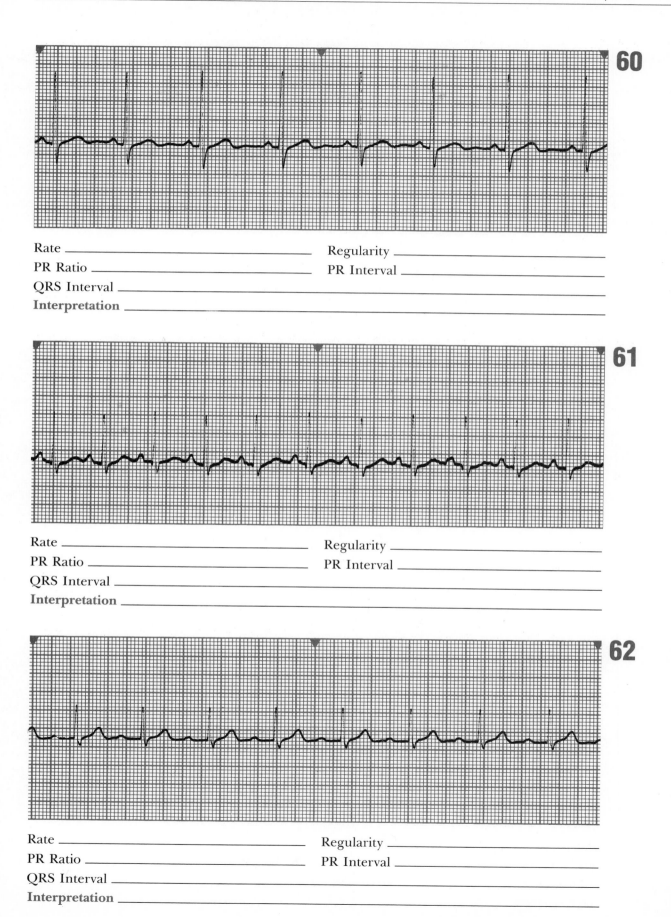

60

Rate _____   Regularity _____

PR Ratio _____   PR Interval _____

QRS Interval _____

Interpretation _____

61

Rate _____   Regularity _____

PR Ratio _____   PR Interval _____

QRS Interval _____

Interpretation _____

62

Rate _____   Regularity _____

PR Ratio _____   PR Interval _____

QRS Interval _____

Interpretation _____

63

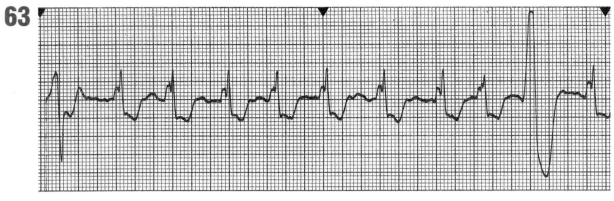

Rate _____ Regularity _____

PR Ratio _____ PR Interval _____

QRS Interval _____

Interpretation _____

64

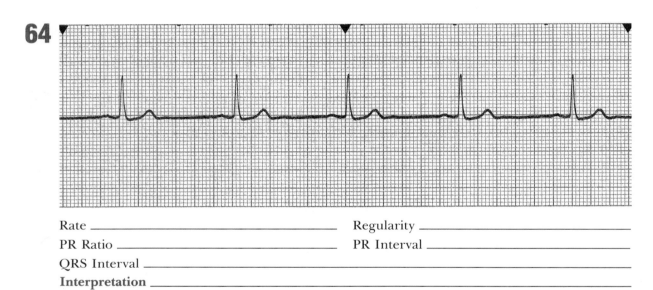

Rate _____ Regularity _____

PR Ratio _____ PR Interval _____

QRS Interval _____

Interpretation _____

65

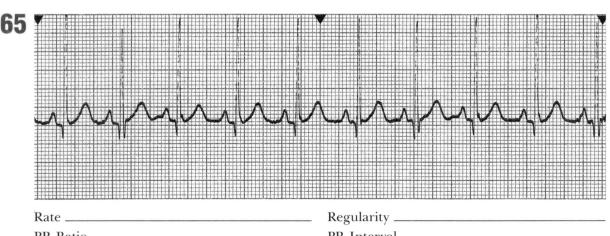

Rate _____ Regularity _____

PR Ratio _____ PR Interval _____

QRS Interval _____

Interpretation _____

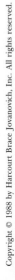

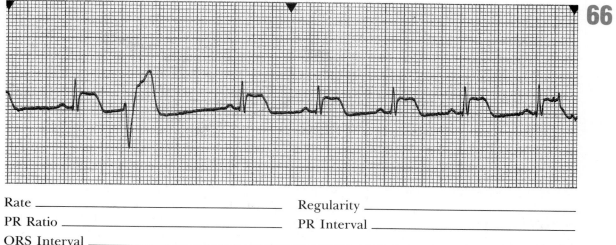

66

Rate _____ Regularity _____
PR Ratio _____ PR Interval _____
QRS Interval _____
Interpretation _____

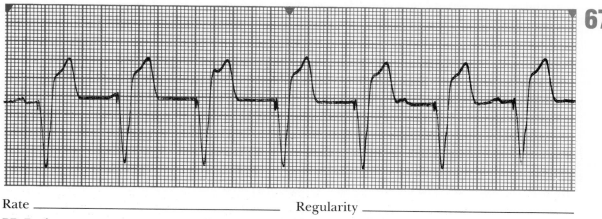

67

Rate _____ Regularity _____
PR Ratio _____ PR Interval _____
QRS Interval _____
Interpretation _____

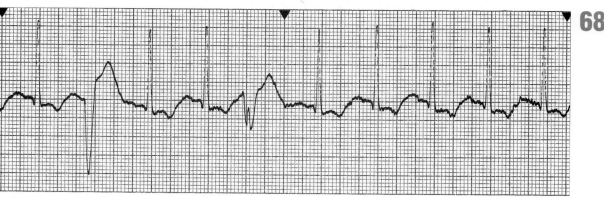

68

Rate _____ Regularity _____
PR Ratio _____ PR Interval _____
QRS Interval _____
Interpretation _____

69

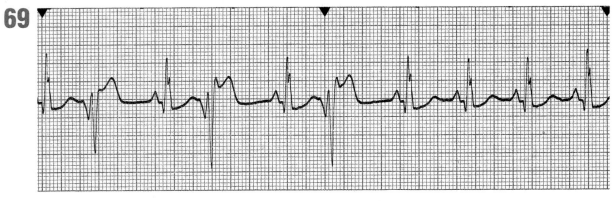

Rate _____   Regularity _____

PR Ratio _____   PR Interval _____

QRS Interval _____

Interpretation _____

70

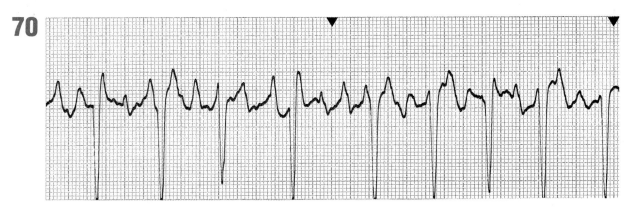

Rate _____   Regularity _____

PR Ratio _____   PR Interval _____

QRS Interval _____

Interpretation _____

71

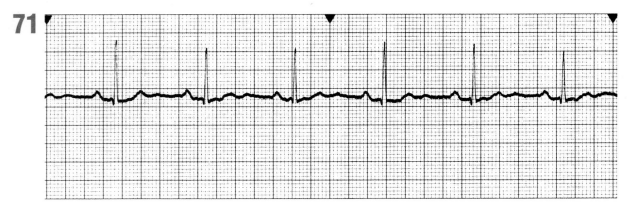

Rate _____   Regularity _____

PR Ratio _____   PR Interval _____

QRS Interval _____

Interpretation _____

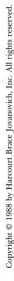

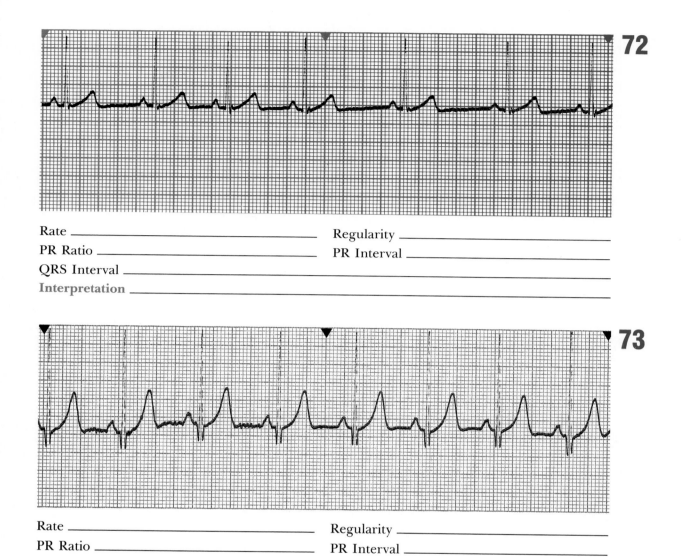

72

Rate _____ Regularity _____
PR Ratio _____ PR Interval _____
QRS Interval _____
Interpretation _____

73

Rate _____ Regularity _____
PR Ratio _____ PR Interval _____
QRS Interval _____
Interpretation _____

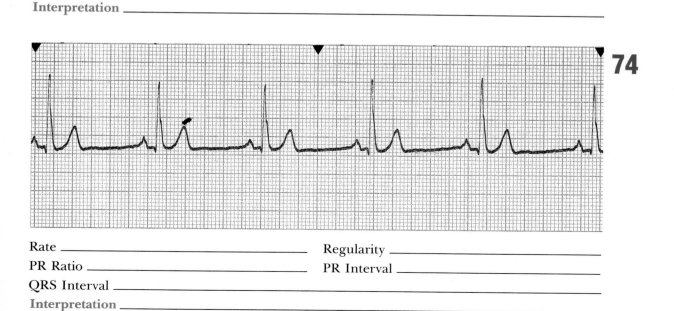

74

Rate _____ Regularity _____
PR Ratio _____ PR Interval _____
QRS Interval _____
Interpretation _____

75

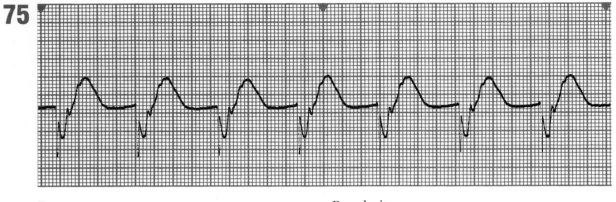

Rate _____   Regularity _____

PR Ratio _____   PR Interval _____

QRS Interval _____

Interpretation _____

76

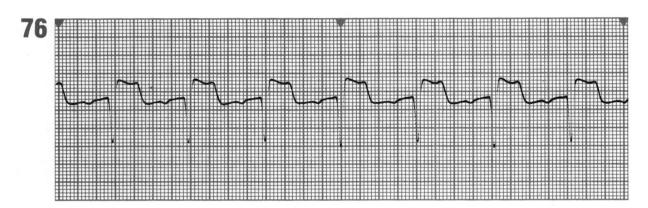

Rate _____   Regularity _____

PR Ratio _____   PR Interval _____

QRS Interval _____

Interpretation _____

77

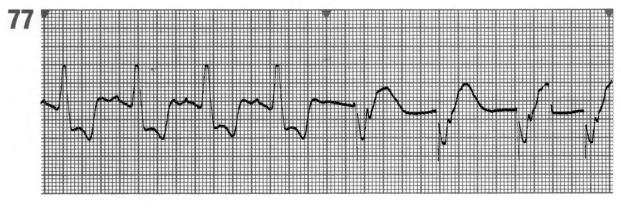

Rate _____   Regularity _____

PR Ratio _____   PR Interval _____

QRS Interval _____

Interpretation _____

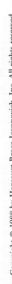

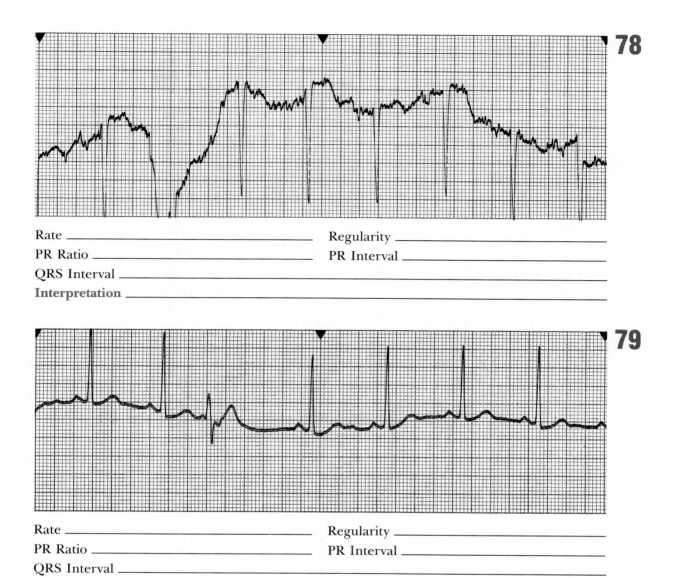

78

Rate _____ Regularity _____

PR Ratio _____ PR Interval _____

QRS Interval _____

Interpretation _____

79

Rate _____ Regularity _____

PR Ratio _____ PR Interval _____

QRS Interval _____

Interpretation _____

80

Rate _____ Regularity _____

PR Ratio _____ PR Interval _____

QRS Interval _____

Interpretation _____

81

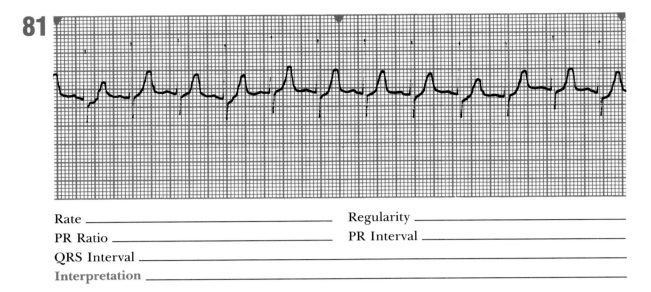

Rate _____   Regularity _____

PR Ratio _____   PR Interval _____

QRS Interval _____

Interpretation _____

82

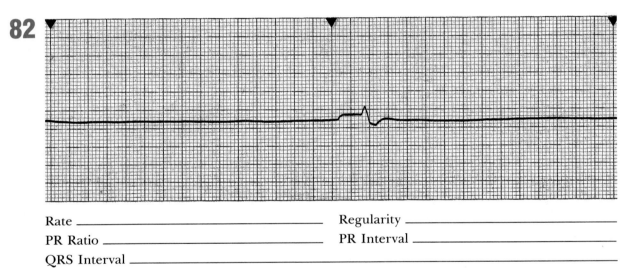

Rate _____   Regularity _____

PR Ratio _____   PR Interval _____

QRS Interval _____

Interpretation _____

83

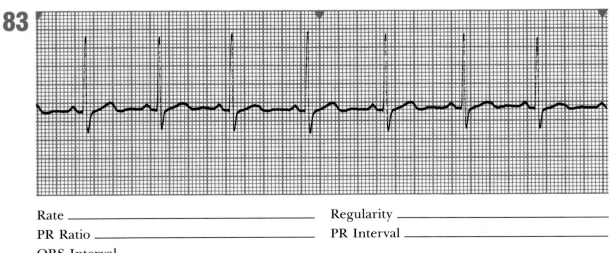

Rate _____   Regularity _____

PR Ratio _____   PR Interval _____

QRS Interval _____

Interpretation _____

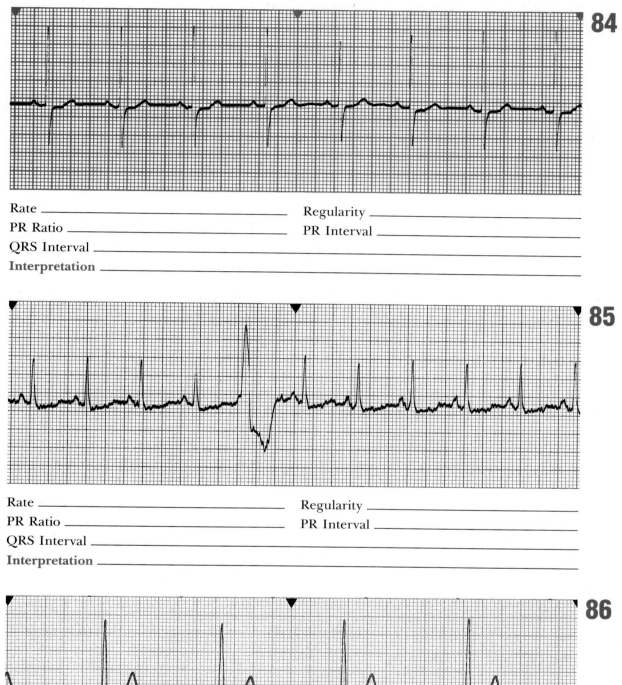

84

Rate _____ Regularity _____

PR Ratio _____ PR Interval _____

QRS Interval _____

Interpretation _____

85

Rate _____ Regularity _____

PR Ratio _____ PR Interval _____

QRS Interval _____

Interpretation _____

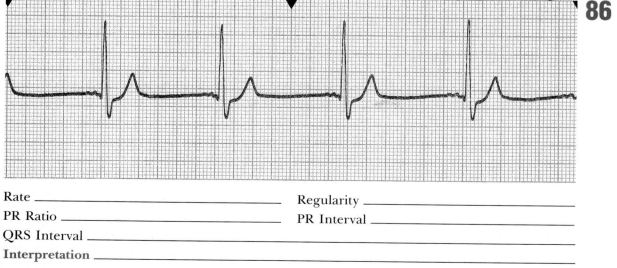

86

Rate _____ Regularity _____

PR Ratio _____ PR Interval _____

QRS Interval _____

Interpretation _____

87

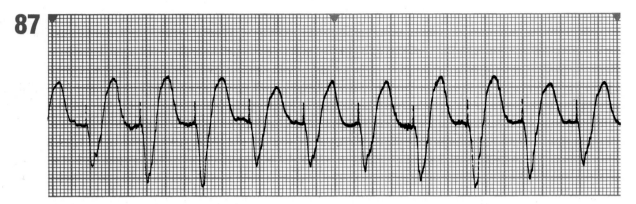

Rate _____ Regularity _____

PR Ratio _____ PR Interval _____

QRS Interval _____

Interpretation _____

88

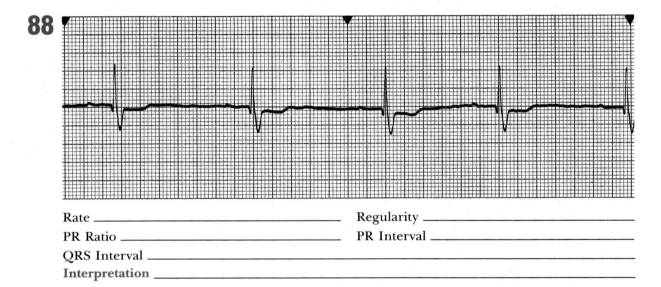

Rate _____ Regularity _____

PR Ratio _____ PR Interval _____

QRS Interval _____

Interpretation _____

89

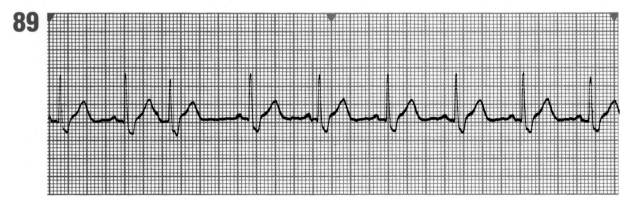

Rate _____ Regularity _____

PR Ratio _____ PR Interval _____

QRS Interval _____

Interpretation _____

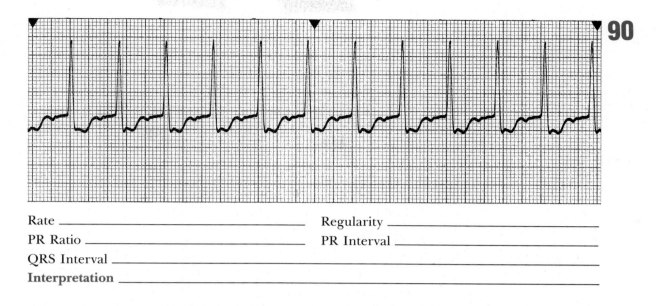

90

Rate _____ Regularity _____

PR Ratio _____ PR Interval _____

QRS Interval _____

Interpretation _____

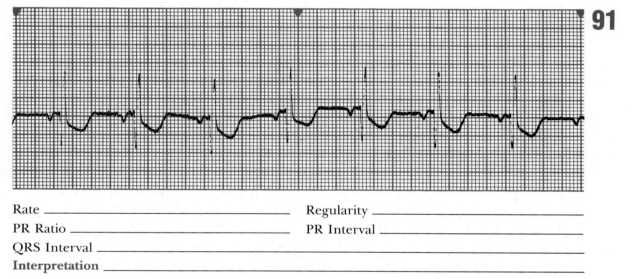

91

Rate _____ Regularity _____

PR Ratio _____ PR Interval _____

QRS Interval _____

Interpretation _____

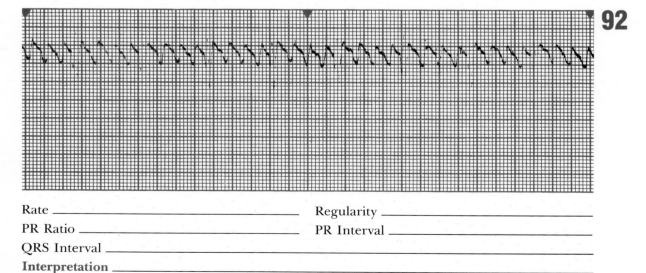

92

Rate _____ Regularity _____

PR Ratio _____ PR Interval _____

QRS Interval _____

Interpretation _____

93

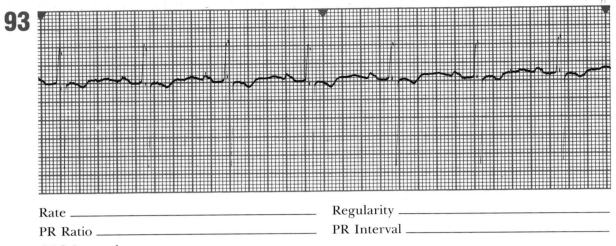

Rate _____   Regularity _____

PR Ratio _____   PR Interval _____

QRS Interval _____

Interpretation _____

94

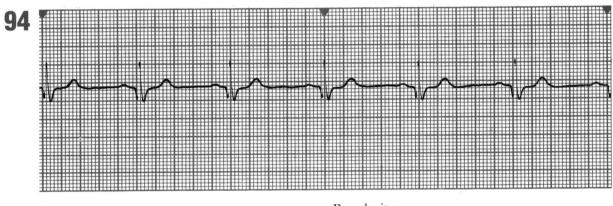

Rate _____   Regularity _____

PR Ratio _____   PR Interval _____

QRS Interval _____

Interpretation _____

95

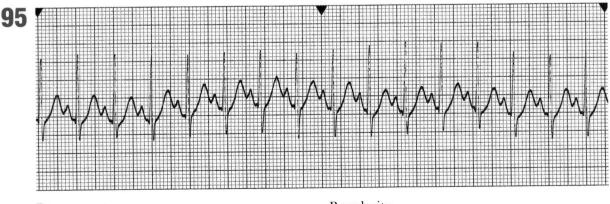

Rate _____   Regularity _____

PR Ratio _____   PR Interval _____

QRS Interval _____

Interpretation _____

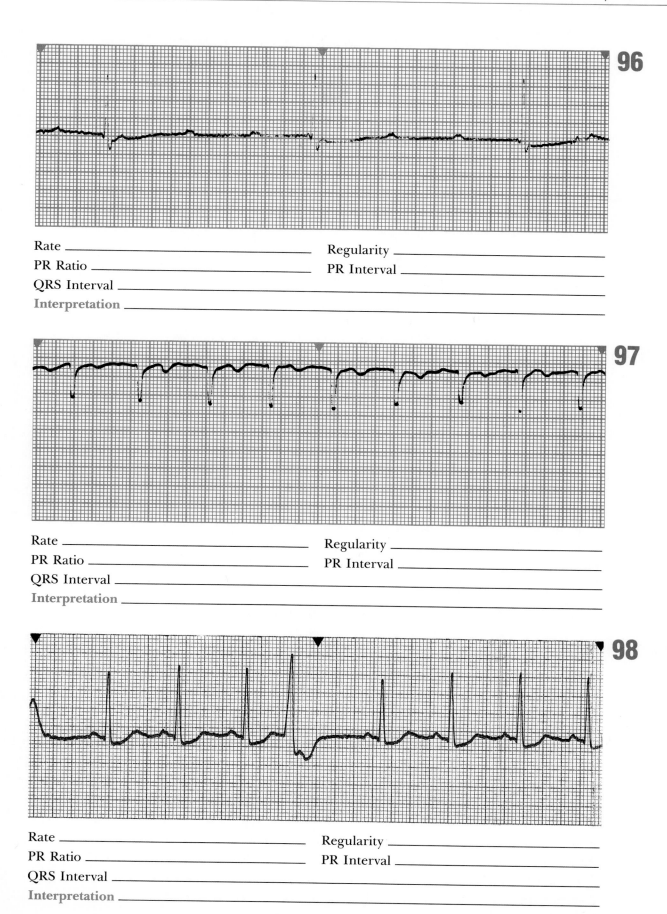

96

Rate _____ Regularity _____

PR Ratio _____ PR Interval _____

QRS Interval _____

Interpretation _____

97

Rate _____ Regularity _____

PR Ratio _____ PR Interval _____

QRS Interval _____

Interpretation _____

98

Rate _____ Regularity _____

PR Ratio _____ PR Interval _____

QRS Interval _____

Interpretation _____

99

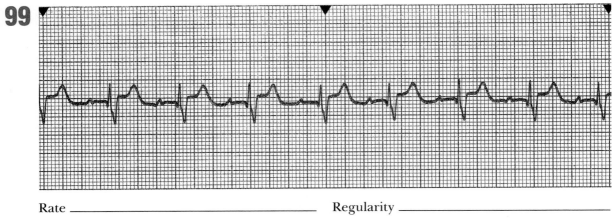

Rate _____   Regularity _____
PR Ratio _____   PR Interval _____
QRS Interval _____
Interpretation _____

100

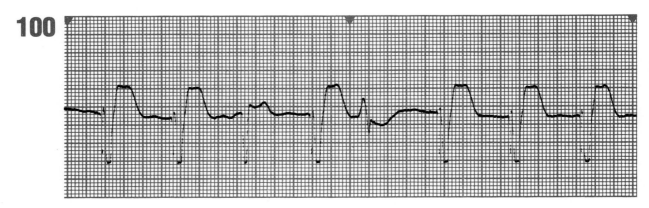

Rate _____   Regularity _____
PR Ratio _____   PR Interval _____
QRS Interval _____
Interpretation _____

101

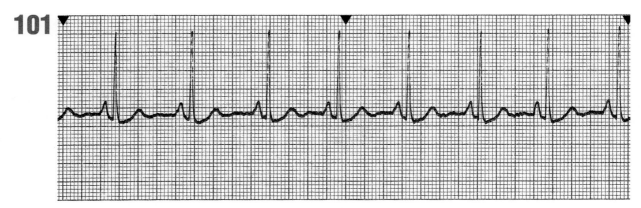

Rate _____   Regularity _____
PR Ratio _____   PR Interval _____
QRS Interval _____
Interpretation _____

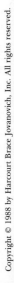

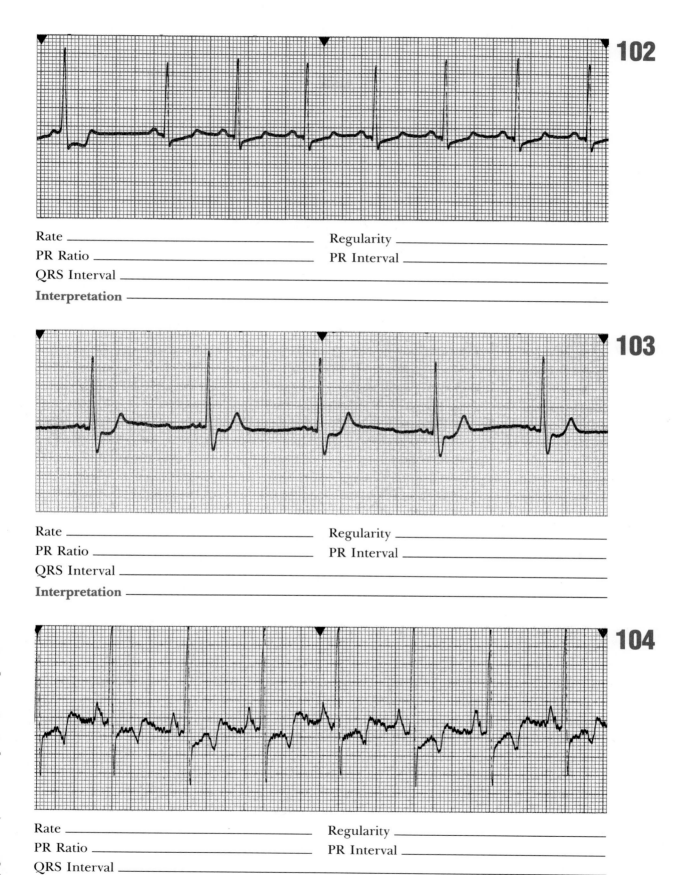

102

Rate _____ Regularity _____

PR Ratio _____ PR Interval _____

QRS Interval _____

Interpretation _____

103

Rate _____ Regularity _____

PR Ratio _____ PR Interval _____

QRS Interval _____

Interpretation _____

104

Rate _____ Regularity _____

PR Ratio _____ PR Interval _____

QRS Interval _____

Interpretation _____

105

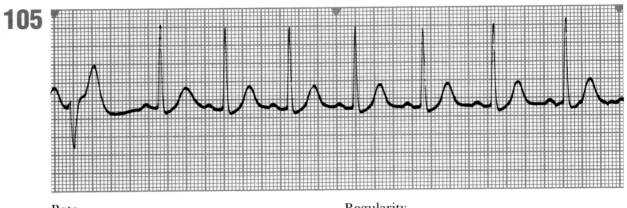

Rate _____ Regularity _____

PR Ratio _____ PR Interval _____

QRS Interval _____

Interpretation _____

106

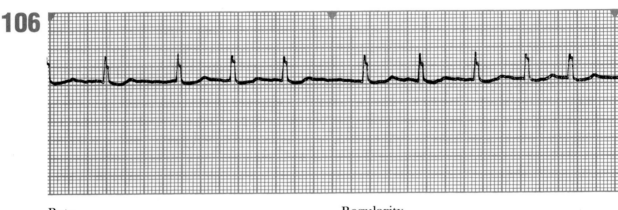

Rate _____ Regularity _____

PR Ratio _____ PR Interval _____

QRS Interval _____

Interpretation _____

107

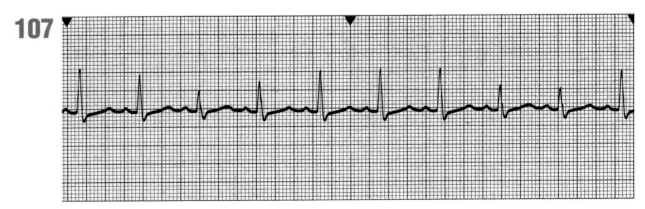

Rate _____ Regularity _____

PR Ratio _____ PR Interval _____

QRS Interval _____

Interpretation _____

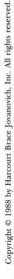

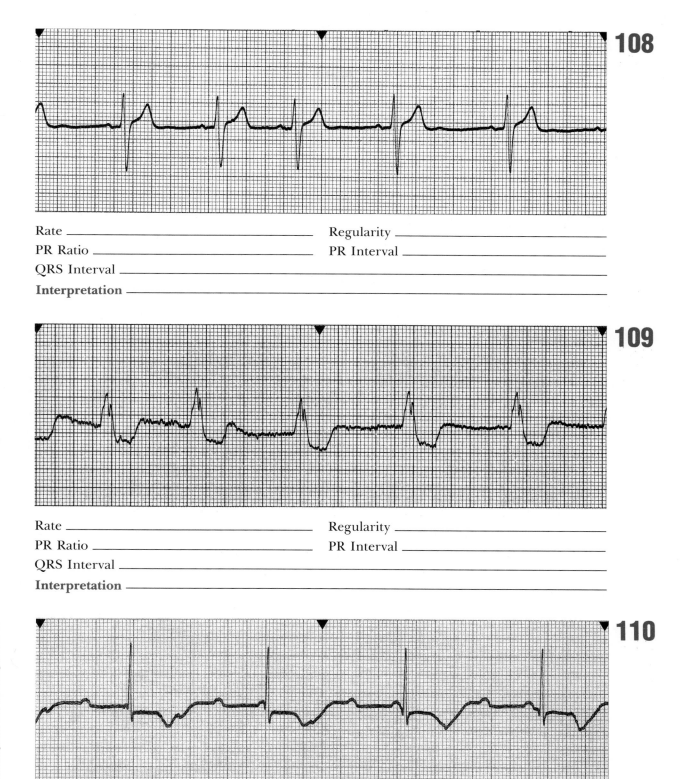

108

Rate _____   Regularity _____

PR Ratio _____   PR Interval _____

QRS Interval _____

Interpretation _____

109

Rate _____   Regularity _____

PR Ratio _____   PR Interval _____

QRS Interval _____

Interpretation _____

110

Rate _____   Regularity _____

PR Ratio _____   PR Interval _____

QRS Interval _____

Interpretation _____

111

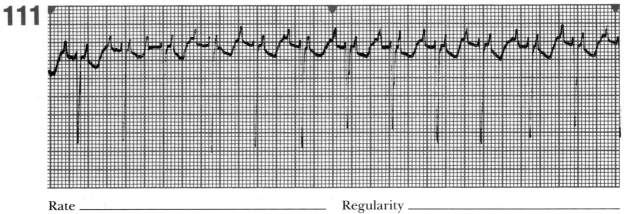

Rate _____   Regularity _____

PR Ratio _____   PR Interval _____

QRS Interval _____

Interpretation _____

112

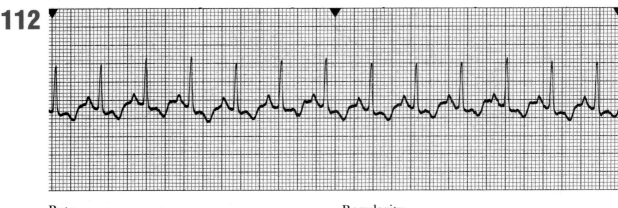

Rate _____   Regularity _____

PR Ratio _____   PR Interval _____

QRS Interval _____

Interpretation _____

113

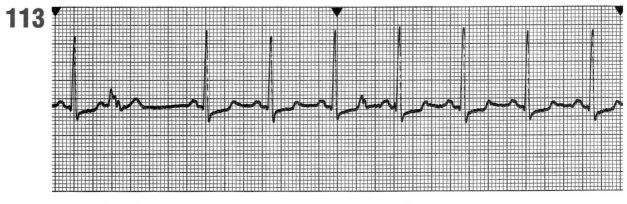

Rate _____   Regularity _____

PR Ratio _____   PR Interval _____

QRS Interval _____

Interpretation _____

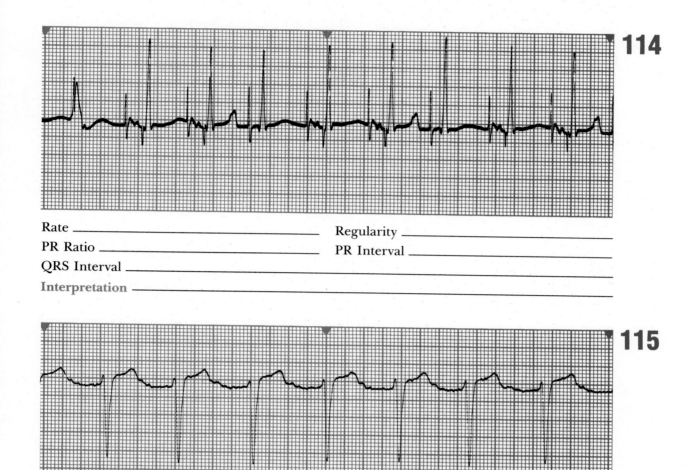

114

Rate _____ Regularity _____

PR Ratio _____ PR Interval _____

QRS Interval _____

Interpretation _____

115

Rate _____ Regularity _____

PR Ratio _____ PR Interval _____

QRS Interval _____

Interpretation _____

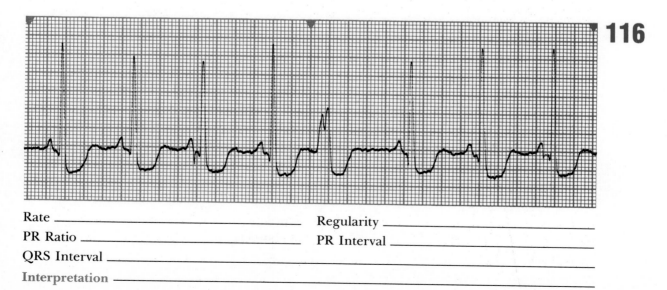

116

Rate _____ Regularity _____

PR Ratio _____ PR Interval _____

QRS Interval _____

Interpretation _____

117

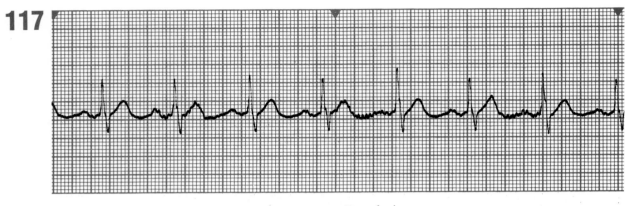

Rate _____ Regularity _____

PR Ratio _____ PR Interval _____

QRS Interval _____

Interpretation _____

118

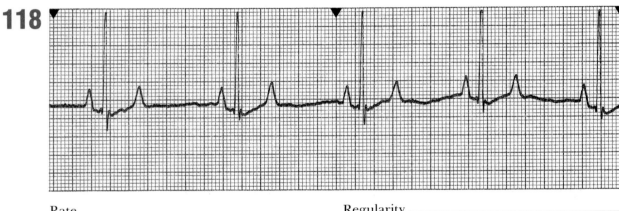

Rate _____ Regularity _____

PR Ratio _____ PR Interval _____

QRS Interval _____

Interpretation _____

119

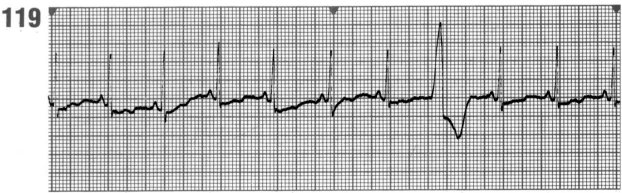

Rate _____ Regularity _____

PR Ratio _____ PR Interval _____

QRS Interval _____

Interpretation _____

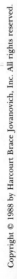

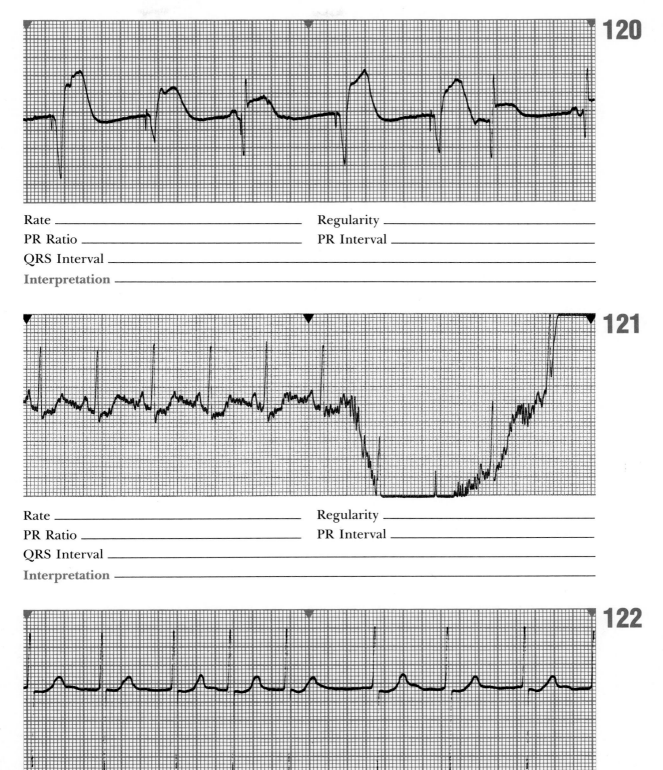

120

Rate _____   Regularity _____

PR Ratio _____   PR Interval _____

QRS Interval _____

Interpretation _____

121

Rate _____   Regularity _____

PR Ratio _____   PR Interval _____

QRS Interval _____

Interpretation _____

122

Rate _____   Regularity _____

PR Ratio _____   PR Interval _____

QRS Interval _____

Interpretation _____

123

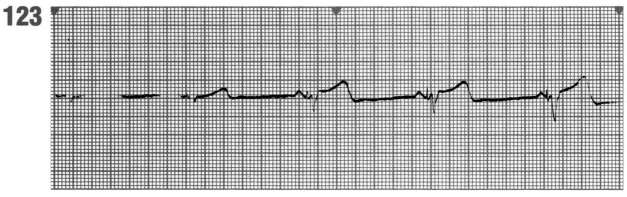

Rate _____ Regularity _____
PR Ratio _____ PR Interval _____
QRS Interval _____
Interpretation _____

124

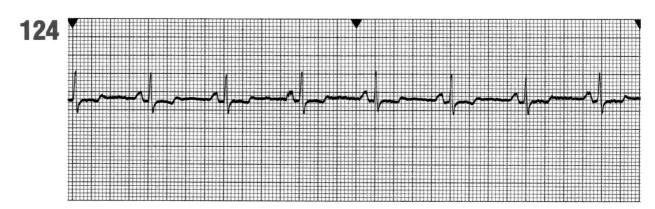

Rate _____ Regularity _____
PR Ratio _____ PR Interval _____
QRS Interval _____
Interpretation _____

125

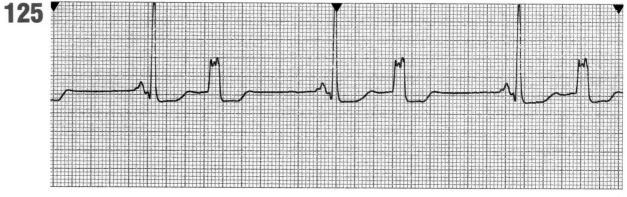

Rate _____ Regularity _____
PR Ratio _____ PR Interval _____
QRS Interval _____
Interpretation _____

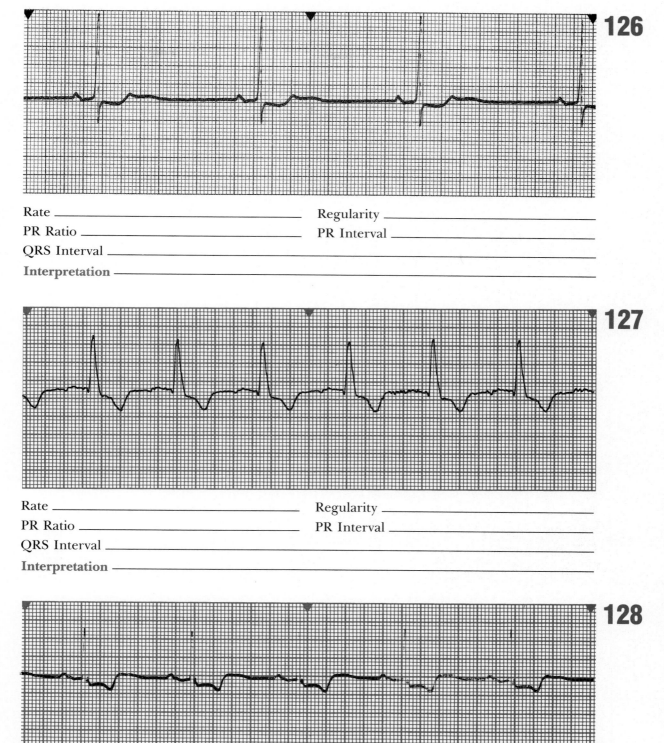

126

Rate _____   Regularity _____
PR Ratio _____   PR Interval _____
QRS Interval _____
Interpretation _____

127

Rate _____   Regularity _____
PR Ratio _____   PR Interval _____
QRS Interval _____
Interpretation _____

128

Rate _____   Regularity _____
PR Ratio _____   PR Interval _____
QRS Interval _____
Interpretation _____

129

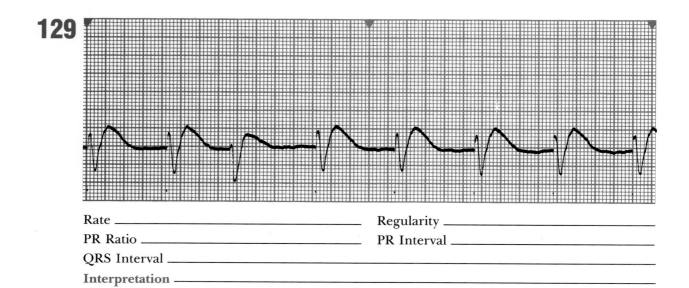

Rate _____   Regularity _____

PR Ratio _____   PR Interval _____

QRS Interval _____

Interpretation _____

130

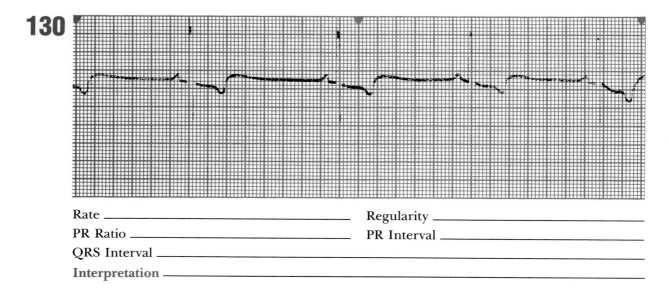

Rate _____   Regularity _____

PR Ratio _____   PR Interval _____

QRS Interval _____

Interpretation _____

131

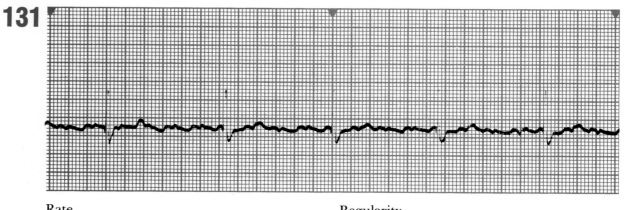

Rate _____   Regularity _____

PR Ratio _____   PR Interval _____

QRS Interval _____

Interpretation _____

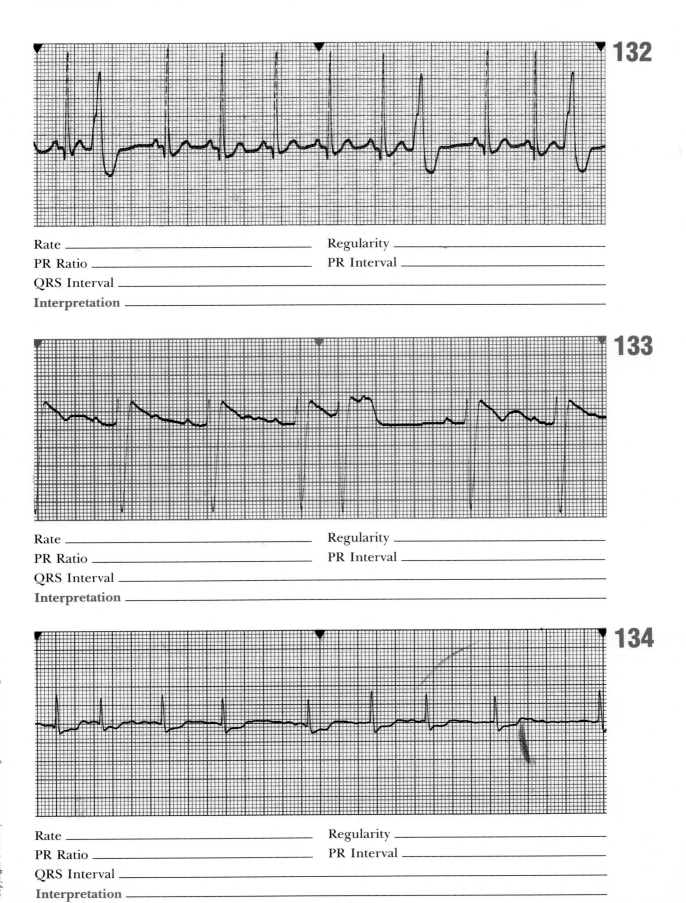

132

Rate _____ Regularity _____
PR Ratio _____ PR Interval _____
QRS Interval _____
Interpretation _____

133

Rate _____ Regularity _____
PR Ratio _____ PR Interval _____
QRS Interval _____
Interpretation _____

134

Rate _____ Regularity _____
PR Ratio _____ PR Interval _____
QRS Interval _____
Interpretation _____

135

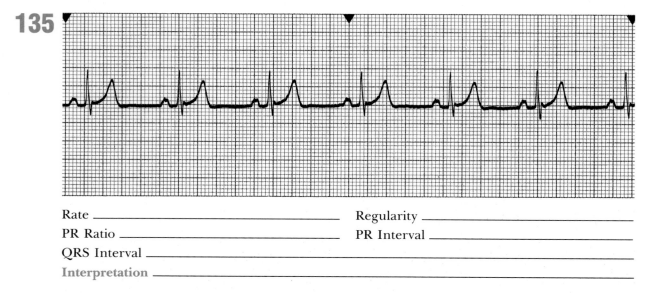

Rate _____   Regularity _____

PR Ratio _____   PR Interval _____

QRS Interval _____

Interpretation _____

136

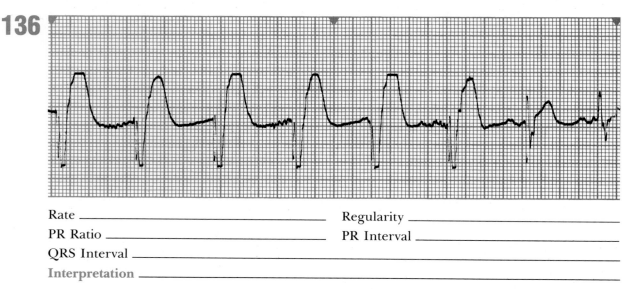

Rate _____   Regularity _____

PR Ratio _____   PR Interval _____

QRS Interval _____

Interpretation _____

137

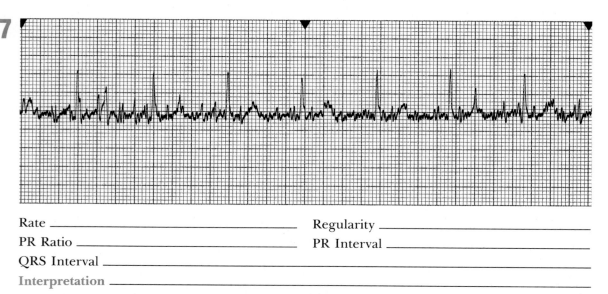

Rate _____   Regularity _____

PR Ratio _____   PR Interval _____

QRS Interval _____

Interpretation _____

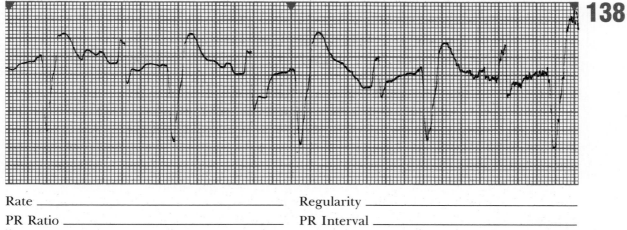

138

Rate _____ Regularity _____

PR Ratio _____ PR Interval _____

QRS Interval _____

Interpretation _____

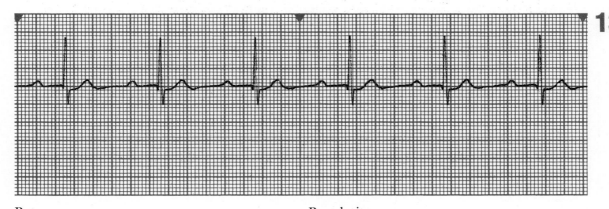

139

Rate _____ Regularity _____

PR Ratio _____ PR Interval _____

QRS Interval _____

Interpretation _____

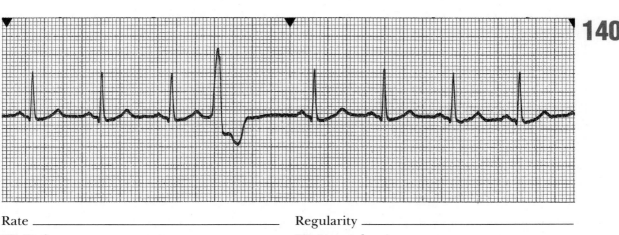

140

Rate _____ Regularity _____

PR Ratio _____ PR Interval _____

QRS Interval _____

Interpretation _____

141

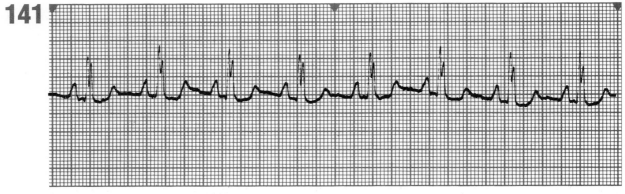

Rate _____   Regularity _____

PR Ratio _____   PR Interval _____

QRS Interval _____

Interpretation _____

142

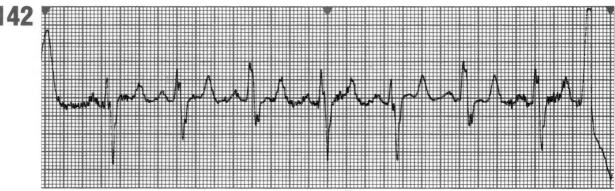

Rate _____   Regularity _____

PR Ratio _____   PR Interval _____

QRS Interval _____

Interpretation _____

143

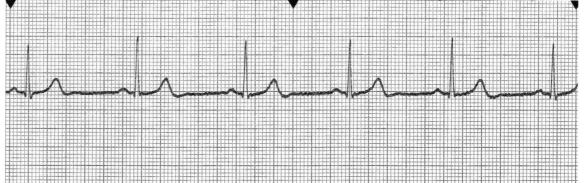

Rate _____   Regularity _____

PR Ratio _____   PR Interval _____

QRS Interval _____

Interpretation _____

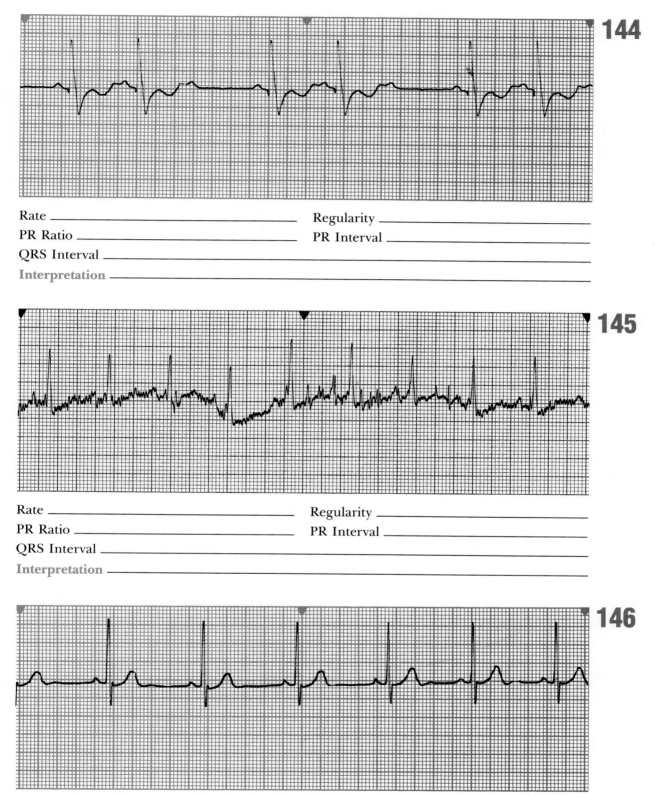

144

Rate _____ Regularity _____

PR Ratio _____ PR Interval _____

QRS Interval _____

Interpretation _____

145

Rate _____ Regularity _____

PR Ratio _____ PR Interval _____

QRS Interval _____

Interpretation _____

146

Rate _____ Regularity _____

PR Ratio _____ PR Interval _____

QRS Interval _____

Interpretation _____

147

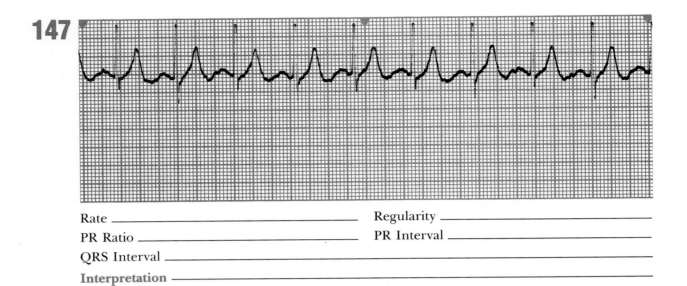

Rate _____ Regularity _____

PR Ratio _____ PR Interval _____

QRS Interval _____

Interpretation _____

148

Rate _____ Regularity _____

PR Ratio _____ PR Interval _____

QRS Interval _____

Interpretation _____

149

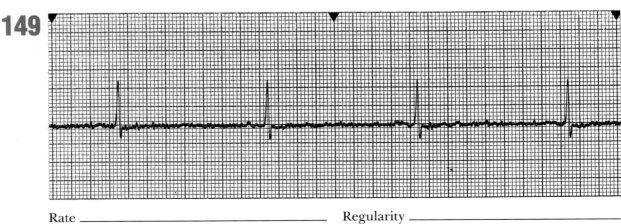

Rate _____ Regularity _____

PR Ratio _____ PR Interval _____

QRS Interval _____

Interpretation _____

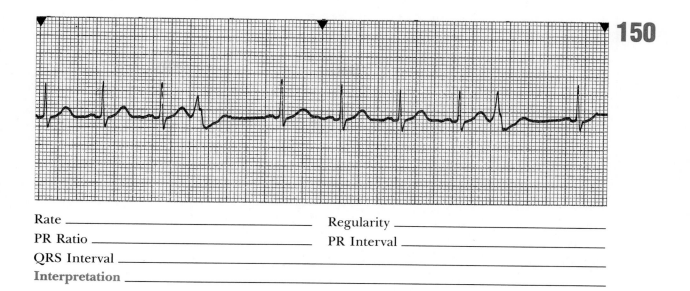

150

Rate _____ Regularity _____
PR Ratio _____ PR Interval _____
QRS Interval _____
Interpretation _____

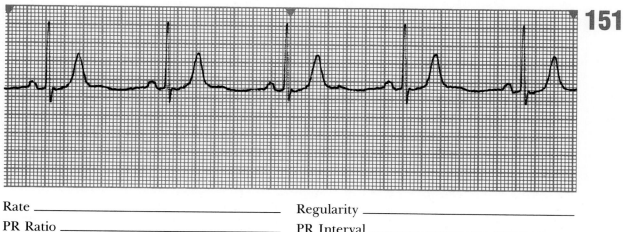

151

Rate _____ Regularity _____
PR Ratio _____ PR Interval _____
QRS Interval _____
Interpretation _____

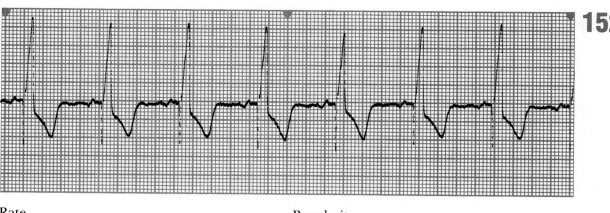

152

Rate _____ Regularity _____
PR Ratio _____ PR Interval _____
QRS Interval _____
Interpretation _____

153

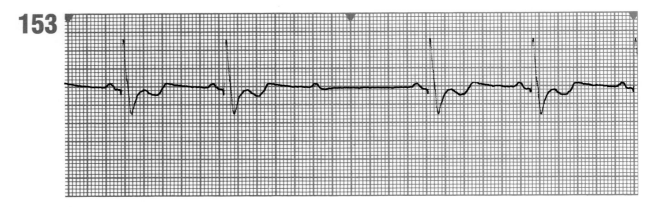

Rate _____ Regularity _____

PR Ratio _____ PR Interval _____

QRS Interval _____

Interpretation _____

154

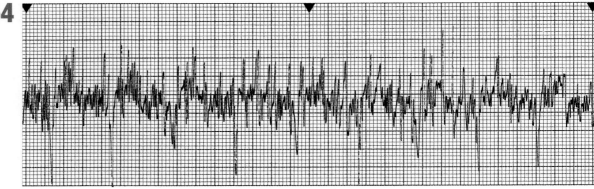

Rate _____ Regularity _____

PR Ratio _____ PR Interval _____

QRS Interval _____

Interpretation _____

155

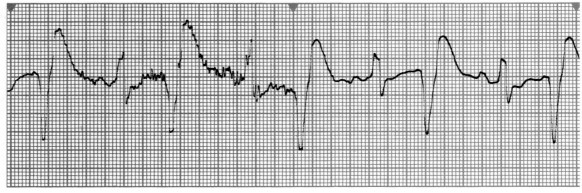

Rate _____ Regularity _____

PR Ratio _____ PR Interval _____

QRS Interval _____

Interpretation _____

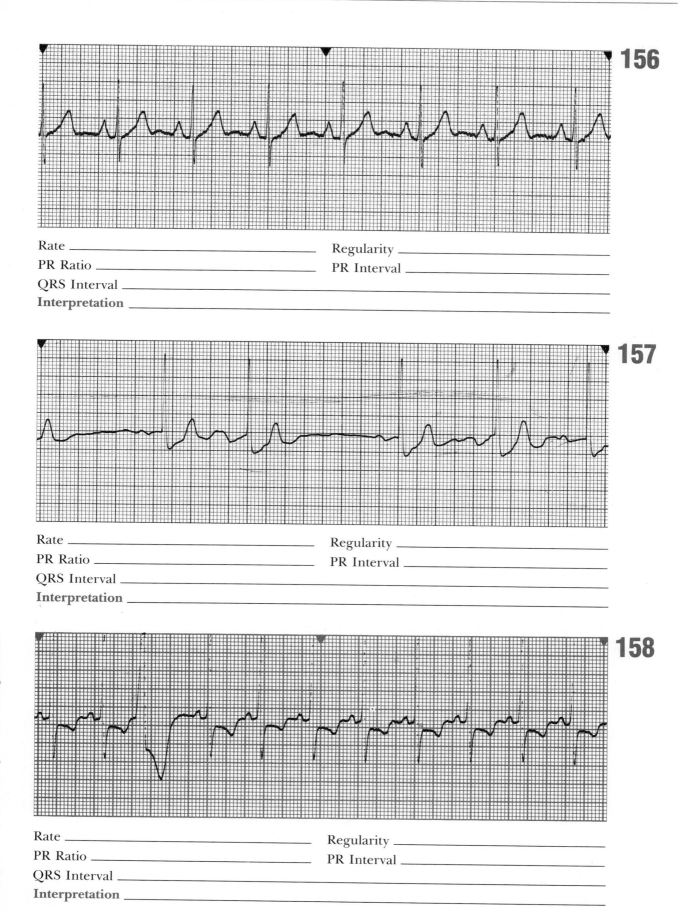

156

Rate _____ Regularity _____
PR Ratio _____ PR Interval _____
QRS Interval _____
Interpretation _____

157

Rate _____ Regularity _____
PR Ratio _____ PR Interval _____
QRS Interval _____
Interpretation _____

158

Rate _____ Regularity _____
PR Ratio _____ PR Interval _____
QRS Interval _____
Interpretation _____

159

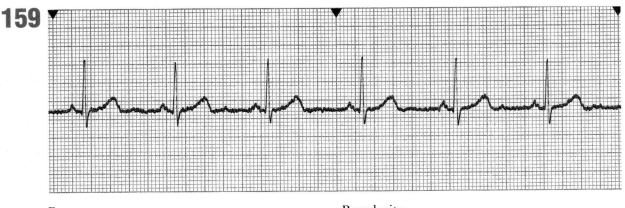

Rate _____   Regularity _____
PR Ratio _____   PR Interval _____
QRS Interval _____
Interpretation _____

160

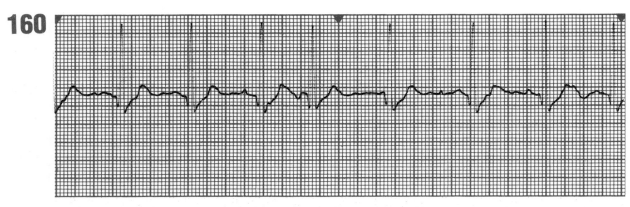

Rate _____   Regularity _____
PR Ratio _____   PR Interval _____
QRS Interval _____
Interpretation _____

161

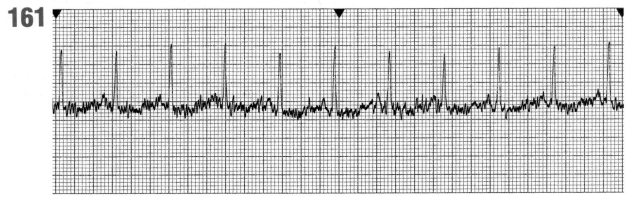

Rate _____   Regularity _____
PR Ratio _____   PR Interval _____
QRS Interval _____
Interpretation _____

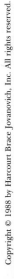

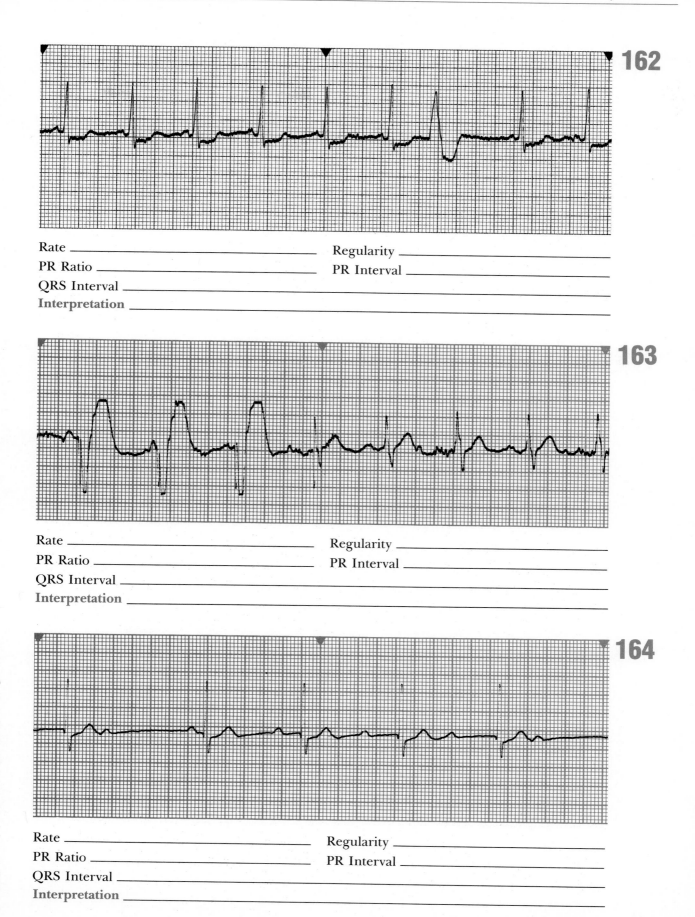

162

Rate _____   Regularity _____

PR Ratio _____   PR Interval _____

QRS Interval _____

Interpretation _____

163

Rate _____   Regularity _____

PR Ratio _____   PR Interval _____

QRS Interval _____

Interpretation _____

164

Rate _____   Regularity _____

PR Ratio _____   PR Interval _____

QRS Interval _____

Interpretation _____

165

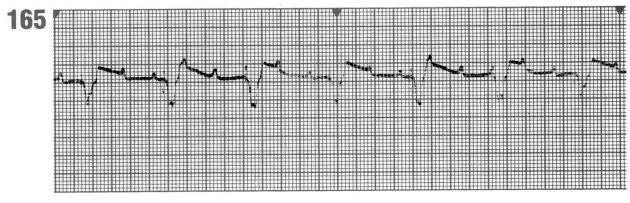

Rate _____   Regularity _____

PR Ratio _____   PR Interval _____

QRS Interval _____

Interpretation _____

166

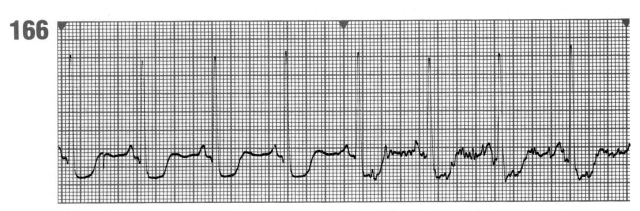

Rate _____   Regularity _____

PR Ratio _____   PR Interval _____

QRS Interval _____

Interpretation _____

167

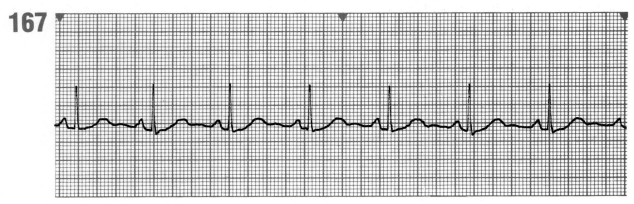

Rate _____   Regularity _____

PR Ratio _____   PR Interval _____

QRS Interval _____

Interpretation _____

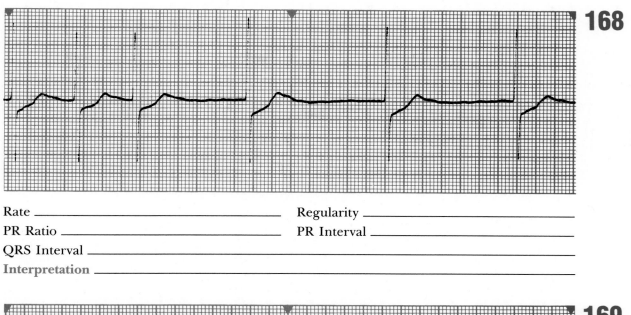

Rate _____ Regularity _____
PR Ratio _____ PR Interval _____
QRS Interval _____
Interpretation _____

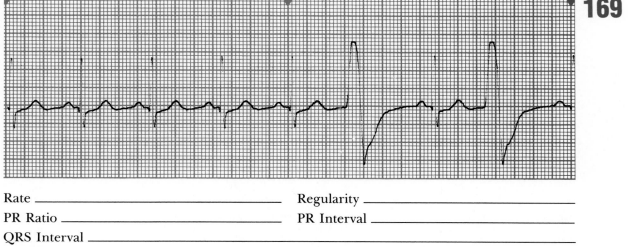

Rate _____ Regularity _____
PR Ratio _____ PR Interval _____
QRS Interval _____
Interpretation _____

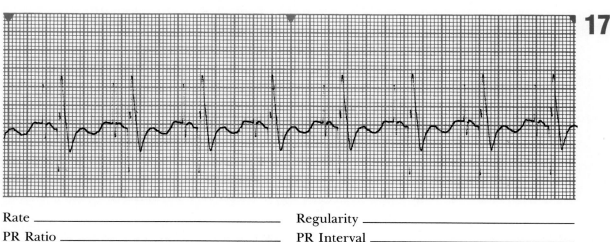

Rate _____ Regularity _____
PR Ratio _____ PR Interval _____
QRS Interval _____
Interpretation _____

171

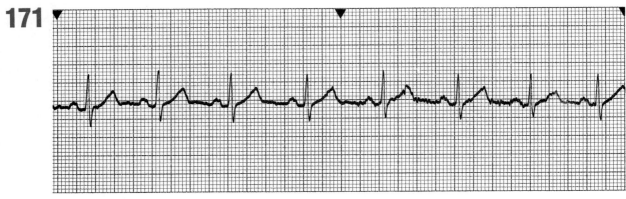

Rate _____   Regularity _____
PR Ratio _____   PR Interval _____
QRS Interval _____
Interpretation _____

172

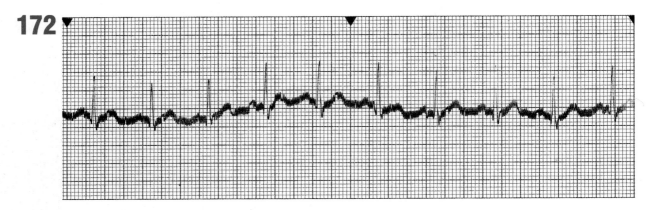

Rate _____   Regularity _____
PR Ratio _____   PR Interval _____
QRS Interval _____
Interpretation _____

173

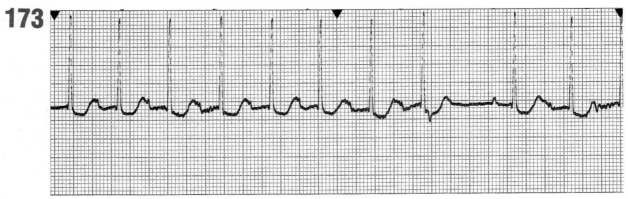

Rate _____   Regularity _____
PR Ratio _____   PR Interval _____
QRS Interval _____
Interpretation _____

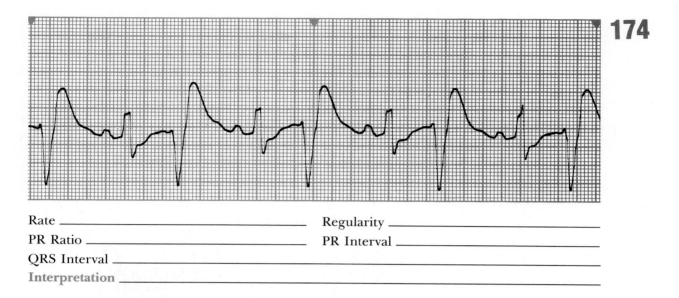

174

Rate _____   Regularity _____

PR Ratio _____   PR Interval _____

QRS Interval _____

Interpretation _____

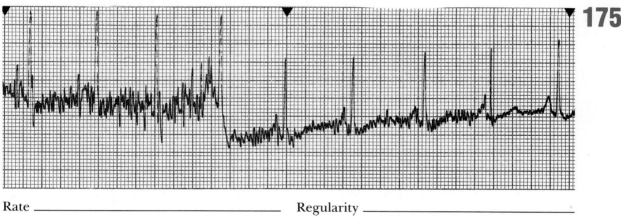

175

Rate _____   Regularity _____

PR Ratio _____   PR Interval _____

QRS Interval _____

Interpretation _____

176

Rate _____   Regularity _____

PR Ratio _____   PR Interval _____

QRS Interval _____

Interpretation _____

177

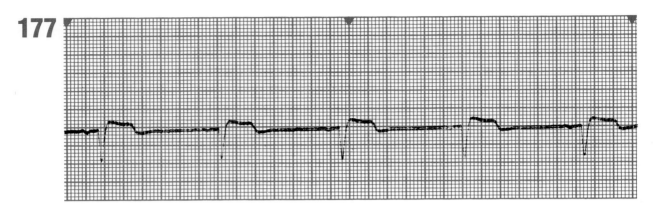

Rate _____   Regularity _____

PR Ratio _____   PR Interval _____

QRS Interval _____

Interpretation _____

178

Rate _____   Regularity _____

PR Ratio _____   PR Interval _____

QRS Interval _____

Interpretation _____

179

Rate _____   Regularity _____

PR Ratio _____   PR Interval _____

QRS Interval _____

Interpretation _____

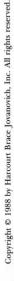

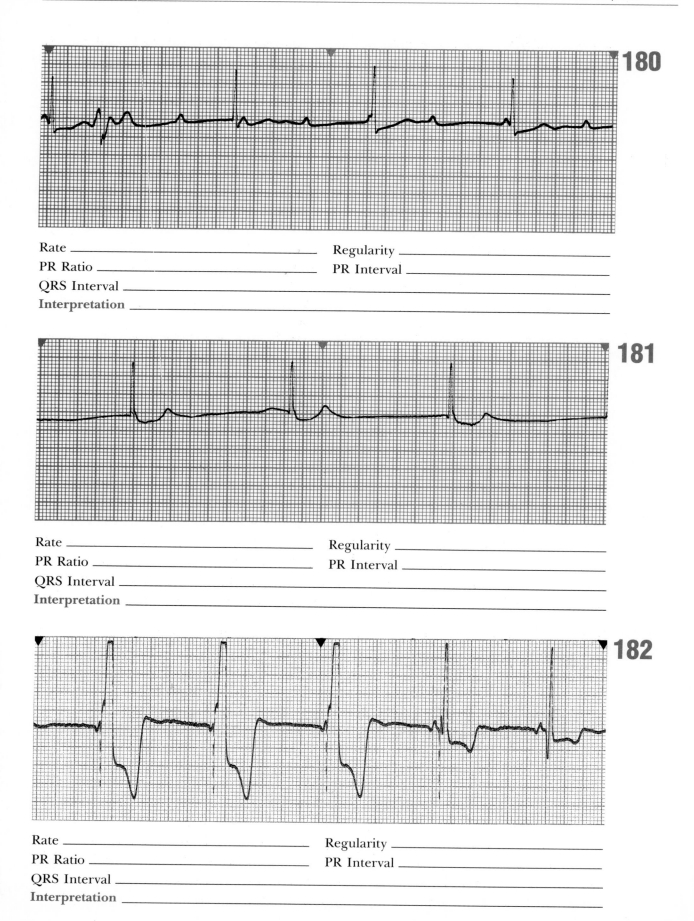

180

Rate _____ Regularity _____

PR Ratio _____ PR Interval _____

QRS Interval _____

Interpretation _____

181

Rate _____ Regularity _____

PR Ratio _____ PR Interval _____

QRS Interval _____

Interpretation _____

182

Rate _____ Regularity _____

PR Ratio _____ PR Interval _____

QRS Interval _____

Interpretation _____

183

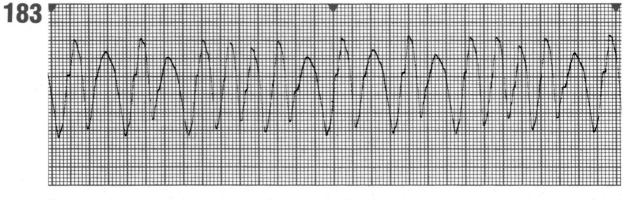

Rate _____   Regularity _____

PR Ratio _____   PR Interval _____

QRS Interval _____

Interpretation _____

184

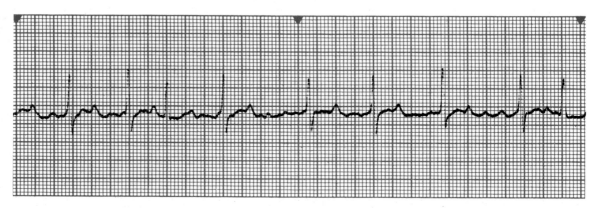

Rate _____   Regularity _____

PR Ratio _____   PR Interval _____

QRS Interval _____

Interpretation _____

185

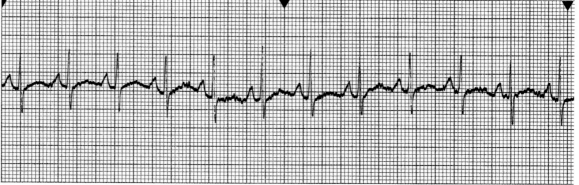

Rate _____   Regularity _____

PR Ratio _____   PR Interval _____

QRS Interval _____

Interpretation _____

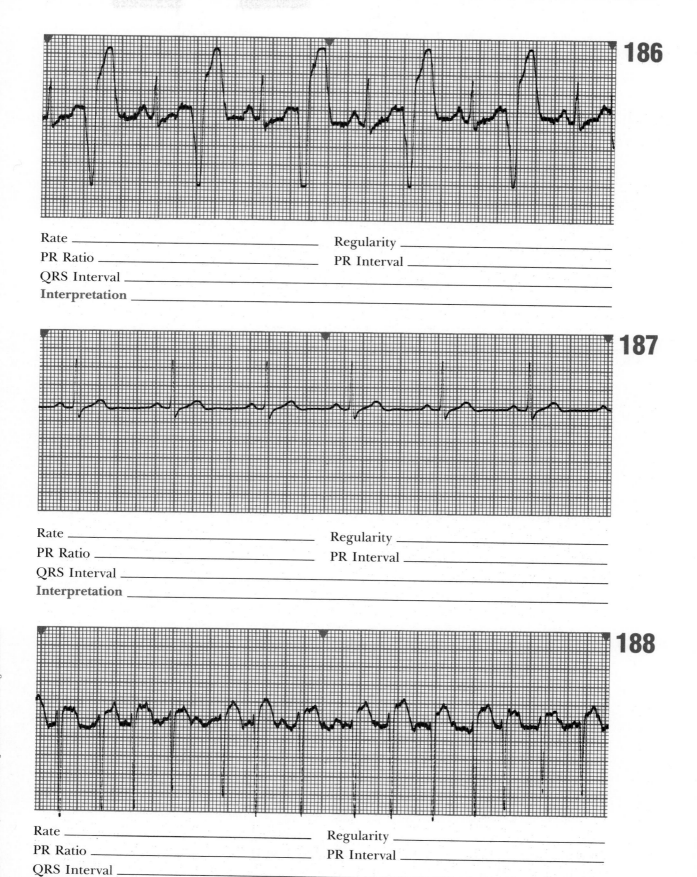

186

Rate _____ Regularity _____

PR Ratio _____ PR Interval _____

QRS Interval _____

Interpretation _____

187

Rate _____ Regularity _____

PR Ratio _____ PR Interval _____

QRS Interval _____

Interpretation _____

188

Rate _____ Regularity _____

PR Ratio _____ PR Interval _____

QRS Interval _____

Interpretation _____

189

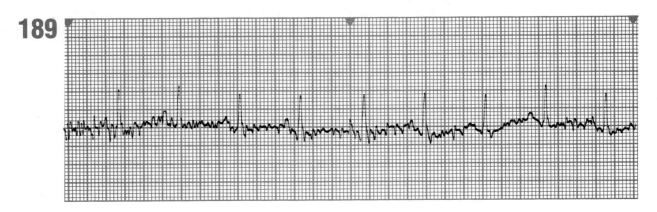

Rate _____   Regularity _____

PR Ratio _____   PR Interval _____

QRS Interval _____

Interpretation _____

190

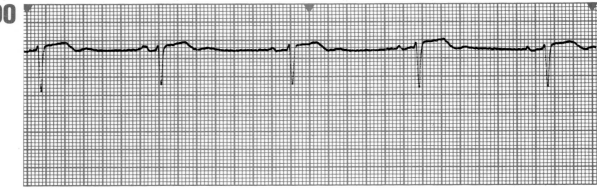

Rate _____   Regularity _____

PR Ratio _____   PR Interval _____

QRS Interval _____

Interpretation _____

191

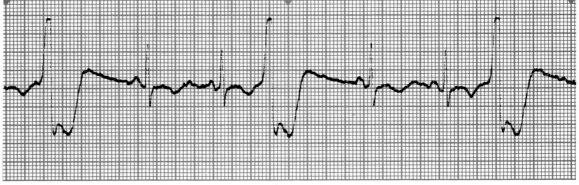

Rate _____   Regularity _____

PR Ratio _____   PR Interval _____

QRS Interval _____

Interpretation _____

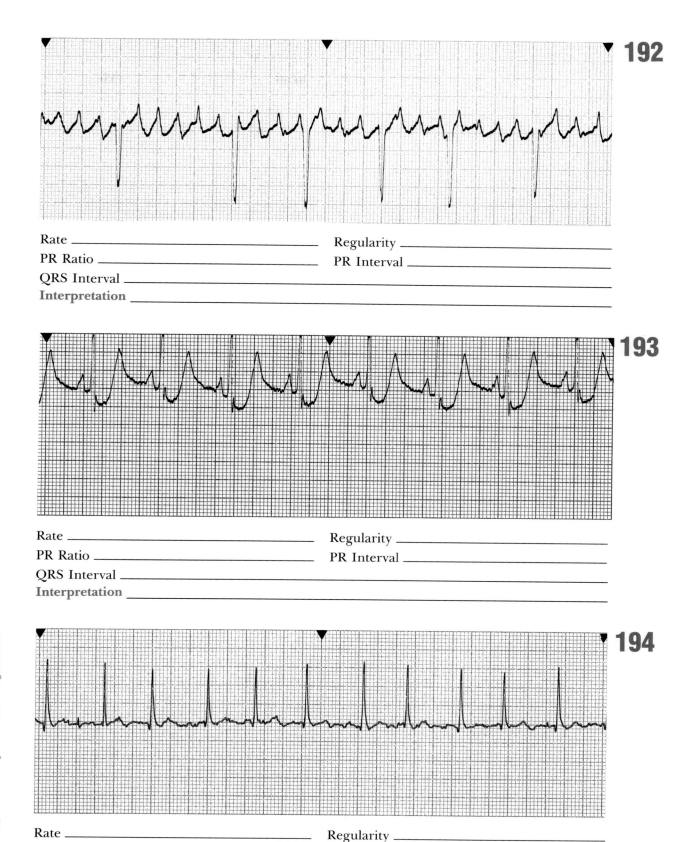

192

Rate _____   Regularity _____

PR Ratio _____   PR Interval _____

QRS Interval _____

Interpretation _____

193

Rate _____   Regularity _____

PR Ratio _____   PR Interval _____

QRS Interval _____

Interpretation _____

194

Rate _____   Regularity _____

PR Ratio _____   PR Interval _____

QRS Interval _____

Interpretation _____

195

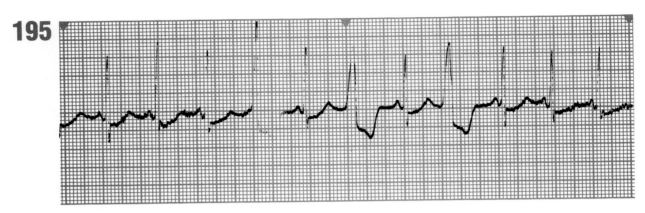

Rate _____   Regularity _____

PR Ratio _____   PR Interval _____

QRS Interval _____

Interpretation _____

196

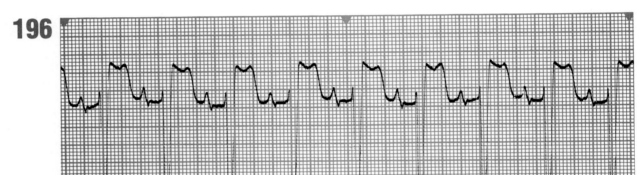

Rate _____   Regularity _____

PR Ratio _____   PR Interval _____

QRS Interval _____

Interpretation _____

197

Rate _____   Regularity _____

PR Ratio _____   PR Interval _____

QRS Interval _____

Interpretation _____

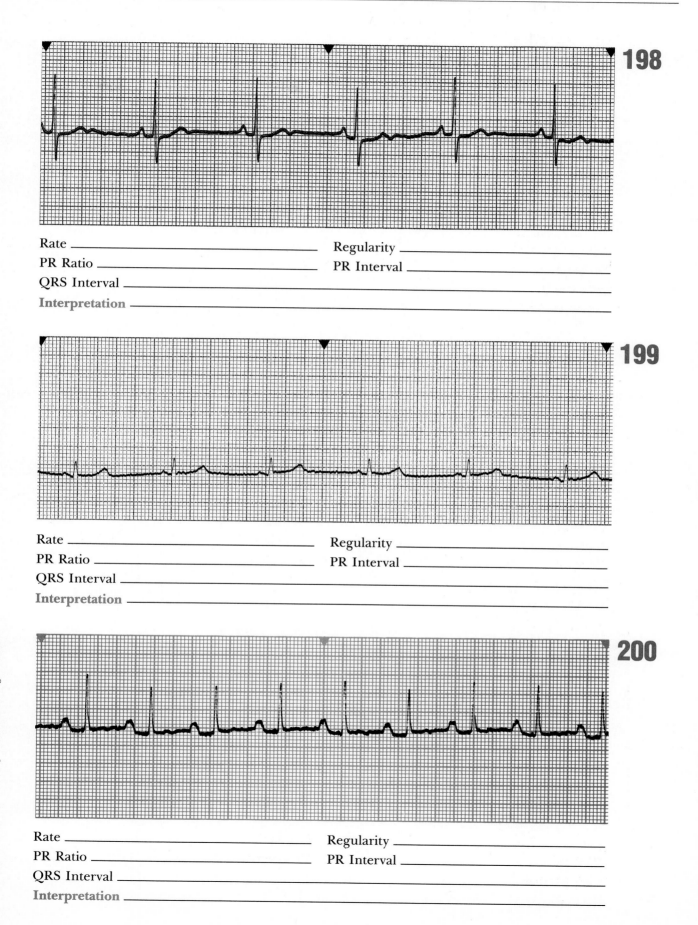

198

Rate _____ Regularity _____

PR Ratio _____ PR Interval _____

QRS Interval _____

Interpretation _____

199

Rate _____ Regularity _____

PR Ratio _____ PR Interval _____

QRS Interval _____

Interpretation _____

200

Rate _____ Regularity _____

PR Ratio _____ PR Interval _____

QRS Interval _____

Interpretation _____

201

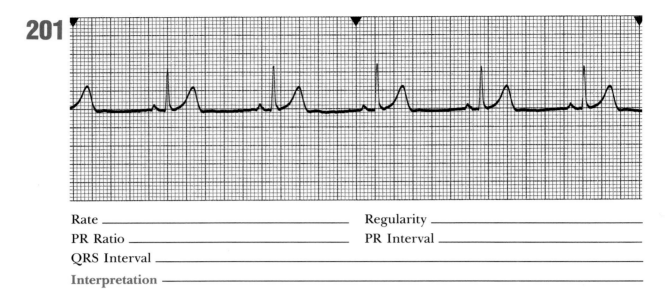

Rate _____ Regularity _____

PR Ratio _____ PR Interval _____

QRS Interval _____

Interpretation _____

202

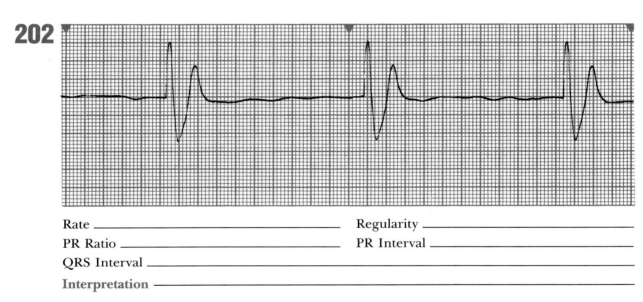

Rate _____ Regularity _____

PR Ratio _____ PR Interval _____

QRS Interval _____

Interpretation _____

203

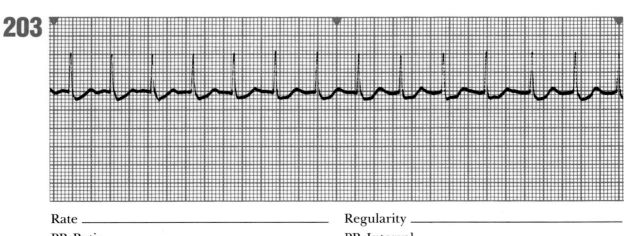

Rate _____ Regularity _____

PR Ratio _____ PR Interval _____

QRS Interval _____

Interpretation _____

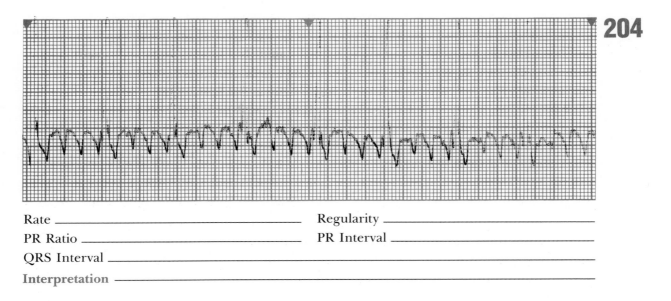

204

Rate _____ Regularity _____

PR Ratio _____ PR Interval _____

QRS Interval _____

Interpretation _____

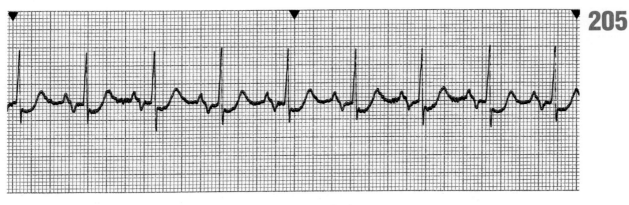

205

Rate _____ Regularity _____

PR Ratio _____ PR Interval _____

QRS Interval _____

Interpretation _____

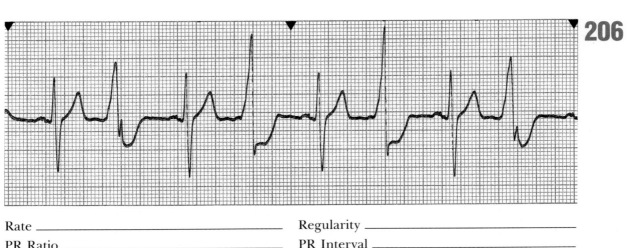

206

Rate _____ Regularity _____

PR Ratio _____ PR Interval _____

QRS Interval _____

Interpretation _____

207

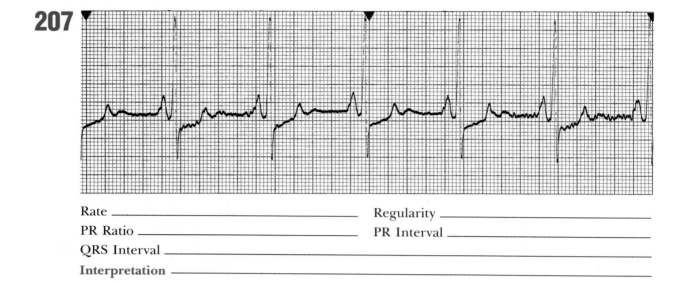

Rate _____   Regularity _____

PR Ratio _____   PR Interval _____

QRS Interval _____

Interpretation _____

208

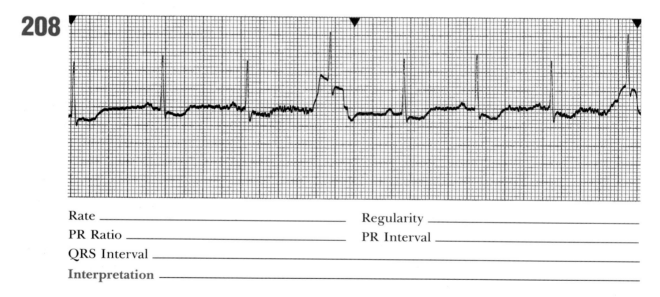

Rate _____   Regularity _____

PR Ratio _____   PR Interval _____

QRS Interval _____

Interpretation _____

209

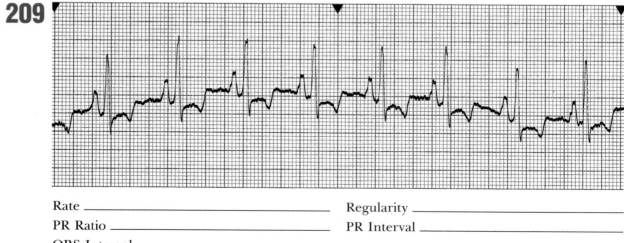

Rate _____   Regularity _____

PR Ratio _____   PR Interval _____

QRS Interval _____

Interpretation _____

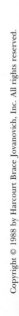

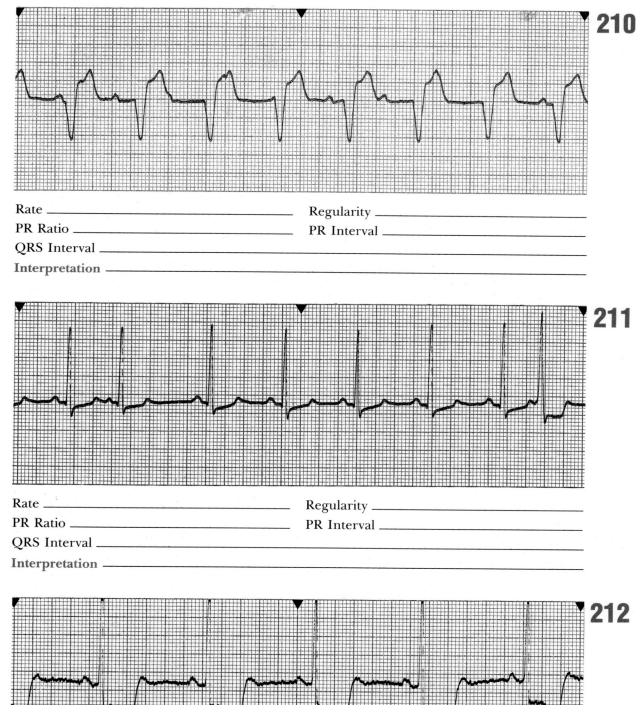

210

Rate _____ Regularity _____
PR Ratio _____ PR Interval _____
QRS Interval _____
Interpretation _____

211

Rate _____ Regularity _____
PR Ratio _____ PR Interval _____
QRS Interval _____
Interpretation _____

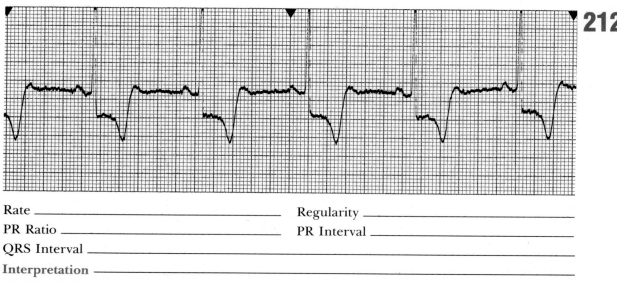

212

Rate _____ Regularity _____
PR Ratio _____ PR Interval _____
QRS Interval _____
Interpretation _____

213

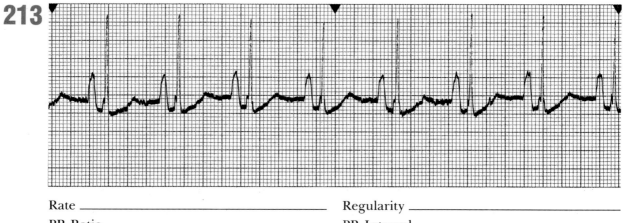

Rate _____   Regularity _____

PR Ratio _____   PR Interval _____

QRS Interval _____

Interpretation _____

214

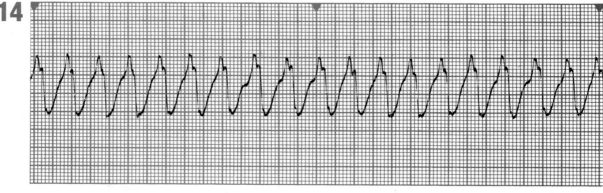

Rate _____   Regularity _____

PR Ratio _____   PR Interval _____

QRS Interval _____

Interpretation _____

215

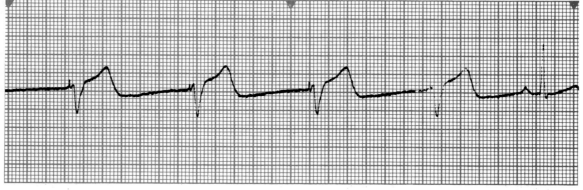

Rate _____   Regularity _____

PR Ratio _____   PR Interval _____

QRS Interval _____

Interpretation _____

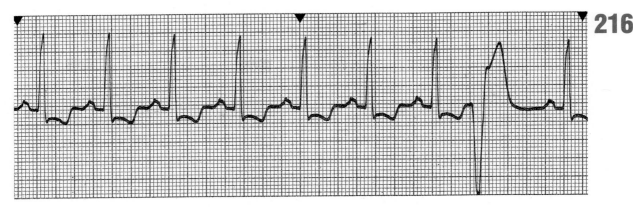

216

Rate _____ Regularity _____

PR Ratio _____ PR Interval _____

QRS Interval _____

Interpretation _____

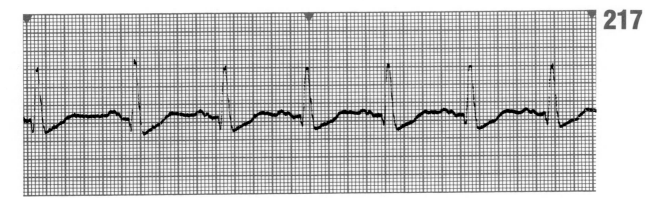

217

Rate _____ Regularity _____

PR Ratio _____ PR Interval _____

QRS Interval _____

Interpretation _____

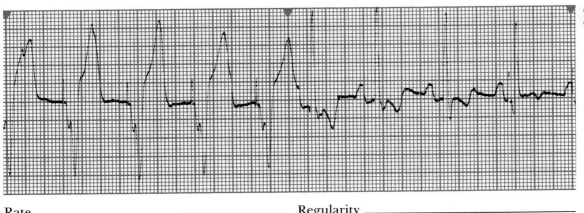

218

Rate _____ Regularity _____

PR Ratio _____ PR Interval _____

QRS Interval _____

Interpretation _____

219

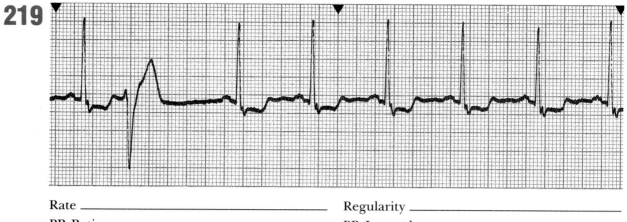

Rate _____   Regularity _____
PR Ratio _____   PR Interval _____
QRS Interval _____
Interpretation _____

220

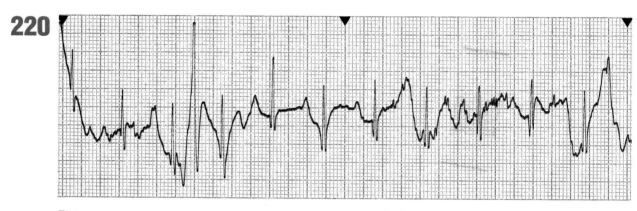

Rate _____   Regularity _____
PR Ratio _____   PR Interval _____
QRS Interval _____
Interpretation _____

221

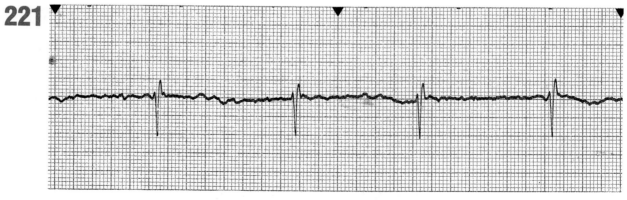

Rate _____   Regularity _____
PR Ratio _____   PR Interval _____
QRS Interval _____
Interpretation _____

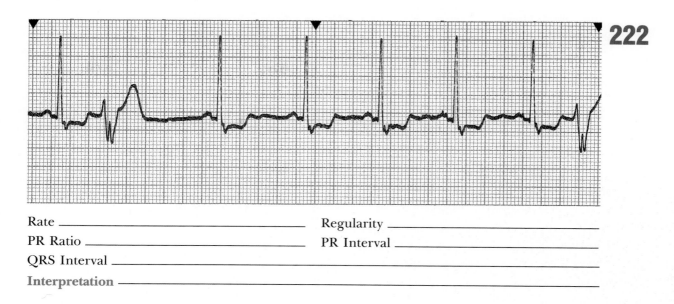

222

Rate _____   Regularity _____

PR Ratio _____   PR Interval _____

QRS Interval _____

Interpretation _____

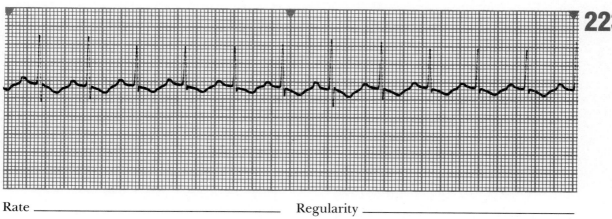

223

Rate _____   Regularity _____

PR Ratio _____   PR Interval _____

QRS Interval _____

Interpretation _____

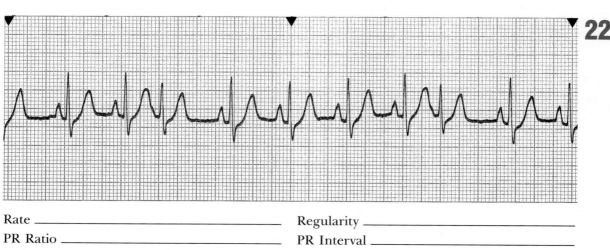

224

Rate _____   Regularity _____

PR Ratio _____   PR Interval _____

QRS Interval _____

Interpretation _____

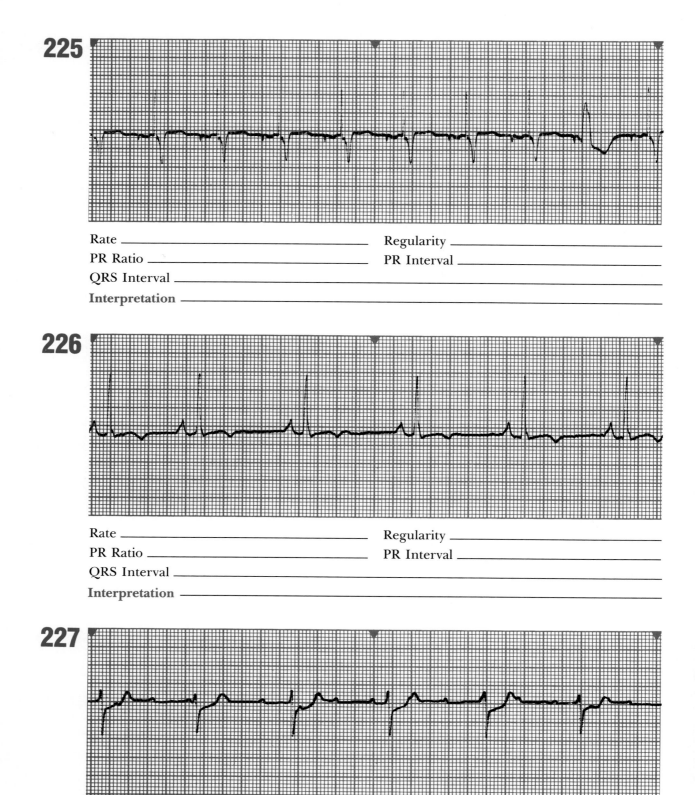

225

Rate _____ Regularity _____
PR Ratio _____ PR Interval _____
QRS Interval _____
Interpretation _____

226

Rate _____ Regularity _____
PR Ratio _____ PR Interval _____
QRS Interval _____
Interpretation _____

227

Rate _____ Regularity _____
PR Ratio _____ PR Interval _____
QRS Interval _____
Interpretation _____

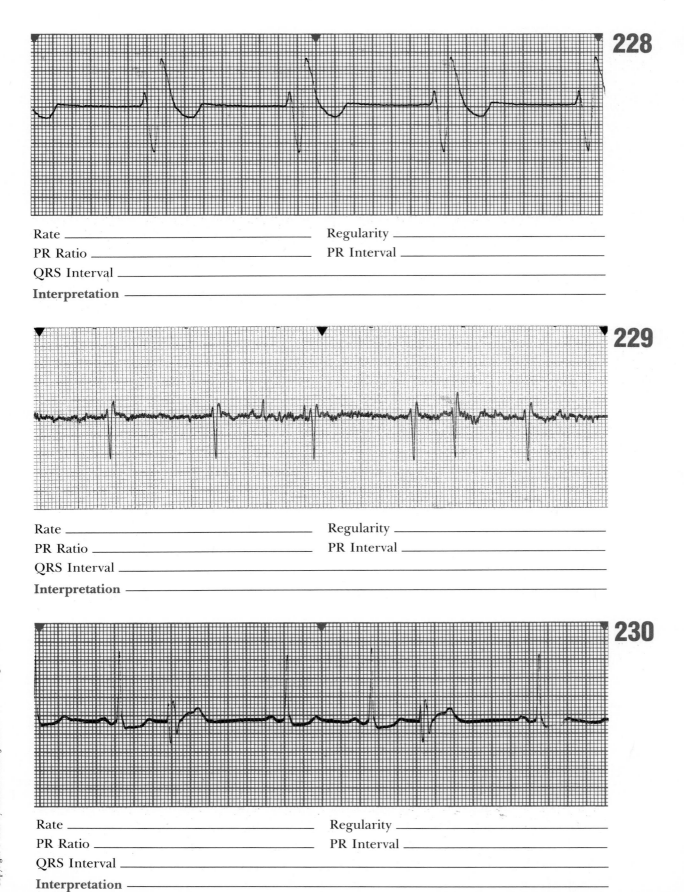

228

Rate _____ Regularity _____

PR Ratio _____ PR Interval _____

QRS Interval _____

Interpretation _____

229

Rate _____ Regularity _____

PR Ratio _____ PR Interval _____

QRS Interval _____

Interpretation _____

230

Rate _____ Regularity _____

PR Ratio _____ PR Interval _____

QRS Interval _____

Interpretation _____

231

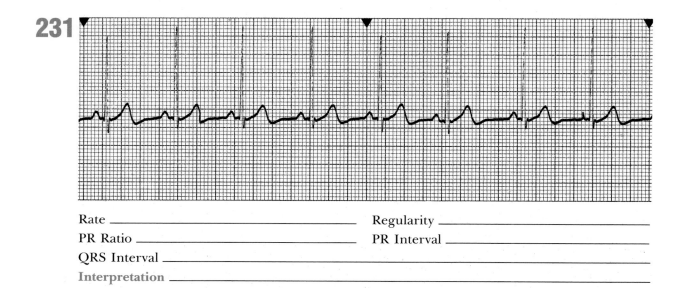

Rate _____ Regularity _____

PR Ratio _____ PR Interval _____

QRS Interval _____

Interpretation _____

232

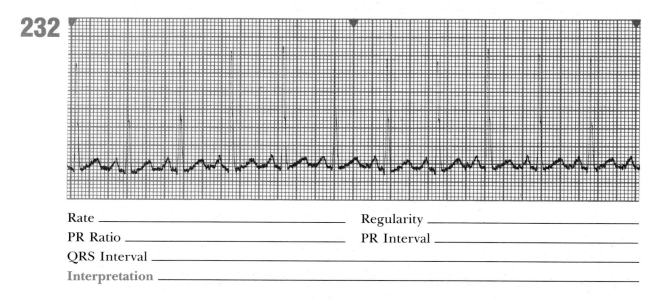

Rate _____ Regularity _____

PR Ratio _____ PR Interval _____

QRS Interval _____

Interpretation _____

233

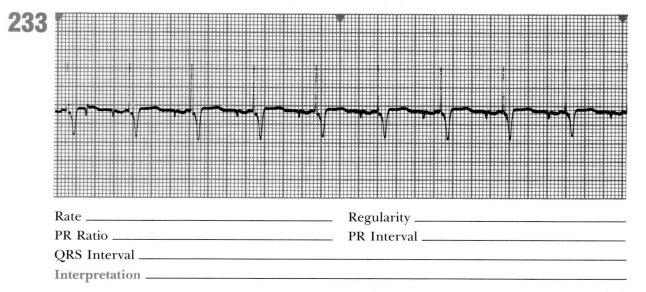

Rate _____ Regularity _____

PR Ratio _____ PR Interval _____

QRS Interval _____

Interpretation _____

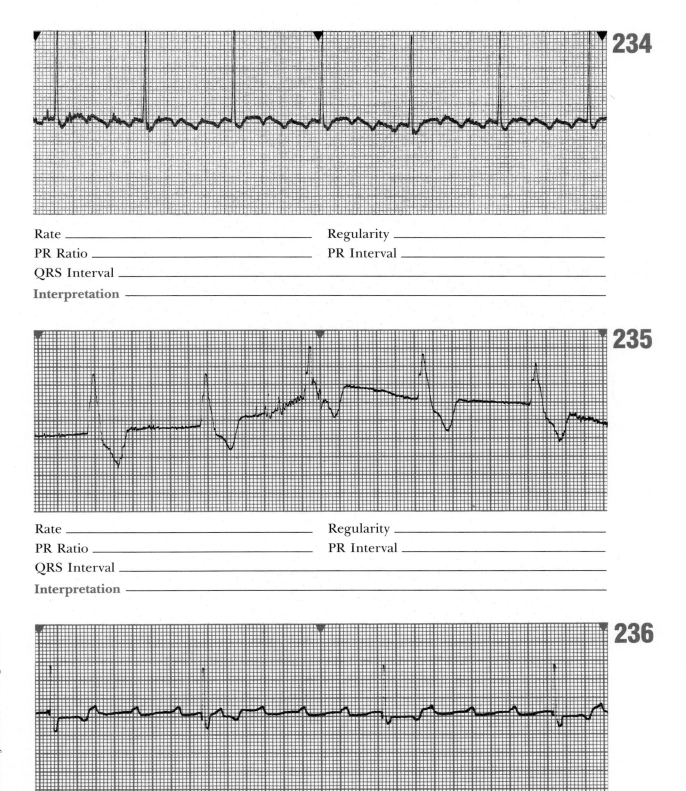

234

Rate _____   Regularity _____

PR Ratio _____   PR Interval _____

QRS Interval _____

Interpretation _____

235

Rate _____   Regularity _____

PR Ratio _____   PR Interval _____

QRS Interval _____

Interpretation _____

236

Rate _____   Regularity _____

PR Ratio _____   PR Interval _____

QRS Interval _____

Interpretation _____

237

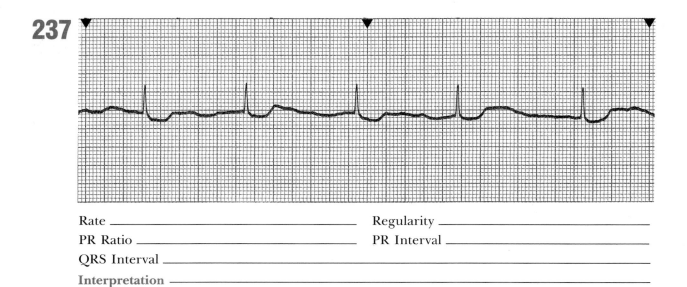

Rate _____ Regularity _____

PR Ratio _____ PR Interval _____

QRS Interval _____

Interpretation _____

238

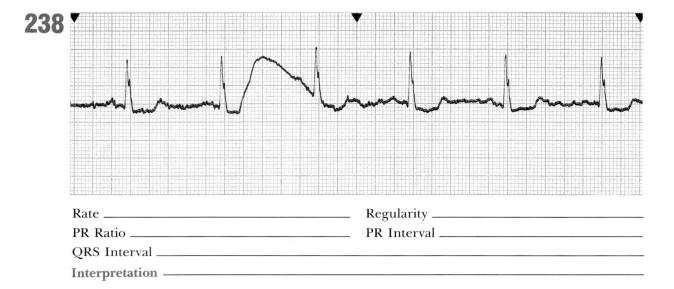

Rate _____ Regularity _____

PR Ratio _____ PR Interval _____

QRS Interval _____

Interpretation _____

239

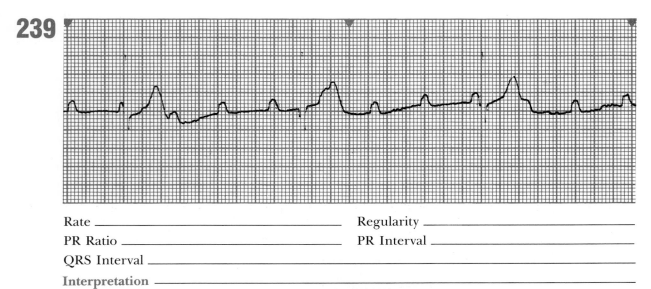

Rate _____ Regularity _____

PR Ratio _____ PR Interval _____

QRS Interval _____

Interpretation _____

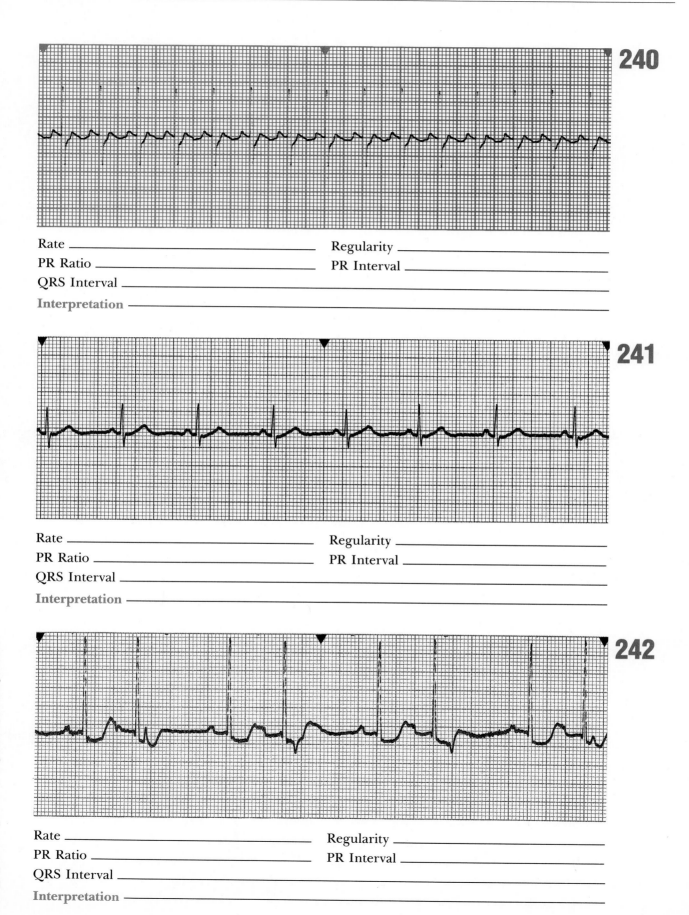

240

Rate _____ Regularity _____

PR Ratio _____ PR Interval _____

QRS Interval _____

Interpretation _____

241

Rate _____ Regularity _____

PR Ratio _____ PR Interval _____

QRS Interval _____

Interpretation _____

242

Rate _____ Regularity _____

PR Ratio _____ PR Interval _____

QRS Interval _____

Interpretation _____

243

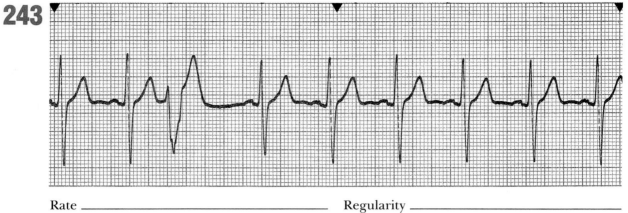

Rate _____   Regularity _____

PR Ratio _____   PR Interval _____

QRS Interval _____

Interpretation _____

244

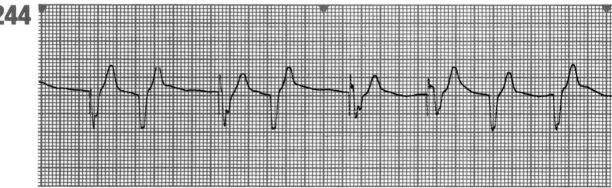

Rate _____   Regularity _____

PR Ratio _____   PR Interval _____

QRS Interval _____

Interpretation _____

245

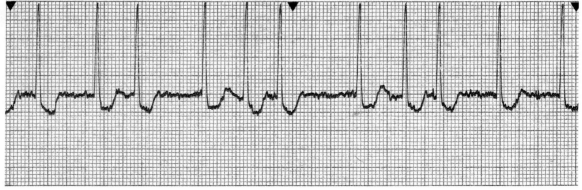

Rate _____   Regularity _____

PR Ratio _____   PR Interval _____

QRS Interval _____

Interpretation _____

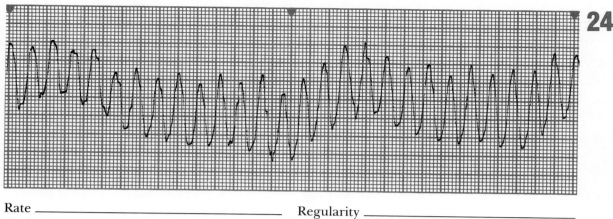

246

Rate _____   Regularity _____

PR Ratio _____   PR Interval _____

QRS Interval _____

Interpretation _____

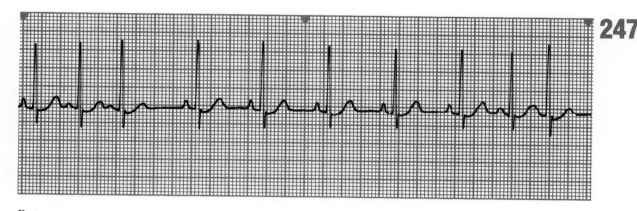

247

Rate _____   Regularity _____

PR Ratio _____   PR Interval _____

QRS Interval _____

Interpretation _____

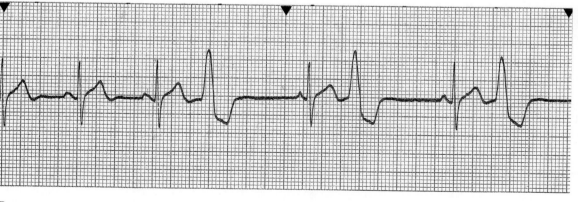

248

Rate _____   Regularity _____

PR Ratio _____   PR Interval _____

QRS Interval _____

Interpretation _____

249

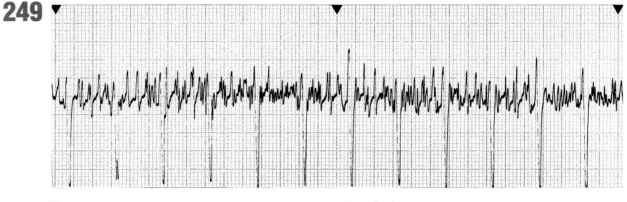

Rate _____ Regularity _____
PR Ratio _____ PR Interval _____
QRS Interval _____
Interpretation _____

250

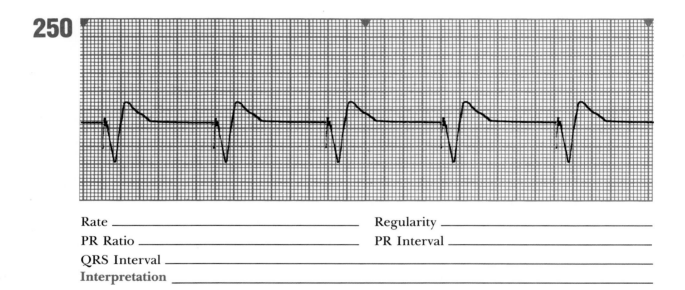

Rate _____ Regularity _____
PR Ratio _____ PR Interval _____
QRS Interval _____
Interpretation _____

251

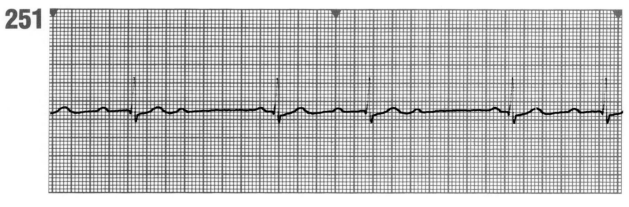

Rate _____ Regularity _____
PR Ratio _____ PR Interval _____
QRS Interval _____
Interpretation _____

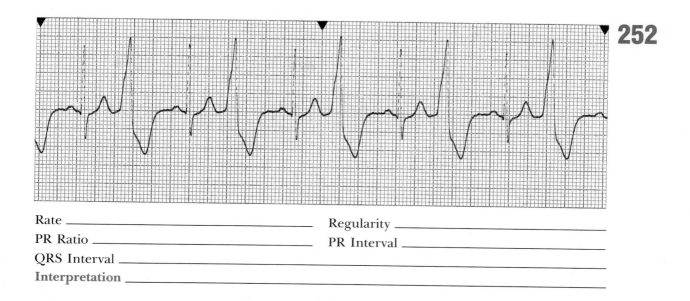

252

Rate _____ Regularity _____

PR Ratio _____ PR Interval _____

QRS Interval _____

Interpretation _____

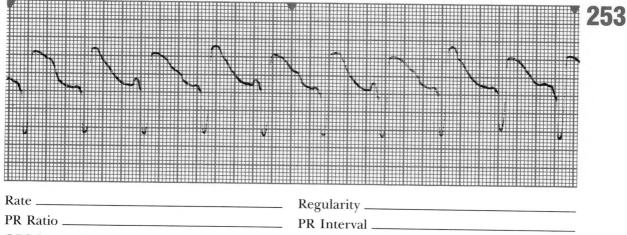

253

Rate _____ Regularity _____

PR Ratio _____ PR Interval _____

QRS Interval _____

Interpretation _____

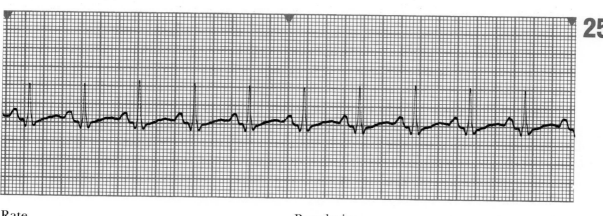

254

Rate _____ Regularity _____

PR Ratio _____ PR Interval _____

QRS Interval _____

Interpretation _____

255

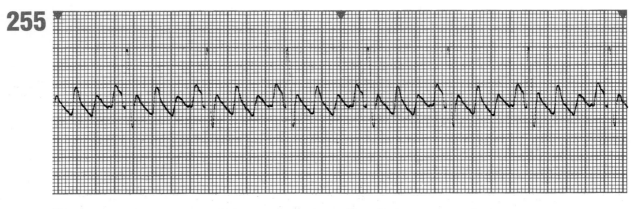

Rate _____ Regularity _____

PR Ratio _____ PR Interval _____

QRS Interval _____

Interpretation _____

256

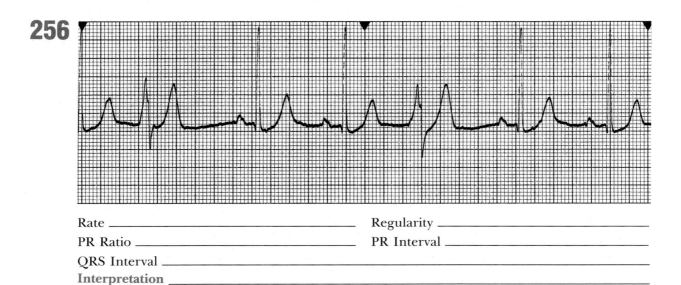

Rate _____ Regularity _____

PR Ratio _____ PR Interval _____

QRS Interval _____

Interpretation _____

257

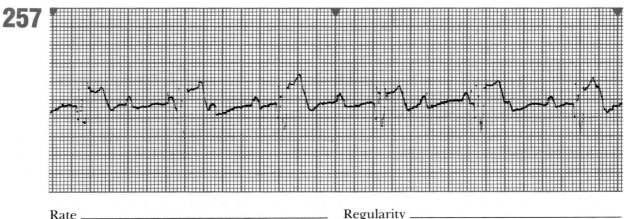

Rate _____ Regularity _____

PR Ratio _____ PR Interval _____

QRS Interval _____

Interpretation _____

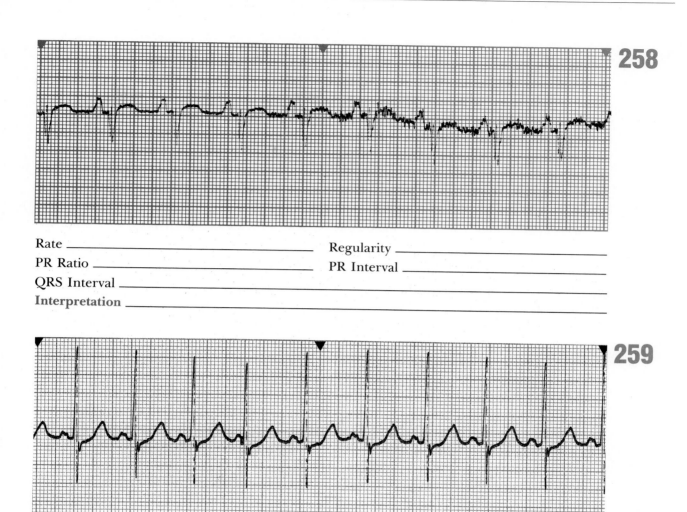

Rate _____   Regularity _____

PR Ratio _____   PR Interval _____

QRS Interval _____

Interpretation _____

Rate _____   Regularity _____

PR Ratio _____   PR Interval _____

QRS Interval _____

Interpretation _____

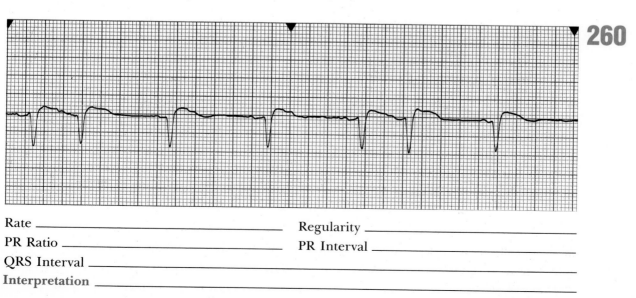

Rate _____   Regularity _____

PR Ratio _____   PR Interval _____

QRS Interval _____

Interpretation _____

261

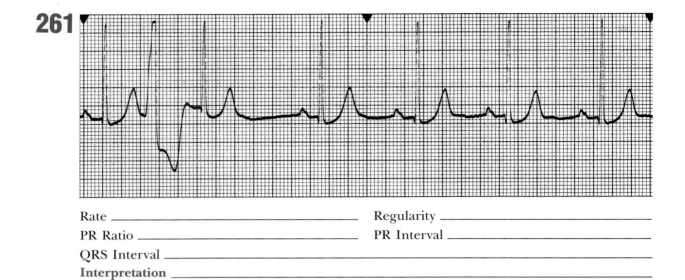

Rate _____   Regularity _____

PR Ratio _____   PR Interval _____

QRS Interval _____

Interpretation _____

262

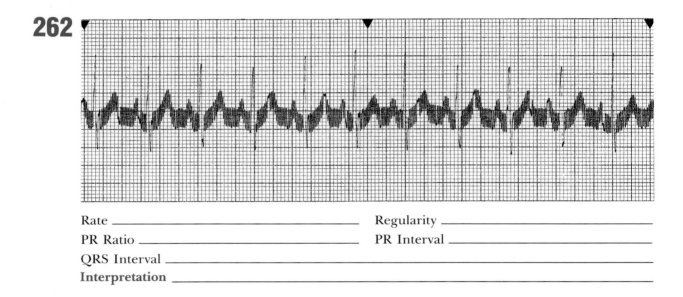

Rate _____   Regularity _____

PR Ratio _____   PR Interval _____

QRS Interval _____

Interpretation _____

263

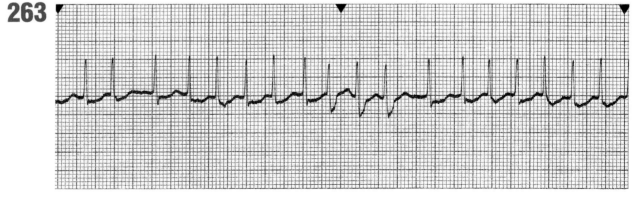

Rate _____   Regularity _____

PR Ratio _____   PR Interval _____

QRS Interval _____

Interpretation _____

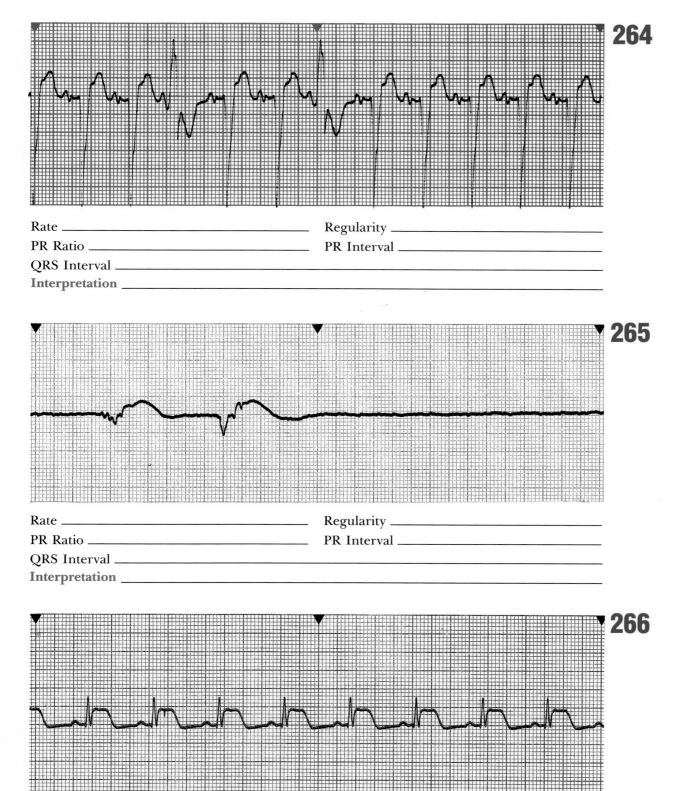

264

Rate _____ Regularity _____

PR Ratio _____ PR Interval _____

QRS Interval _____

Interpretation _____

265

Rate _____ Regularity _____

PR Ratio _____ PR Interval _____

QRS Interval _____

Interpretation _____

266

Rate _____ Regularity _____

PR Ratio _____ PR Interval _____

QRS Interval _____

Interpretation _____

267

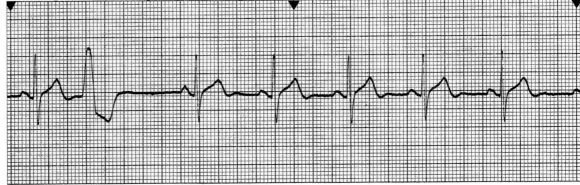

Rate _____   Regularity _____
PR Ratio _____   PR Interval _____
QRS Interval _____
Interpretation _____

268

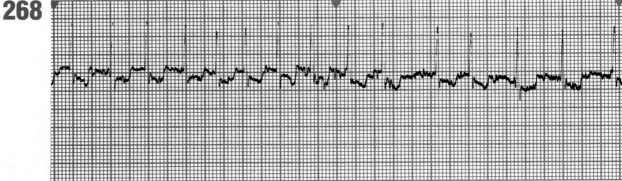

Rate _____   Regularity _____
PR Ratio _____   PR Interval _____
QRS Interval _____
Interpretation _____

269

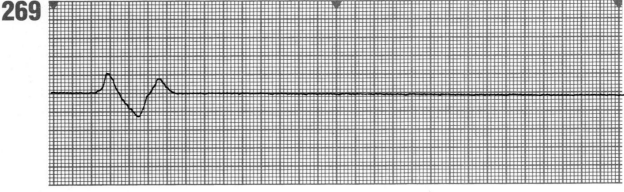

Rate _____   Regularity _____
PR Ratio _____   PR Interval _____
QRS Interval _____
Interpretation _____

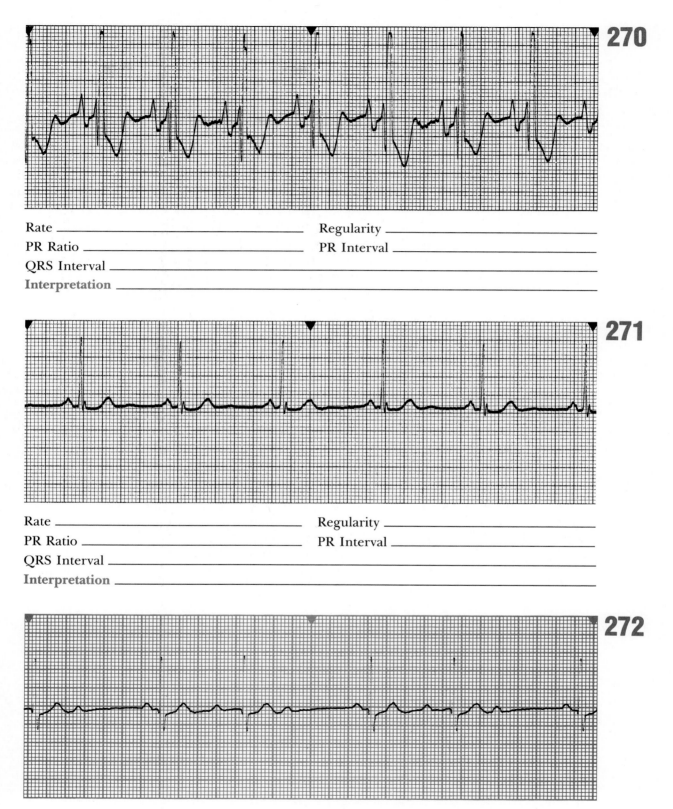

270

Rate _____ Regularity _____

PR Ratio _____ PR Interval _____

QRS Interval _____

Interpretation _____

271

Rate _____ Regularity _____

PR Ratio _____ PR Interval _____

QRS Interval _____

Interpretation _____

272

Rate _____ Regularity _____

PR Ratio _____ PR Interval _____

QRS Interval _____

Interpretation _____

273

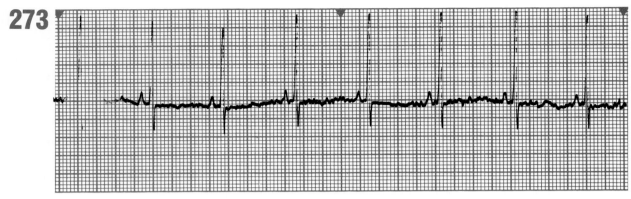

Rate _____   Regularity _____

PR Ratio _____   PR Interval _____

QRS Interval _____

Interpretation _____

274

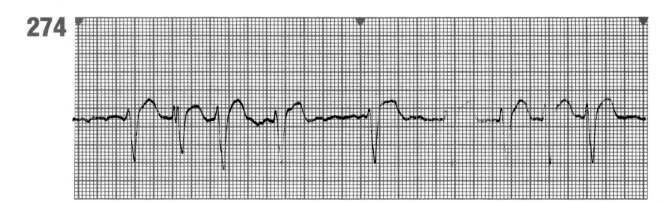

Rate _____   Regularity _____

PR Ratio _____   PR Interval _____

QRS Interval _____

Interpretation _____

275

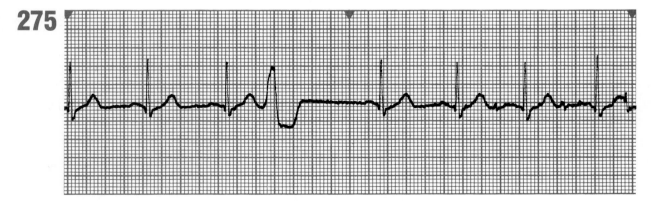

Rate _____   Regularity _____

PR Ratio _____   PR Interval _____

QRS Interval _____

Interpretation _____

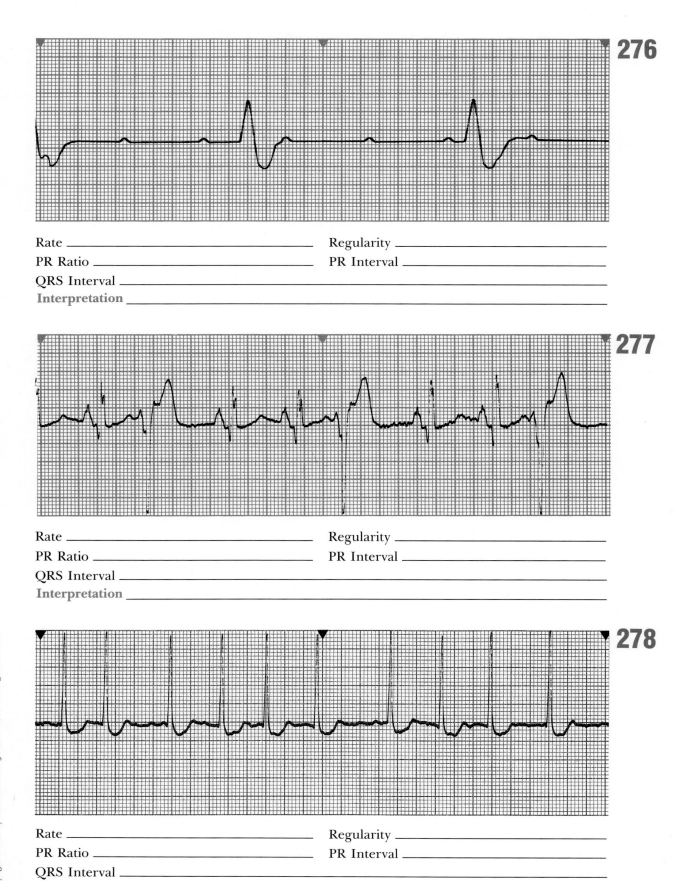

276

Rate _____ Regularity _____

PR Ratio _____ PR Interval _____

QRS Interval _____

Interpretation _____

277

Rate _____ Regularity _____

PR Ratio _____ PR Interval _____

QRS Interval _____

Interpretation _____

278

Rate _____ Regularity _____

PR Ratio _____ PR Interval _____

QRS Interval _____

Interpretation _____

279

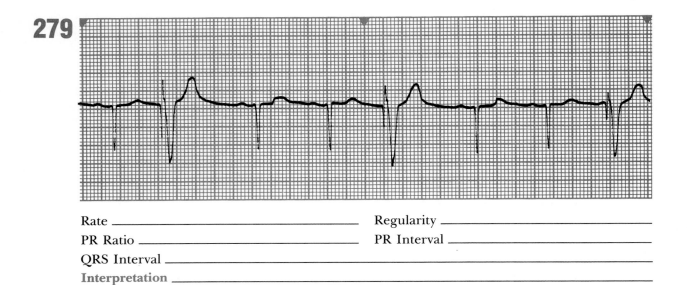

Rate _____   Regularity _____
PR Ratio _____   PR Interval _____
QRS Interval _____
Interpretation _____

280

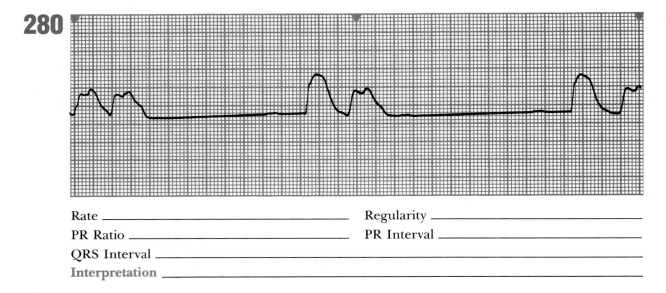

Rate _____   Regularity _____
PR Ratio _____   PR Interval _____
QRS Interval _____
Interpretation _____

281

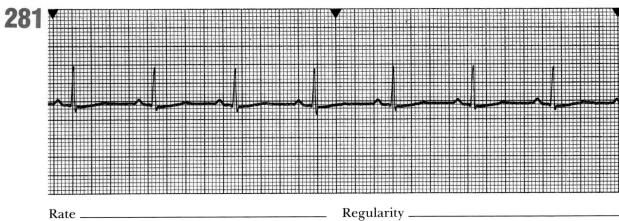

Rate _____   Regularity _____
PR Ratio _____   PR Interval _____
QRS Interval _____
Interpretation _____

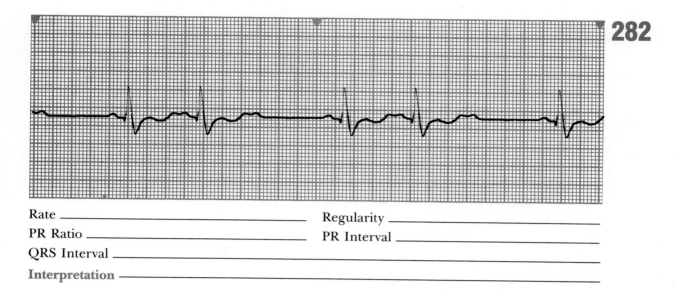

282

Rate _____ Regularity _____

PR Ratio _____ PR Interval _____

QRS Interval _____

Interpretation _____

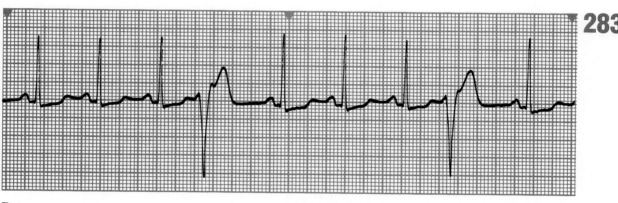

283

Rate _____ Regularity _____

PR Ratio _____ PR Interval _____

QRS Interval _____

Interpretation _____

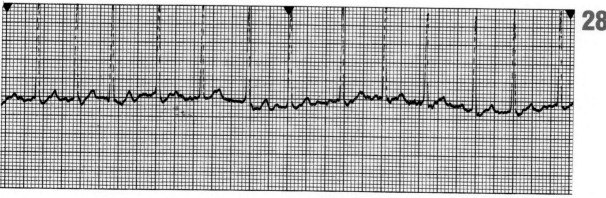

284

Rate _____ Regularity _____

PR Ratio _____ PR Interval _____

QRS Interval _____

Interpretation _____

285

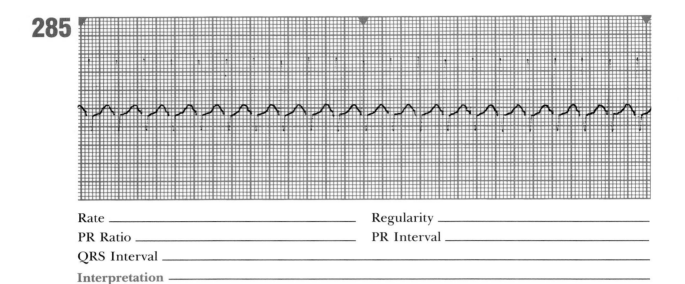

Rate _____   Regularity _____

PR Ratio _____   PR Interval _____

QRS Interval _____

Interpretation _____

286

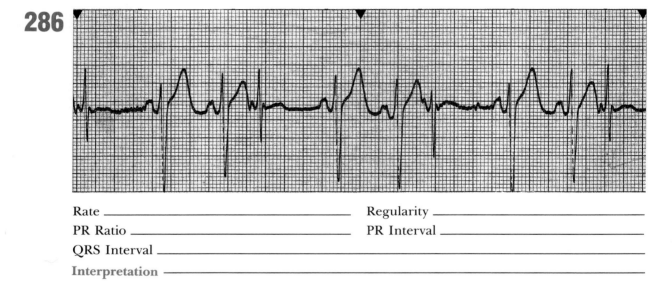

Rate _____   Regularity _____

PR Ratio _____   PR Interval _____

QRS Interval _____

Interpretation _____

287

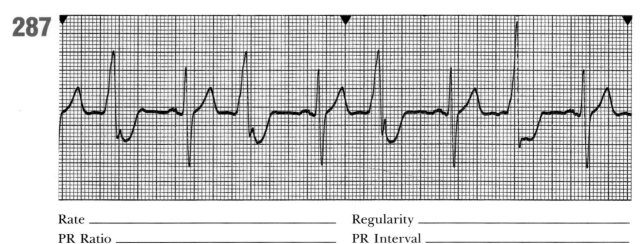

Rate _____   Regularity _____

PR Ratio _____   PR Interval _____

QRS Interval _____

Interpretation _____

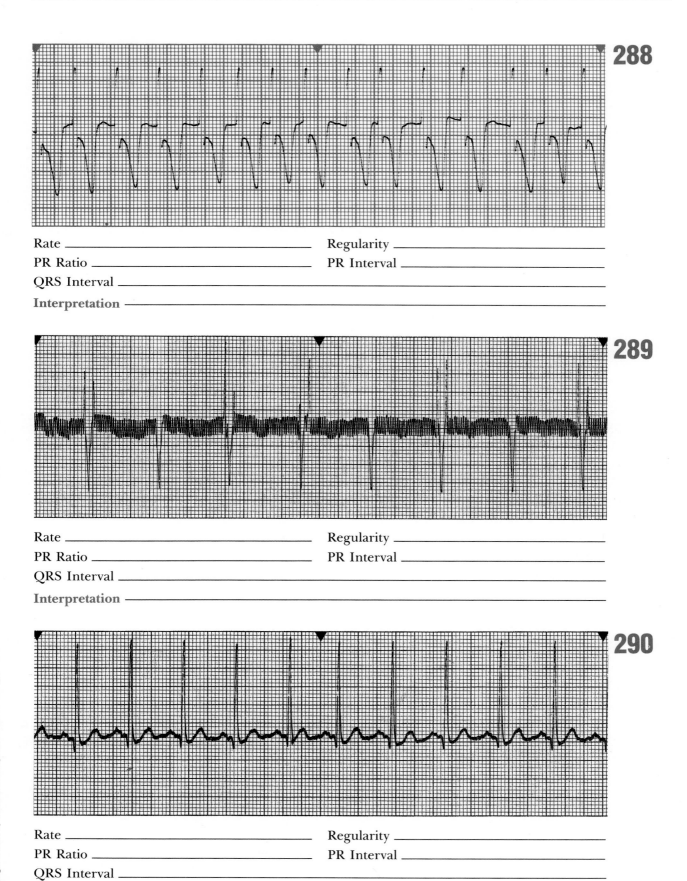

288

Rate _____   Regularity _____

PR Ratio _____   PR Interval _____

QRS Interval _____

Interpretation _____

289

Rate _____   Regularity _____

PR Ratio _____   PR Interval _____

QRS Interval _____

Interpretation _____

290

Rate _____   Regularity _____

PR Ratio _____   PR Interval _____

QRS Interval _____

Interpretation _____

291

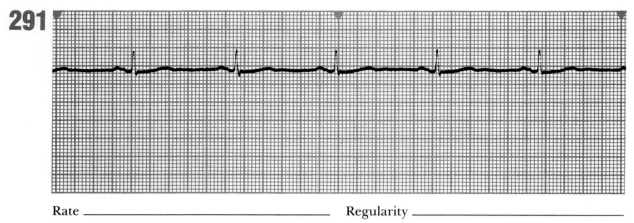

Rate _____   Regularity _____

PR Ratio _____   PR Interval _____

QRS Interval _____

Interpretation _____

292

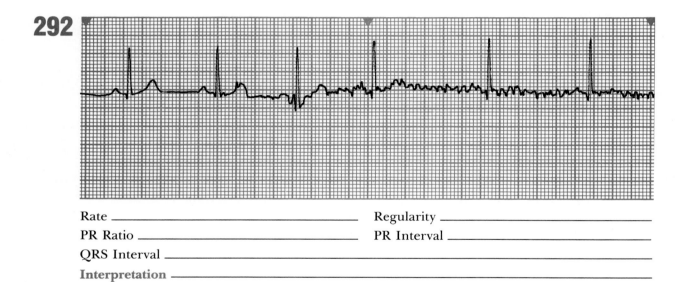

Rate _____   Regularity _____

PR Ratio _____   PR Interval _____

QRS Interval _____

Interpretation _____

293

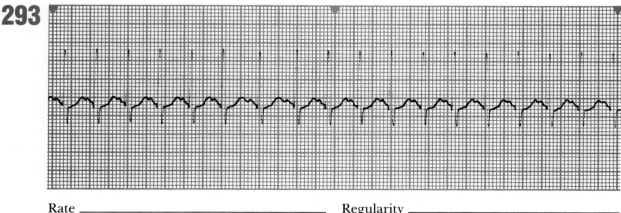

Rate _____   Regularity _____

PR Ratio _____   PR Interval _____

QRS Interval _____

Interpretation _____

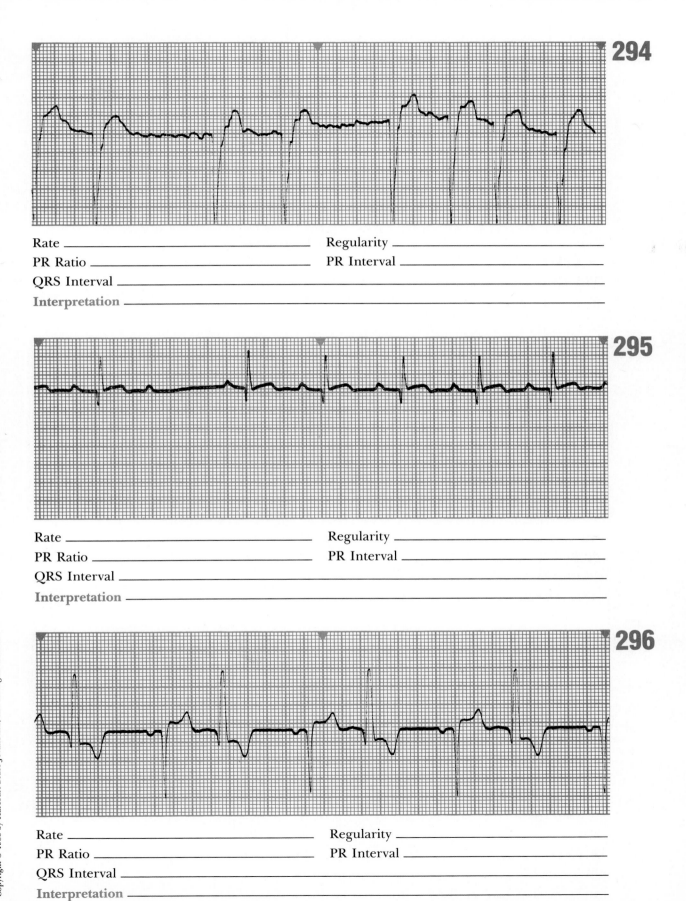

294

Rate _____ Regularity _____

PR Ratio _____ PR Interval _____

QRS Interval _____

Interpretation _____

295

Rate _____ Regularity _____

PR Ratio _____ PR Interval _____

QRS Interval _____

Interpretation _____

296

Rate _____ Regularity _____

PR Ratio _____ PR Interval _____

QRS Interval _____

Interpretation _____

297

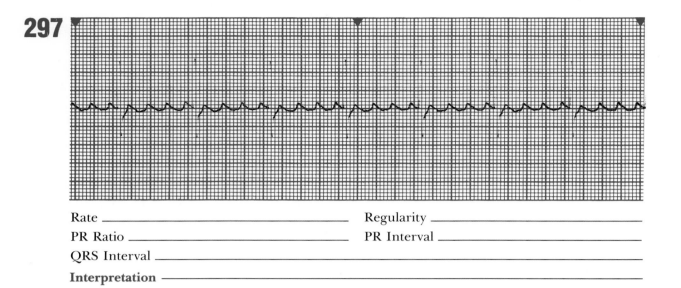

Rate _____   Regularity _____
PR Ratio _____   PR Interval _____
QRS Interval _____
Interpretation _____

298

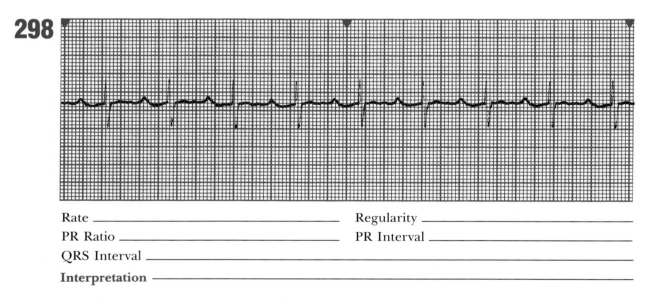

Rate _____   Regularity _____
PR Ratio _____   PR Interval _____
QRS Interval _____
Interpretation _____

299

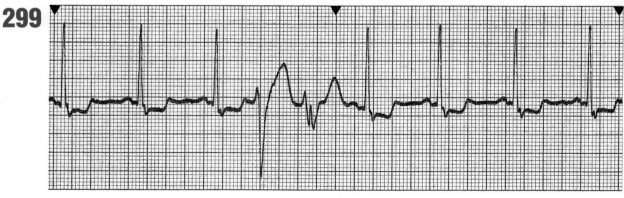

Rate _____   Regularity _____
PR Ratio _____   PR Interval _____
QRS Interval _____
Interpretation _____

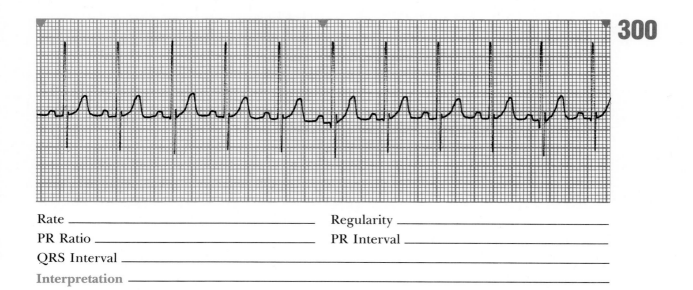

300

Rate _____   Regularity _____

PR Ratio _____   PR Interval _____

QRS Interval _____

Interpretation _____

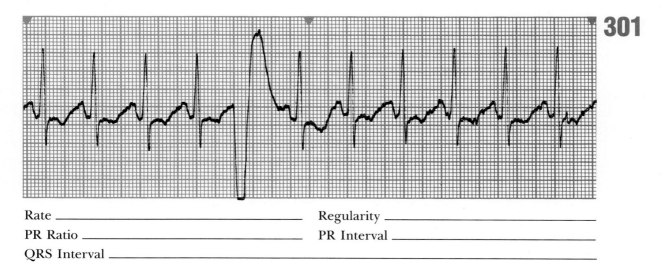

301

Rate _____   Regularity _____

PR Ratio _____   PR Interval _____

QRS Interval _____

Interpretation _____

302

Rate _____   Regularity _____

PR Ratio _____   PR Interval _____

QRS Interval _____

Interpretation _____

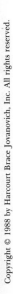

303

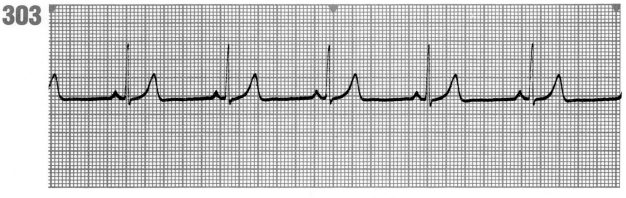

Rate _____ Regularity _____

PR Ratio _____ PR Interval _____

QRS Interval _____

Interpretation _____

304

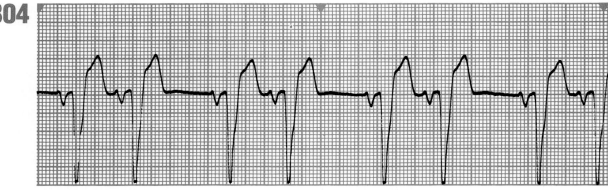

Rate _____ Regularity _____

PR Ratio _____ PR Interval _____

QRS Interval _____

Interpretation _____

305

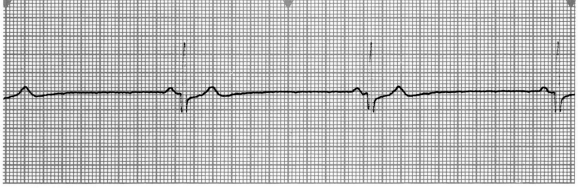

Rate _____ Regularity _____

PR Ratio _____ PR Interval _____

QRS Interval _____

Interpretation _____

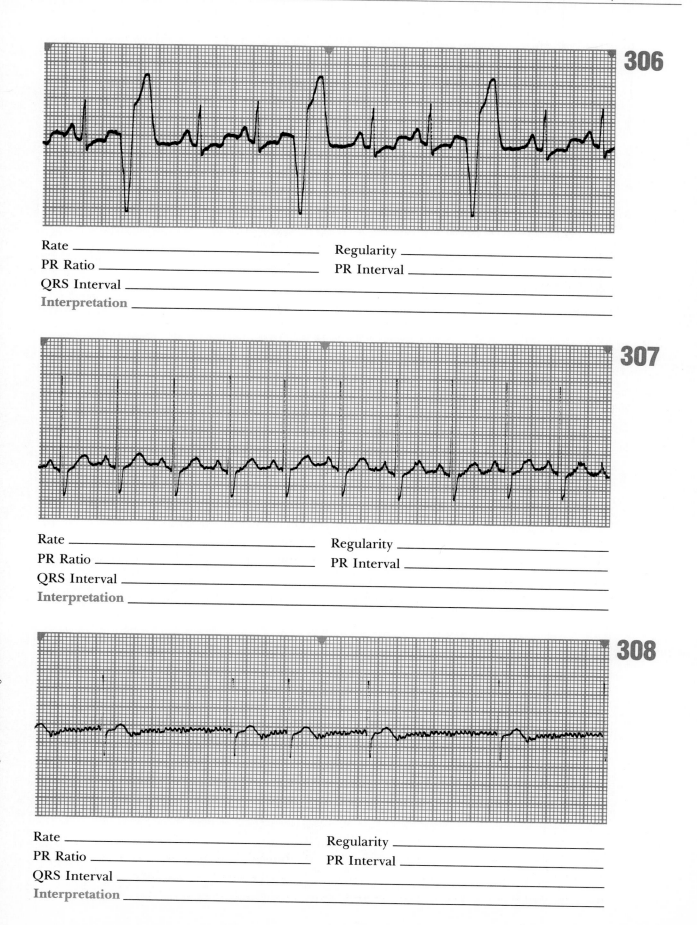

306

Rate _____   Regularity _____

PR Ratio _____   PR Interval _____

QRS Interval _____

Interpretation _____

307

Rate _____   Regularity _____

PR Ratio _____   PR Interval _____

QRS Interval _____

Interpretation _____

308

Rate _____   Regularity _____

PR Ratio _____   PR Interval _____

QRS Interval _____

Interpretation _____

309

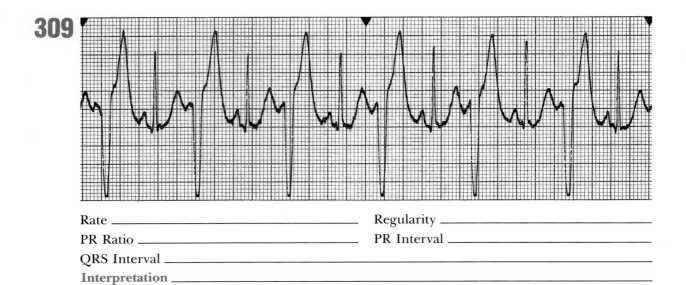

Rate _____   Regularity _____

PR Ratio _____   PR Interval _____

QRS Interval _____

Interpretation _____

310

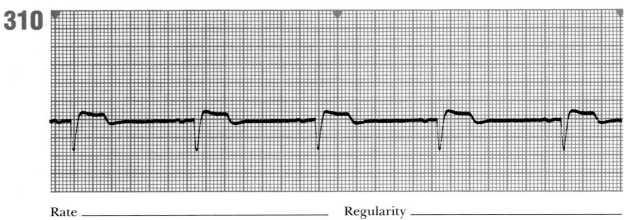

Rate _____   Regularity _____

PR Ratio _____   PR Interval _____

QRS Interval _____

Interpretation _____

311

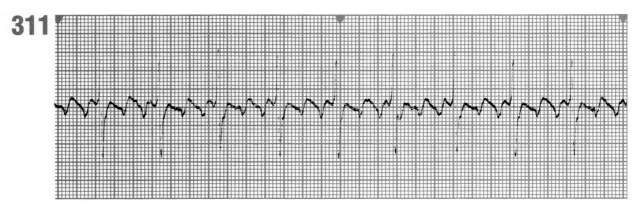

Rate _____   Regularity _____

PR Ratio _____   PR Interval _____

QRS Interval _____

Interpretation _____

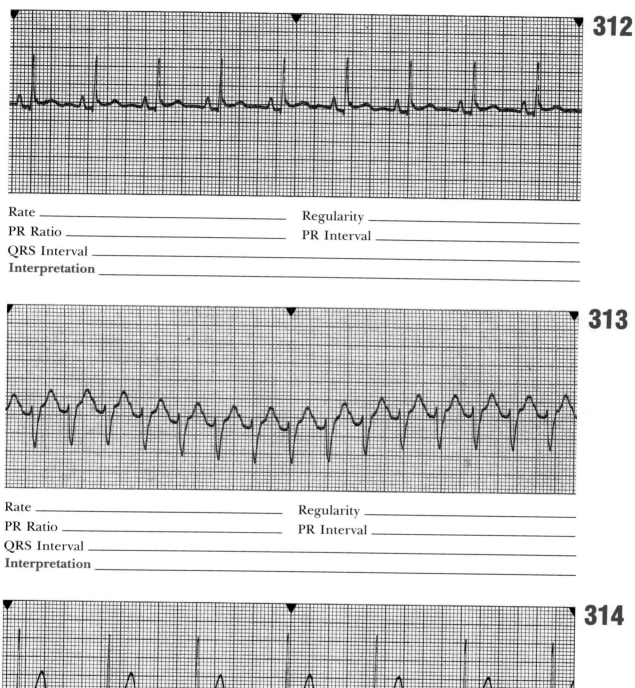

312

Rate _____   Regularity _____

PR Ratio _____   PR Interval _____

QRS Interval _____

Interpretation _____

313

Rate _____   Regularity _____

PR Ratio _____   PR Interval _____

QRS Interval _____

Interpretation _____

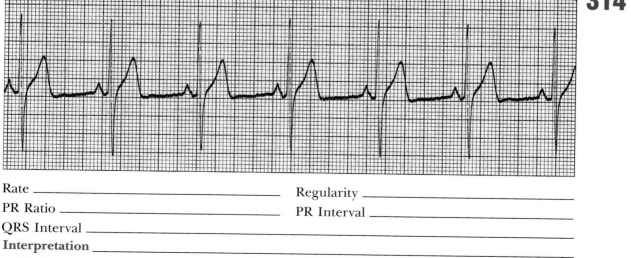

314

Rate _____   Regularity _____

PR Ratio _____   PR Interval _____

QRS Interval _____

Interpretation _____

315

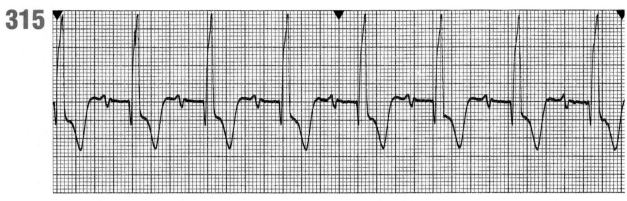

Rate _____ Regularity _____

PR Ratio _____ PR Interval _____

QRS Interval _____

Interpretation _____

316

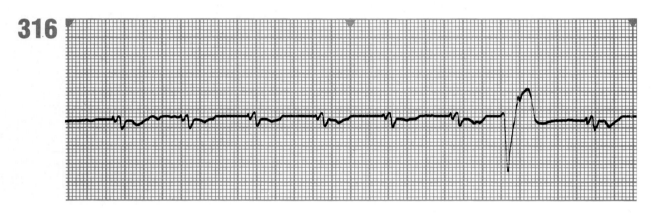

Rate _____ Regularity _____

PR Ratio _____ PR Interval _____

QRS Interval _____

Interpretation _____

317

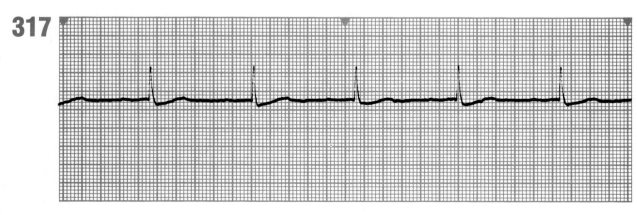

Rate _____ Regularity _____

PR Ratio _____ PR Interval _____

QRS Interval _____

Interpretation _____

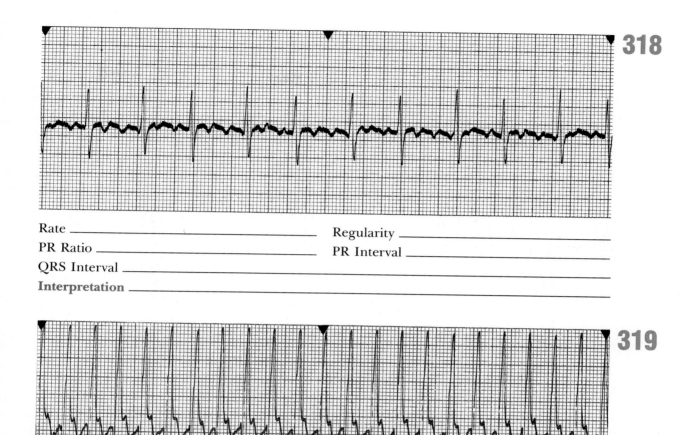

318

Rate _____   Regularity _____

PR Ratio _____   PR Interval _____

QRS Interval _____

Interpretation _____

319

Rate _____   Regularity _____

PR Ratio _____   PR Interval _____

QRS Interval _____

Interpretation _____

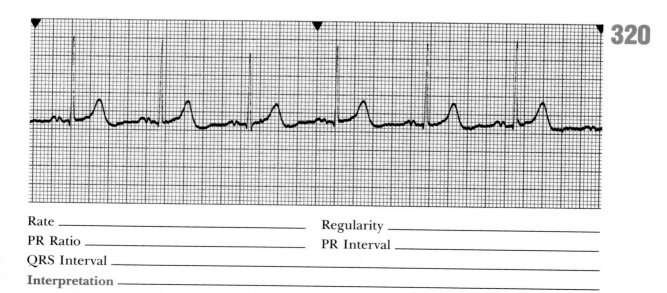

320

Rate _____   Regularity _____

PR Ratio _____   PR Interval _____

QRS Interval _____

Interpretation _____

321

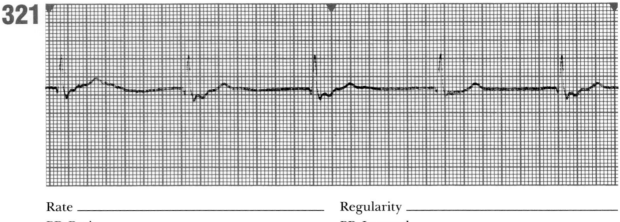

Rate _____   Regularity _____
PR Ratio _____   PR Interval _____
QRS Interval _____
Interpretation _____

322

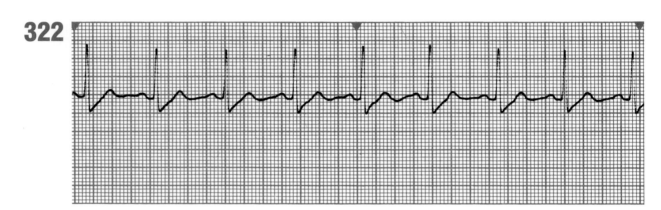

Rate _____   Regularity _____
PR Ratio _____   PR Interval _____
QRS Interval _____
Interpretation _____

323

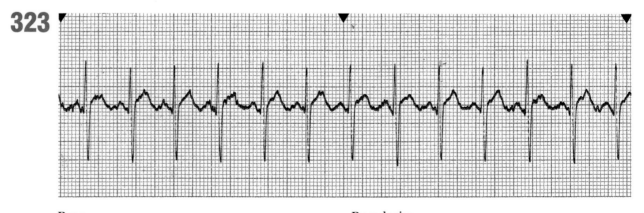

Rate _____   Regularity _____
PR Ratio _____   PR Interval _____
QRS Interval _____
Interpretation _____

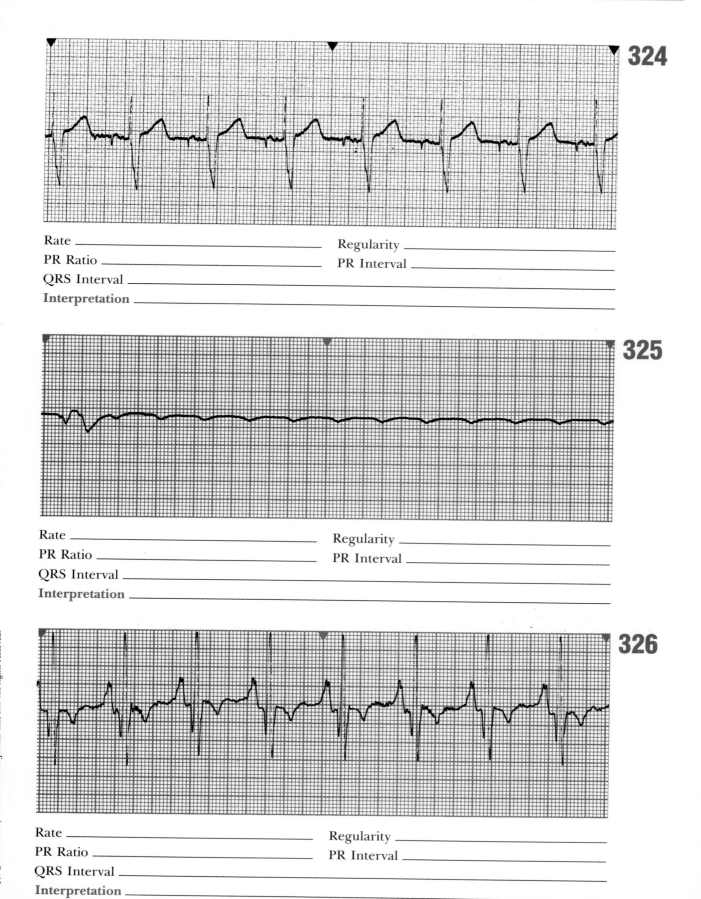

324

Rate _____   Regularity _____

PR Ratio _____   PR Interval _____

QRS Interval _____

Interpretation _____

325

Rate _____   Regularity _____

PR Ratio _____   PR Interval _____

QRS Interval _____

Interpretation _____

326

Rate _____   Regularity _____

PR Ratio _____   PR Interval _____

QRS Interval _____

Interpretation _____

327

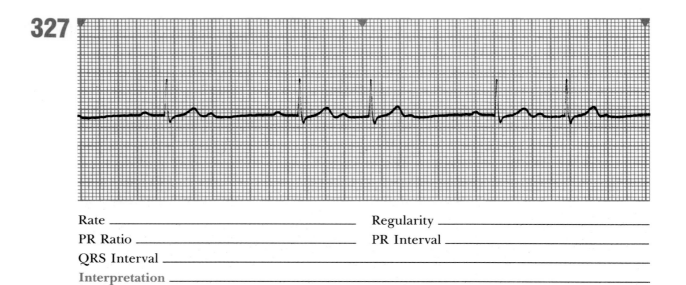

Rate _____ Regularity _____

PR Ratio _____ PR Interval _____

QRS Interval _____

Interpretation _____

328

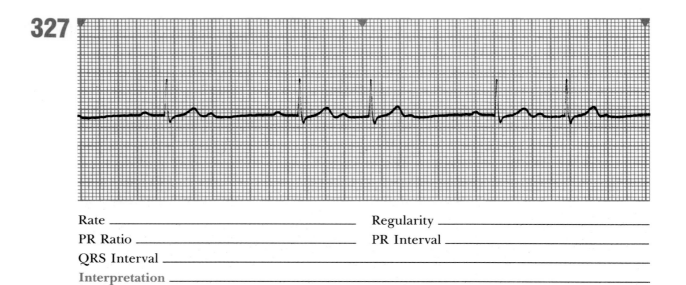

Rate _____ Regularity _____

PR Ratio _____ PR Interval _____

QRS Interval _____

Interpretation _____

329

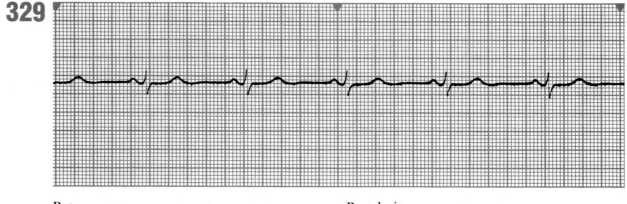

Rate _____ Regularity _____

PR Ratio _____ PR Interval _____

QRS Interval _____

Interpretation _____

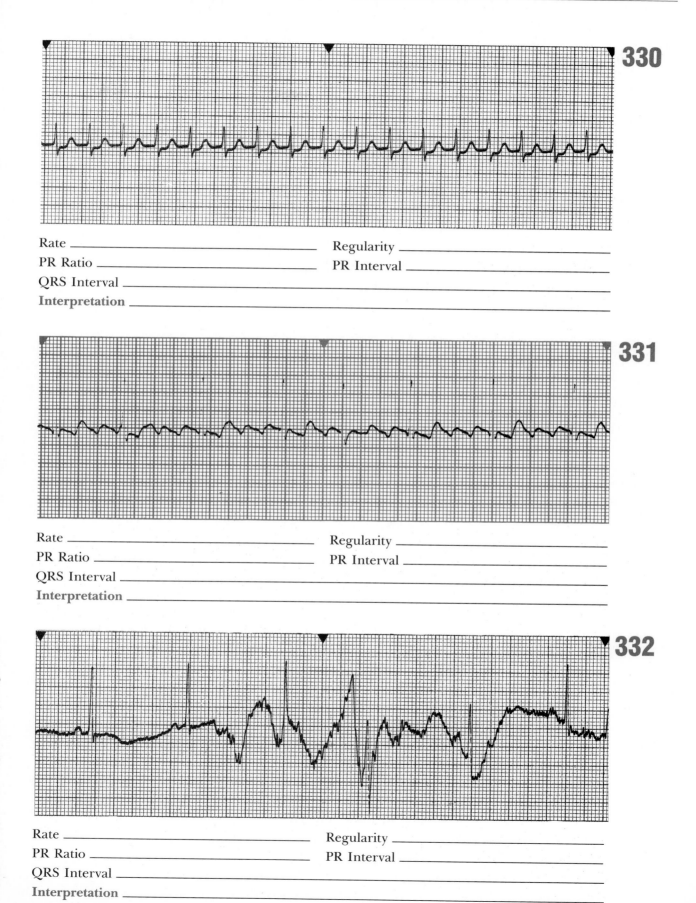

330

Rate _____ Regularity _____

PR Ratio _____ PR Interval _____

QRS Interval _____

Interpretation _____

331

Rate _____ Regularity _____

PR Ratio _____ PR Interval _____

QRS Interval _____

Interpretation _____

332

Rate _____ Regularity _____

PR Ratio _____ PR Interval _____

QRS Interval _____

Interpretation _____

333

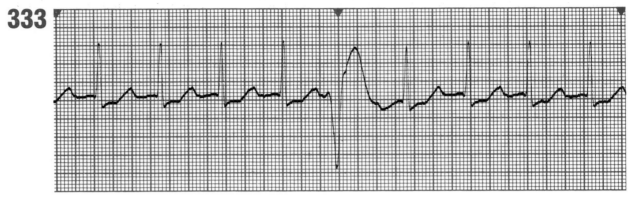

Rate _____   Regularity _____

PR Ratio _____   PR Interval _____

QRS Interval _____

Interpretation _____

334

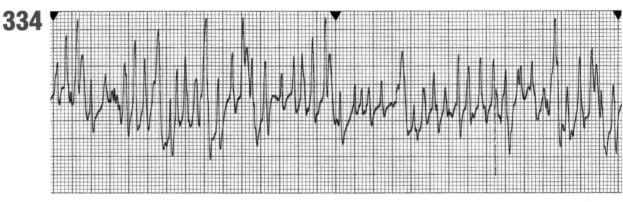

Rate _____   Regularity _____

PR Ratio _____   PR Interval _____

QRS Interval _____

Interpretation _____

335

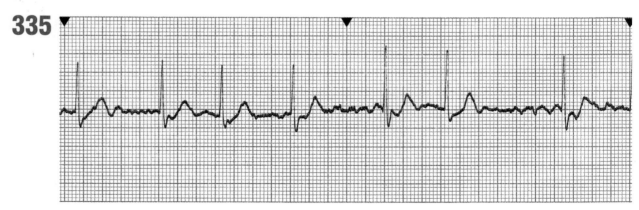

Rate _____   Regularity _____

PR Ratio _____   PR Interval _____

QRS Interval _____

Interpretation _____

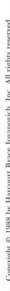

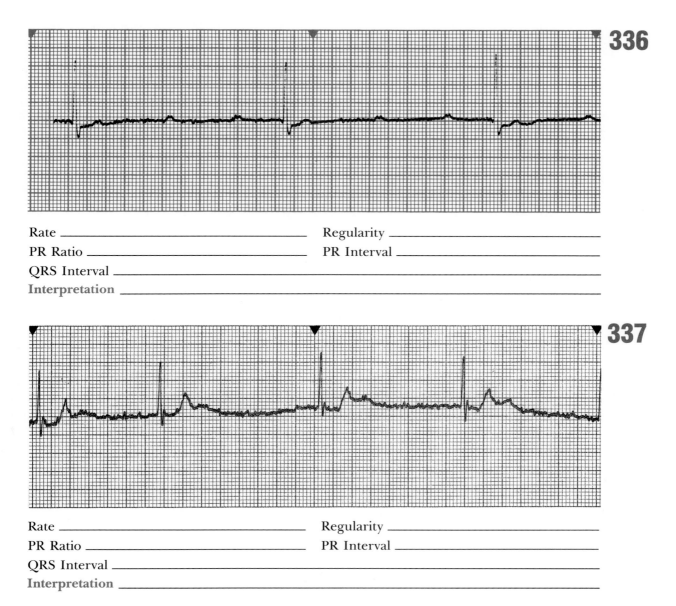

336

Rate _____ Regularity _____
PR Ratio _____ PR Interval _____
QRS Interval _____
Interpretation _____

337

Rate _____ Regularity _____
PR Ratio _____ PR Interval _____
QRS Interval _____
Interpretation _____

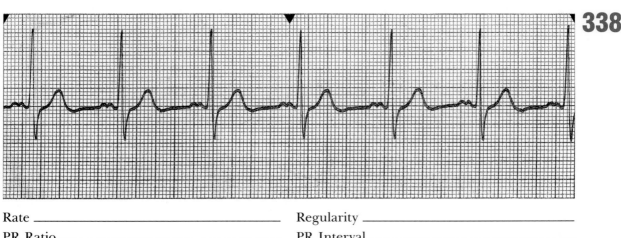

338

Rate _____ Regularity _____
PR Ratio _____ PR Interval _____
QRS Interval _____
Interpretation _____

339

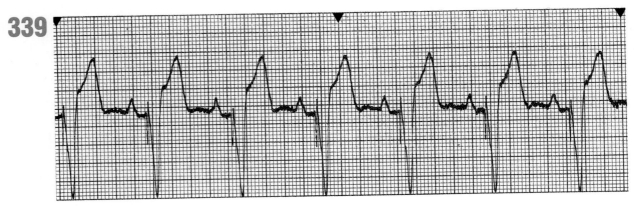

Rate _____   Regularity _____

PR Ratio _____   PR Interval _____

QRS Interval _____

Interpretation _____

340

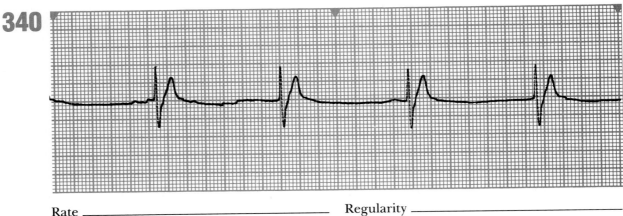

Rate _____   Regularity _____

PR Ratio _____   PR Interval _____

QRS Interval _____

Interpretation _____

341

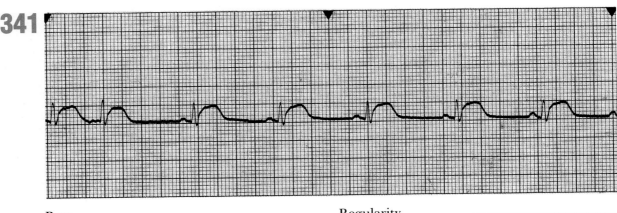

Rate _____   Regularity _____

PR Ratio _____   PR Interval _____

QRS Interval _____

Interpretation _____

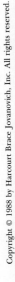

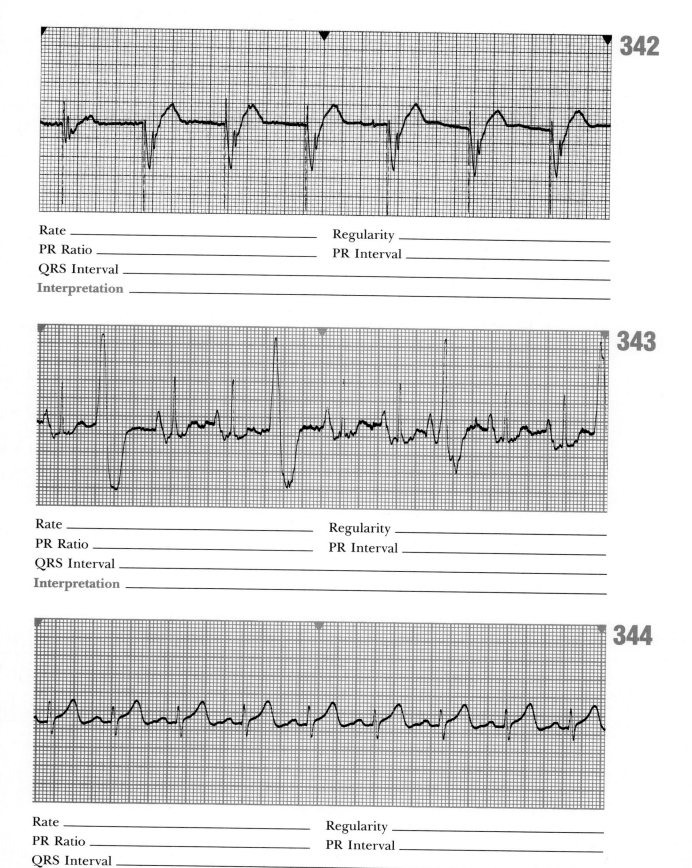

342

Rate _____   Regularity _____

PR Ratio _____   PR Interval _____

QRS Interval _____

Interpretation _____

343

Rate _____   Regularity _____

PR Ratio _____   PR Interval _____

QRS Interval _____

Interpretation _____

344

Rate _____   Regularity _____

PR Ratio _____   PR Interval _____

QRS Interval _____

Interpretation _____

345

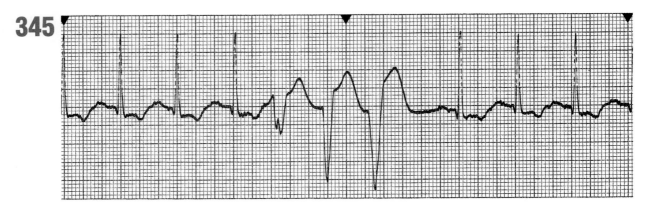

Rate _____ Regularity _____
PR Ratio _____ PR Interval _____
QRS Interval _____
Interpretation _____

346

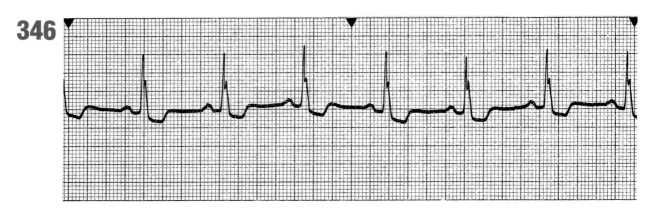

Rate _____ Regularity _____
PR Ratio _____ PR Interval _____
QRS Interval _____
Interpretation _____

347

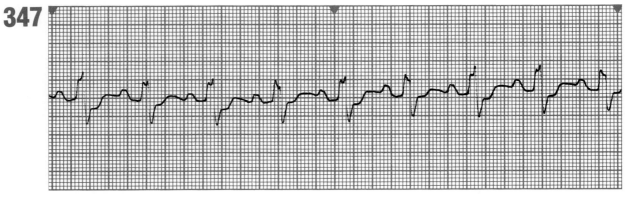

Rate _____ Regularity _____
PR Ratio _____ PR Interval _____
QRS Interval _____
Interpretation _____

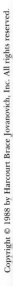

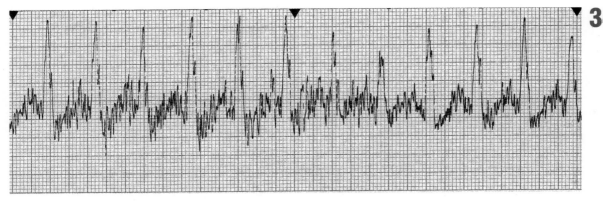

348

Rate _____ Regularity _____

PR Ratio _____ PR Interval _____

QRS Interval _____

Interpretation _____

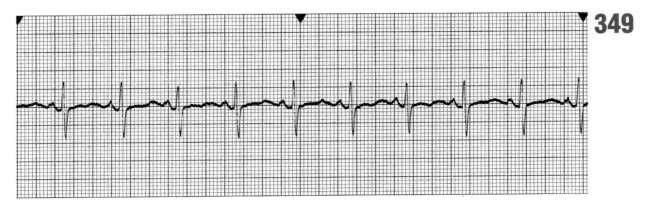

349

Rate _____ Regularity _____

PR Ratio _____ PR Interval _____

QRS Interval _____

Interpretation _____

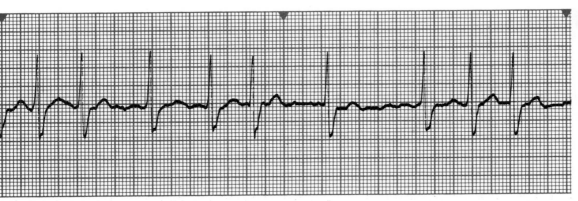

350

Rate _____ Regularity _____

PR Ratio _____ PR Interval _____

QRS Interval _____

Interpretation _____

351

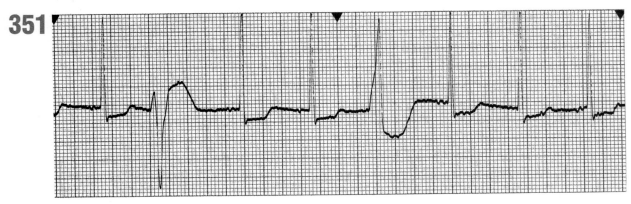

Rate _____   Regularity _____

PR Ratio _____   PR Interval _____

QRS Interval _____

Interpretation _____

352

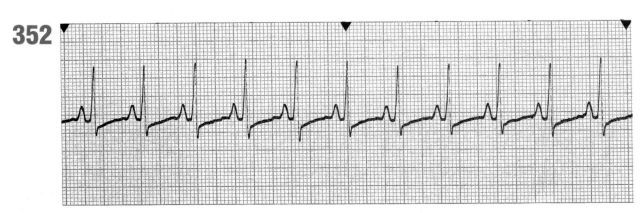

Rate _____   Regularity _____

PR Ratio _____   PR Interval _____

QRS Interval _____

Interpretation _____

353

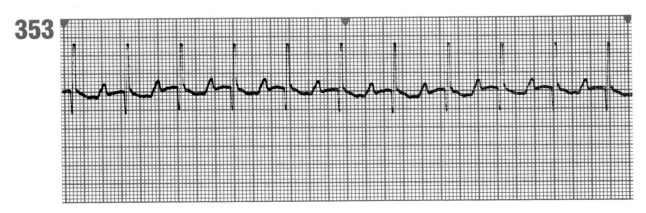

Rate _____   Regularity _____

PR Ratio _____   PR Interval _____

QRS Interval _____

Interpretation _____

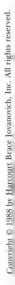

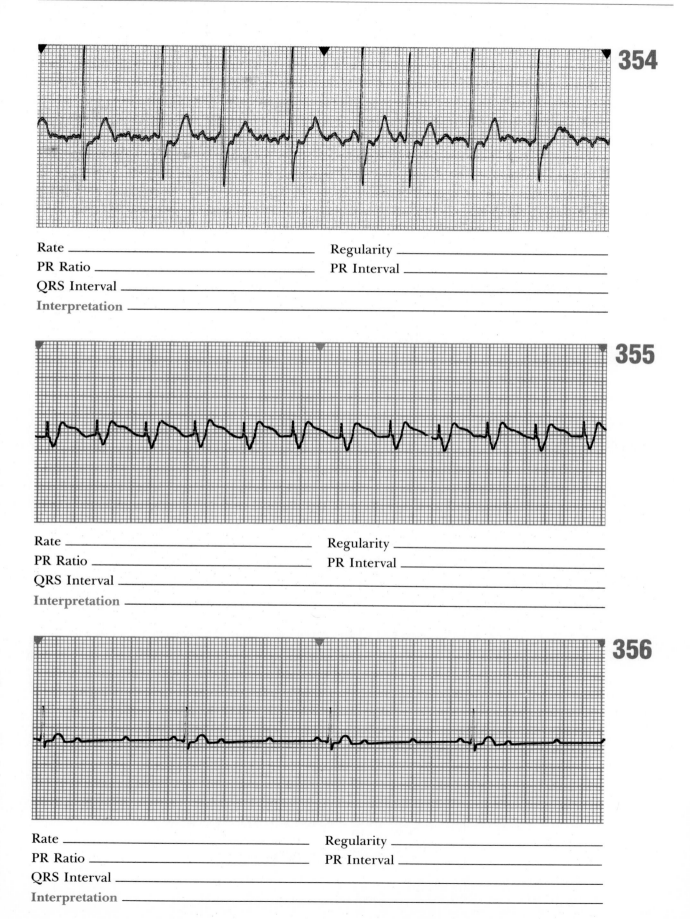

354

Rate _____   Regularity _____

PR Ratio _____   PR Interval _____

QRS Interval _____

Interpretation _____

355

Rate _____   Regularity _____

PR Ratio _____   PR Interval _____

QRS Interval _____

Interpretation _____

356

Rate _____   Regularity _____

PR Ratio _____   PR Interval _____

QRS Interval _____

Interpretation _____

357

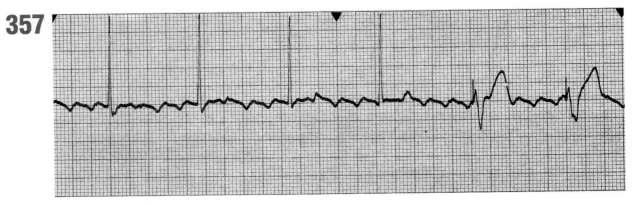

Rate _____ Regularity _____

PR Ratio _____ PR Interval _____

QRS Interval _____

Interpretation _____

358

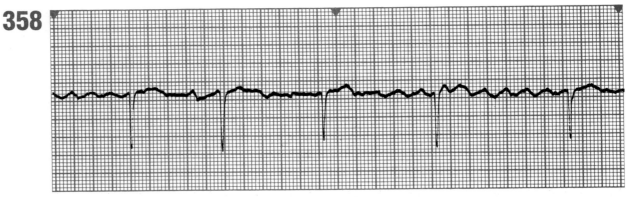

Rate _____ Regularity _____

PR Ratio _____ PR Interval _____

QRS Interval _____

Interpretation _____

359

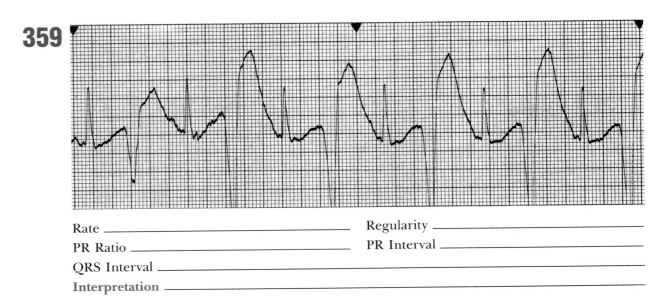

Rate _____ Regularity _____

PR Ratio _____ PR Interval _____

QRS Interval _____

Interpretation _____

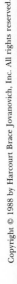

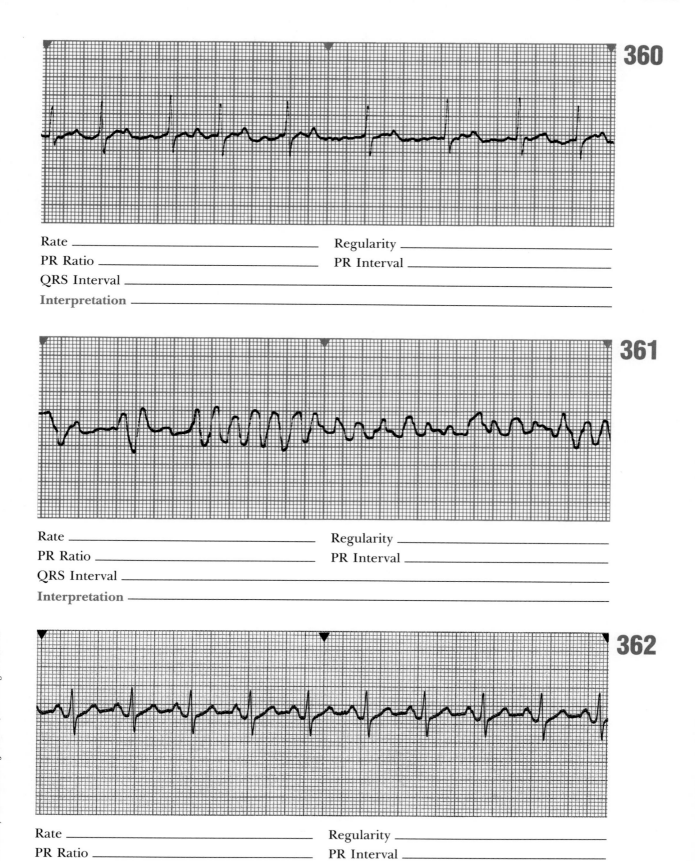

360

Rate _____   Regularity _____

PR Ratio _____   PR Interval _____

QRS Interval _____

Interpretation _____

361

Rate _____   Regularity _____

PR Ratio _____   PR Interval _____

QRS Interval _____

Interpretation _____

362

Rate _____   Regularity _____

PR Ratio _____   PR Interval _____

QRS Interval _____

Interpretation _____

363

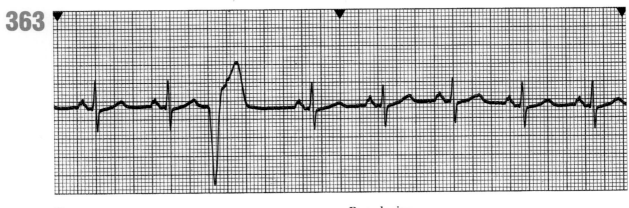

Rate _____ Regularity _____

PR Ratio _____ PR Interval _____

QRS Interval _____

Interpretation _____

364

Rate _____ Regularity _____

PR Ratio _____ PR Interval _____

QRS Interval _____

Interpretation _____

365

Rate _____ Regularity _____

PR Ratio _____ PR Interval _____

QRS Interval _____

Interpretation _____

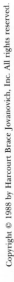

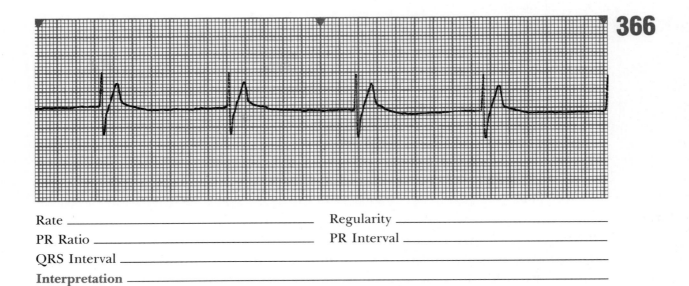

366

Rate _____ Regularity _____

PR Ratio _____ PR Interval _____

QRS Interval _____

Interpretation _____

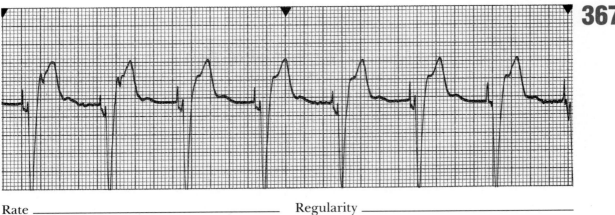

367

Rate _____ Regularity _____

PR Ratio _____ PR Interval _____

QRS Interval _____

Interpretation _____

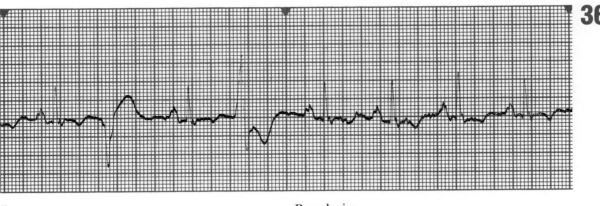

368

Rate _____ Regularity _____

PR Ratio _____ PR Interval _____

QRS Interval _____

Interpretation _____

369

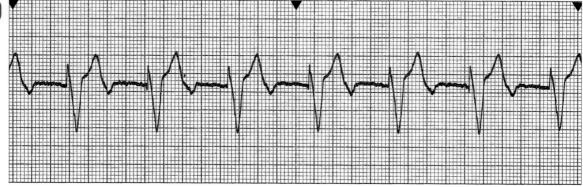

Rate _____ Regularity _____

PR Ratio _____ PR Interval _____

QRS Interval _____

Interpretation _____

370

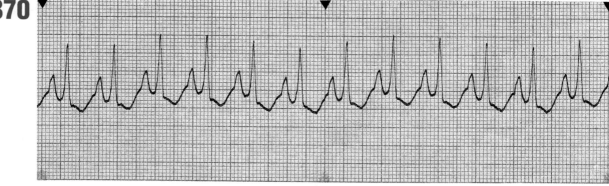

Rate _____ Regularity _____

PR Ratio _____ PR Interval _____

QRS Interval _____

Interpretation _____

371

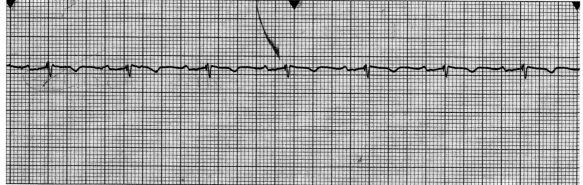

Rate _____ Regularity _____

PR Ratio _____ PR Interval _____

QRS Interval _____

Interpretation _____

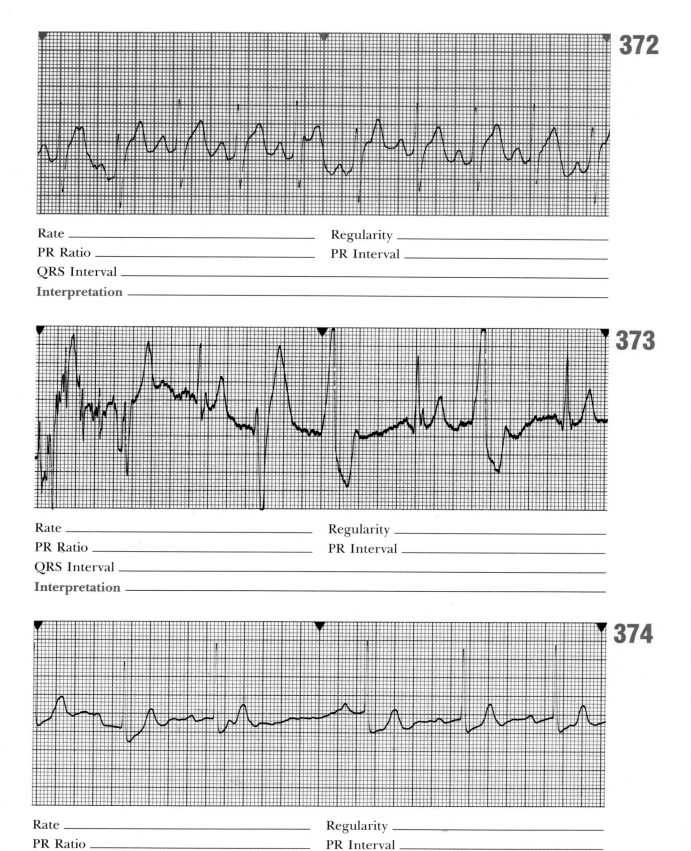

372

Rate _____   Regularity _____

PR Ratio _____   PR Interval _____

QRS Interval _____

Interpretation _____

373

Rate _____   Regularity _____

PR Ratio _____   PR Interval _____

QRS Interval _____

Interpretation _____

374

Rate _____   Regularity _____

PR Ratio _____   PR Interval _____

QRS Interval _____

Interpretation _____

375

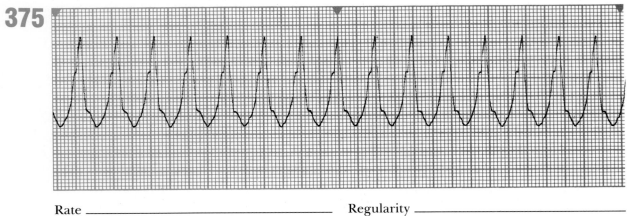

Rate _____   Regularity _____

PR Ratio _____   PR Interval _____

QRS Interval _____

Interpretation _____

376

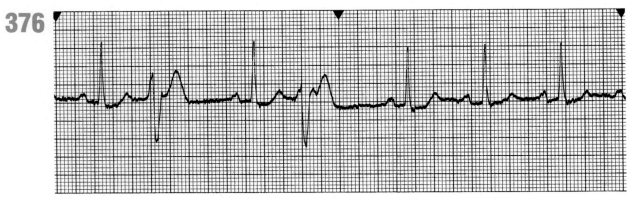

Rate _____   Regularity _____

PR Ratio _____   PR Interval _____

QRS Interval _____

Interpretation _____

377

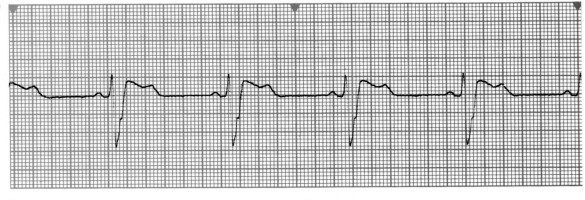

Rate _____   Regularity _____

PR Ratio _____   PR Interval _____

QRS Interval _____

Interpretation _____

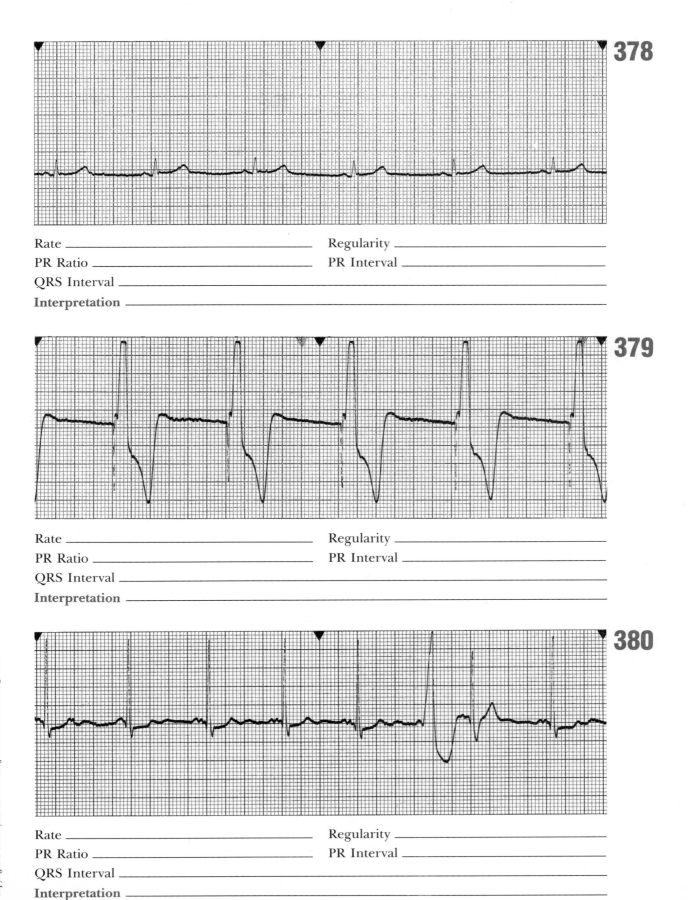

378

Rate ——————————————— Regularity ———————————————

PR Ratio ——————————————— PR Interval ———————————————

QRS Interval ———————————————

Interpretation ———————————————

379

Rate ——————————————— Regularity ———————————————

PR Ratio ——————————————— PR Interval ———————————————

QRS Interval ———————————————

Interpretation ———————————————

380

Rate ——————————————— Regularity ———————————————

PR Ratio ——————————————— PR Interval ———————————————

QRS Interval ———————————————

Interpretation ———————————————

381

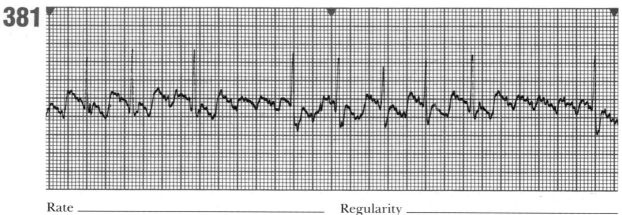

Rate _____   Regularity _____

PR Ratio _____   PR Interval _____

QRS Interval _____

Interpretation _____

382

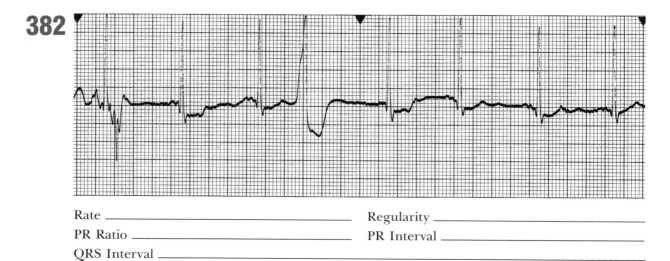

Rate _____   Regularity _____

PR Ratio _____   PR Interval _____

QRS Interval _____

Interpretation _____

383

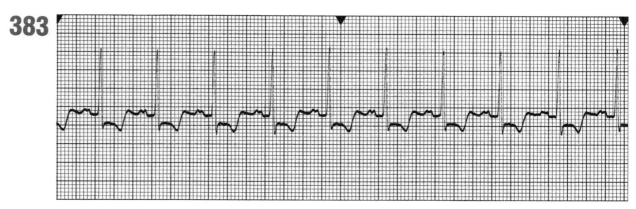

Rate _____   Regularity _____

PR Ratio _____   PR Interval _____

QRS Interval _____

Interpretation _____

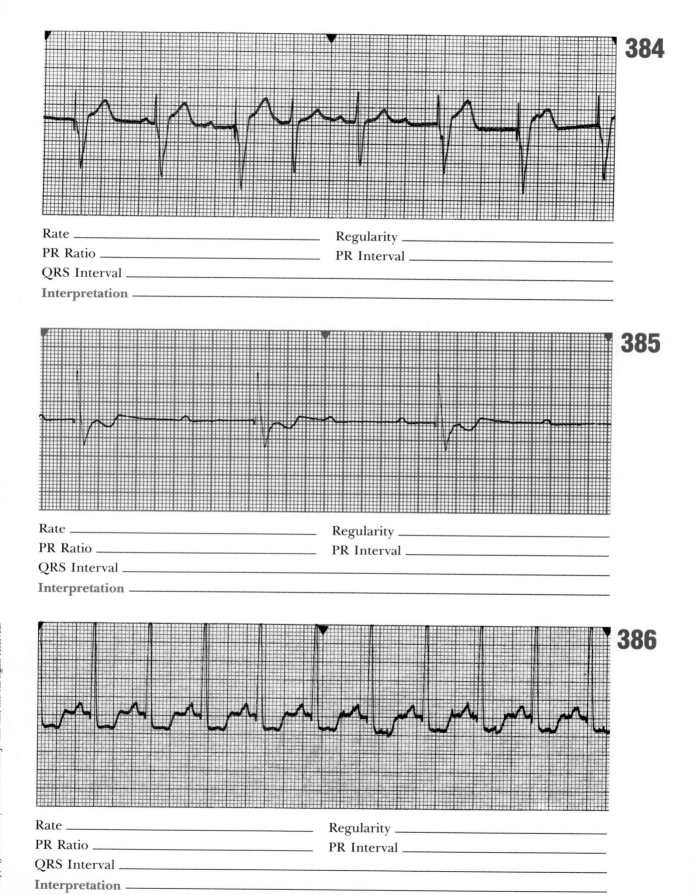

384

Rate _____ Regularity _____
PR Ratio _____ PR Interval _____
QRS Interval _____
Interpretation _____

385

Rate _____ Regularity _____
PR Ratio _____ PR Interval _____
QRS Interval _____
Interpretation _____

386

Rate _____ Regularity _____
PR Ratio _____ PR Interval _____
QRS Interval _____
Interpretation _____

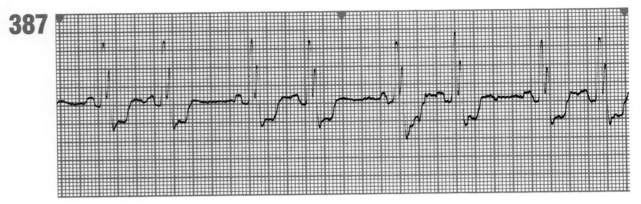

387

Rate _____   Regularity _____
PR Ratio _____   PR Interval _____
QRS Interval _____
Interpretation _____

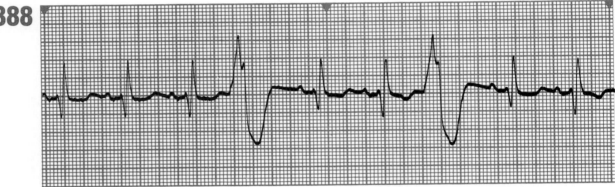

388

Rate _____   Regularity _____
PR Ratio _____   PR Interval _____
QRS Interval _____
Interpretation _____

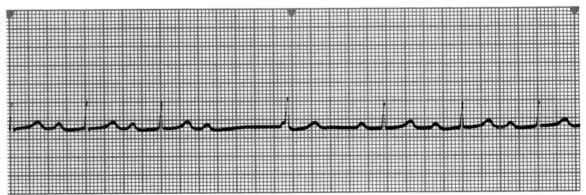

389

Rate _____   Regularity _____
PR Ratio _____   PR Interval _____
QRS Interval _____
Interpretation _____

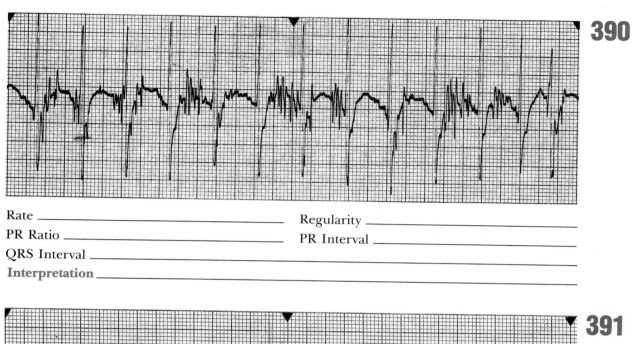

390

Rate _____   Regularity _____

PR Ratio _____   PR Interval _____

QRS Interval _____

Interpretation _____

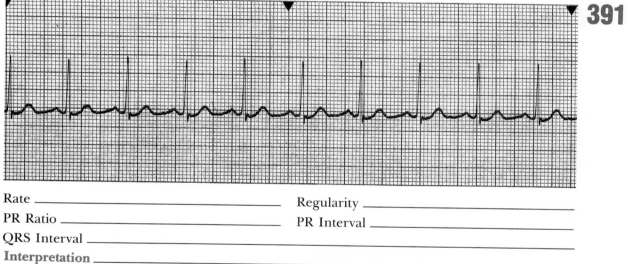

391

Rate _____   Regularity _____

PR Ratio _____   PR Interval _____

QRS Interval _____

Interpretation _____

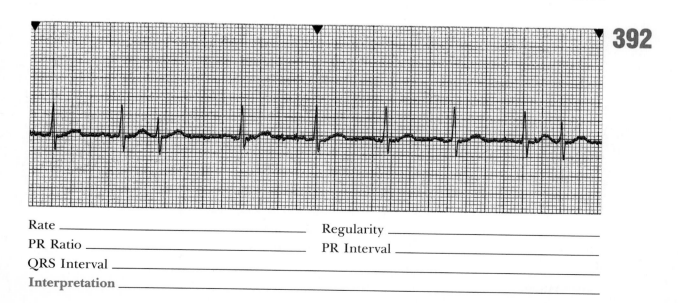

392

Rate _____   Regularity _____

PR Ratio _____   PR Interval _____

QRS Interval _____

Interpretation _____

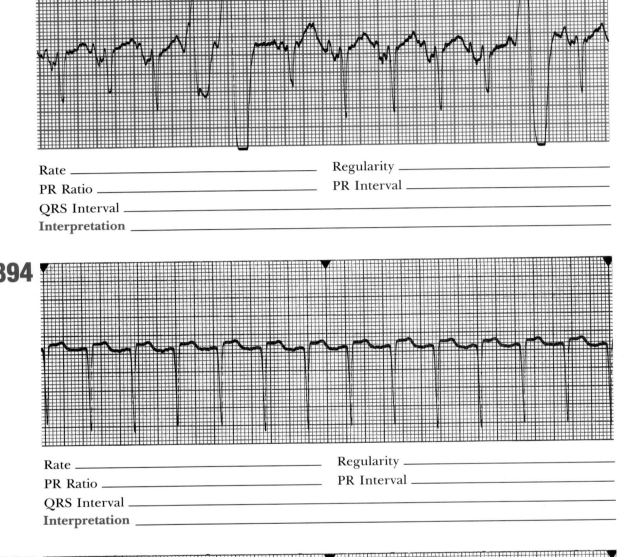

393

Rate _____   Regularity _____

PR Ratio _____   PR Interval _____

QRS Interval _____

Interpretation _____

394

Rate _____   Regularity _____

PR Ratio _____   PR Interval _____

QRS Interval _____

Interpretation _____

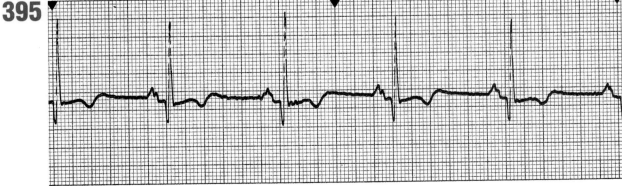

395

Rate _____   Regularity _____

PR Ratio _____   PR Interval _____

QRS Interval _____

Interpretation _____

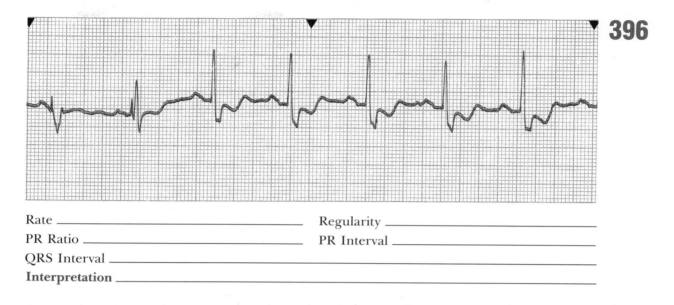

396

Rate _____   Regularity _____

PR Ratio _____   PR Interval _____

QRS Interval _____

Interpretation _____

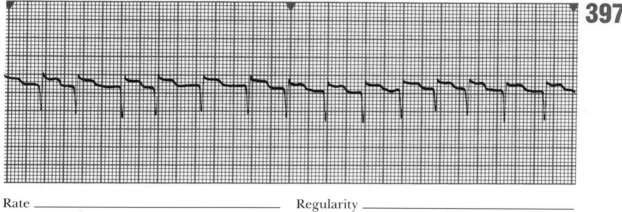

397

Rate _____   Regularity _____

PR Ratio _____   PR Interval _____

QRS Interval _____

Interpretation _____

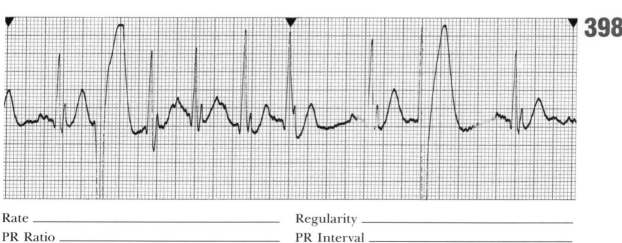

398

Rate _____   Regularity _____

PR Ratio _____   PR Interval _____

QRS Interval _____

Interpretation _____

399

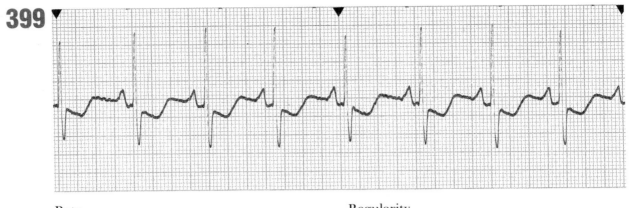

Rate _____ Regularity _____

PR Ratio _____ PR Interval _____

QRS Interval _____

Interpretation _____

400

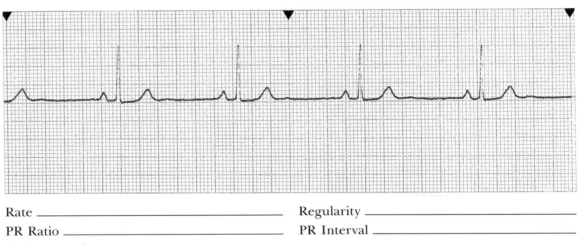

Rate _____ Regularity _____

PR Ratio _____ PR Interval _____

QRS Interval _____

Interpretation _____

401

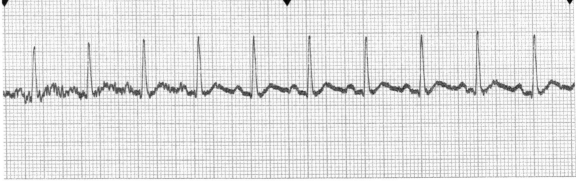

Rate _____ Regularity _____

PR Ratio _____ PR Interval _____

QRS Interval _____

Interpretation _____

402

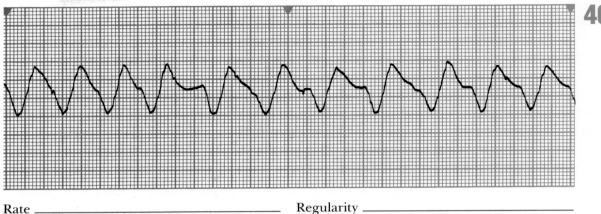

Rate _____   Regularity _____

PR Ratio _____   PR Interval _____

QRS Interval _____

Interpretation _____

403

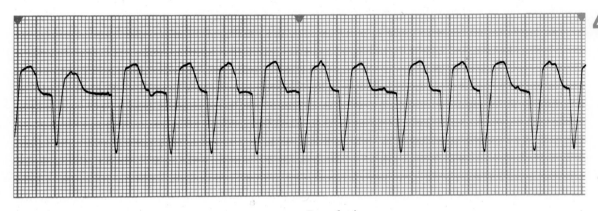

Rate _____   Regularity _____

PR Ratio _____   PR Interval _____

QRS Interval _____

Interpretation _____

404

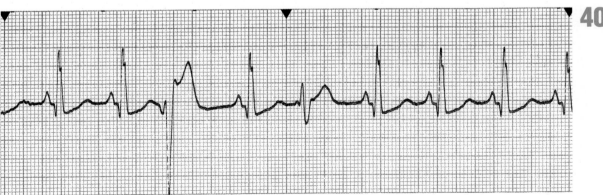

Rate _____   Regularity _____

PR Ratio _____   PR Interval _____

QRS Interval _____

Interpretation _____

405

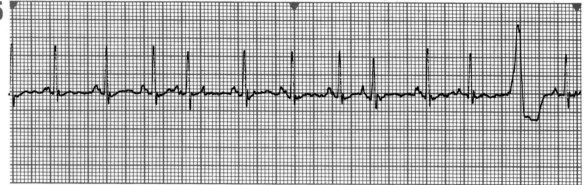

Rate _____ Regularity _____

PR Ratio _____ PR Interval _____

QRS Interval _____

Interpretation _____

406

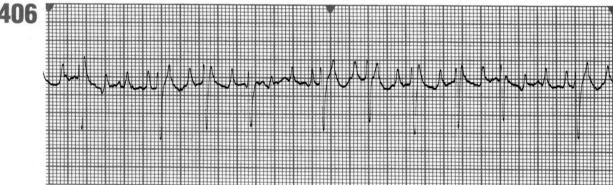

Rate _____ Regularity _____

PR Ratio _____ PR Interval _____

QRS Interval _____

Interpretation _____

407

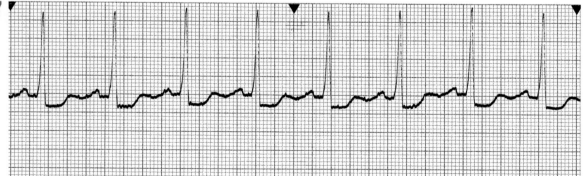

Rate _____ Regularity _____

PR Ratio _____ PR Interval _____

QRS Interval _____

Interpretation _____

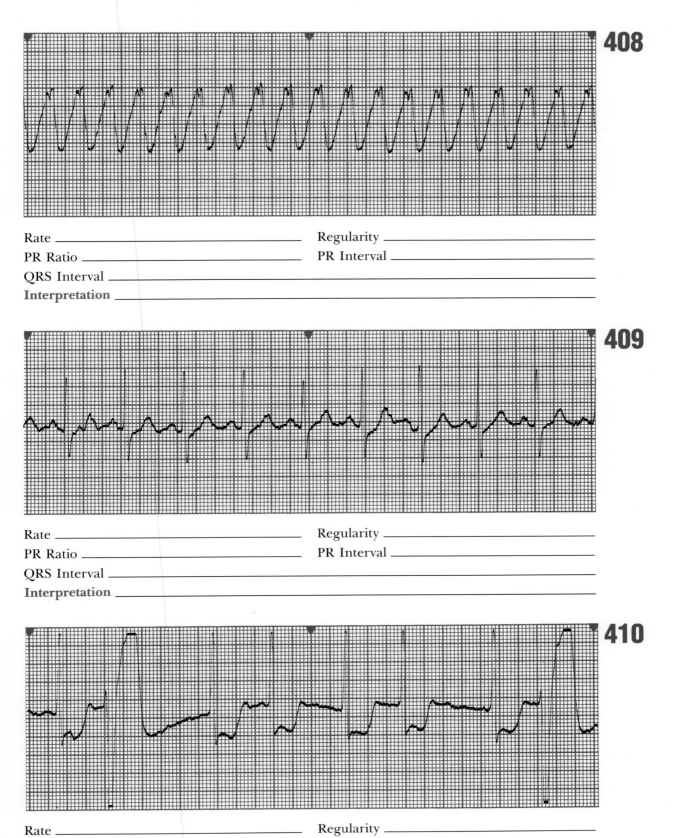

408

Rate _____   Regularity _____
PR Ratio _____   PR Interval _____
QRS Interval _____
Interpretation _____

409

Rate _____   Regularity _____
PR Ratio _____   PR Interval _____
QRS Interval _____
Interpretation _____

410

Rate _____   Regularity _____
PR Ratio _____   PR Interval _____
QRS Interval _____
Interpretation _____

411
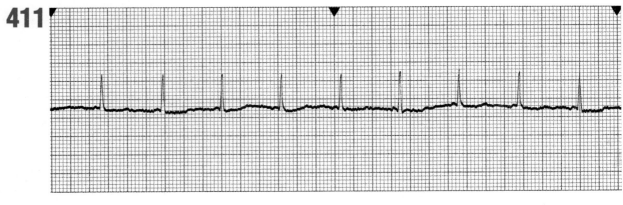

Rate _____   Regularity _____

PR Ratio _____   PR Interval _____

QRS Interval _____

Interpretation _____

412
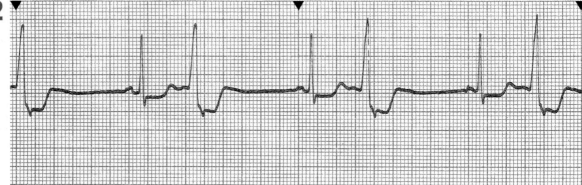

Rate _____   Regularity _____

PR Ratio _____   PR Interval _____

QRS Interval _____

Interpretation _____

413
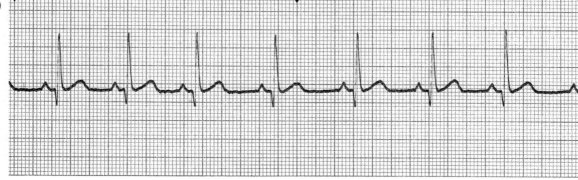

Rate _____   Regularity _____

PR Ratio _____   PR Interval _____

QRS Interval _____

Interpretation _____

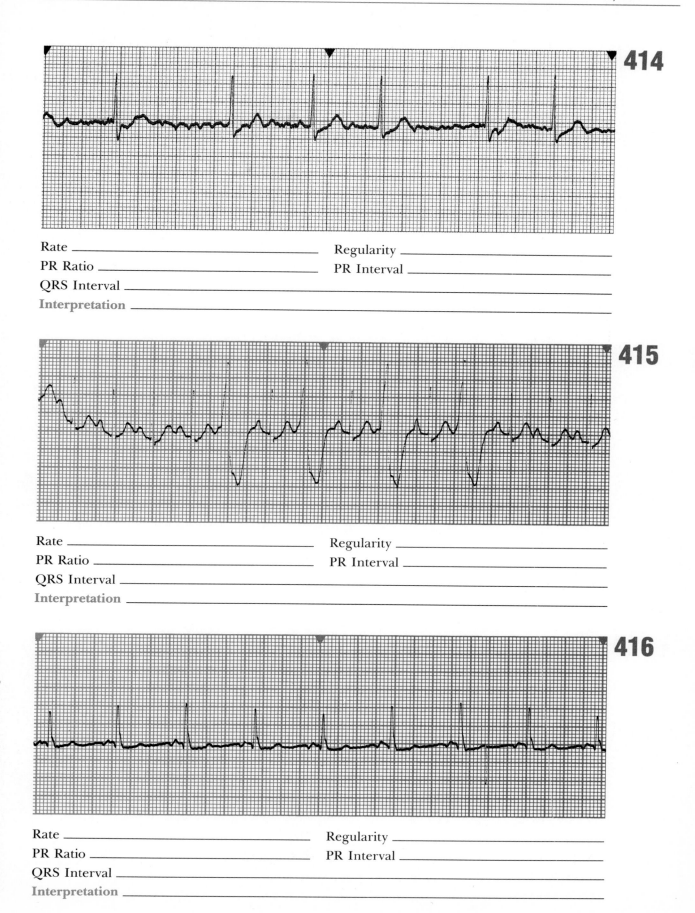

414

Rate _____ Regularity _____

PR Ratio _____ PR Interval _____

QRS Interval _____

Interpretation _____

415

Rate _____ Regularity _____

PR Ratio _____ PR Interval _____

QRS Interval _____

Interpretation _____

416

Rate _____ Regularity _____

PR Ratio _____ PR Interval _____

QRS Interval _____

Interpretation _____

417

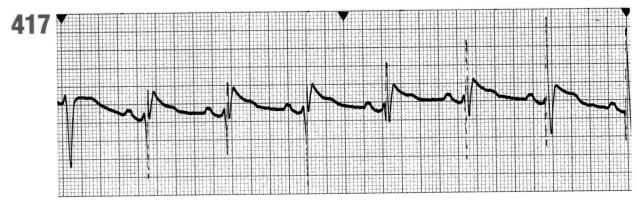

Rate _____ Regularity _____

PR Ratio _____ PR Interval _____

QRS Interval _____

Interpretation _____

418

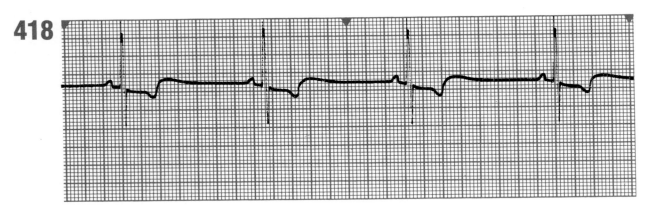

Rate _____ Regularity _____

PR Ratio _____ PR Interval _____

QRS Interval _____

Interpretation _____

419

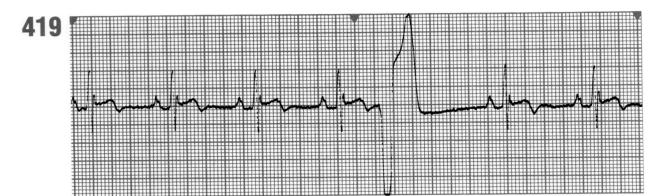

Rate _____ Regularity _____

PR Ratio _____ PR Interval _____

QRS Interval _____

Interpretation _____

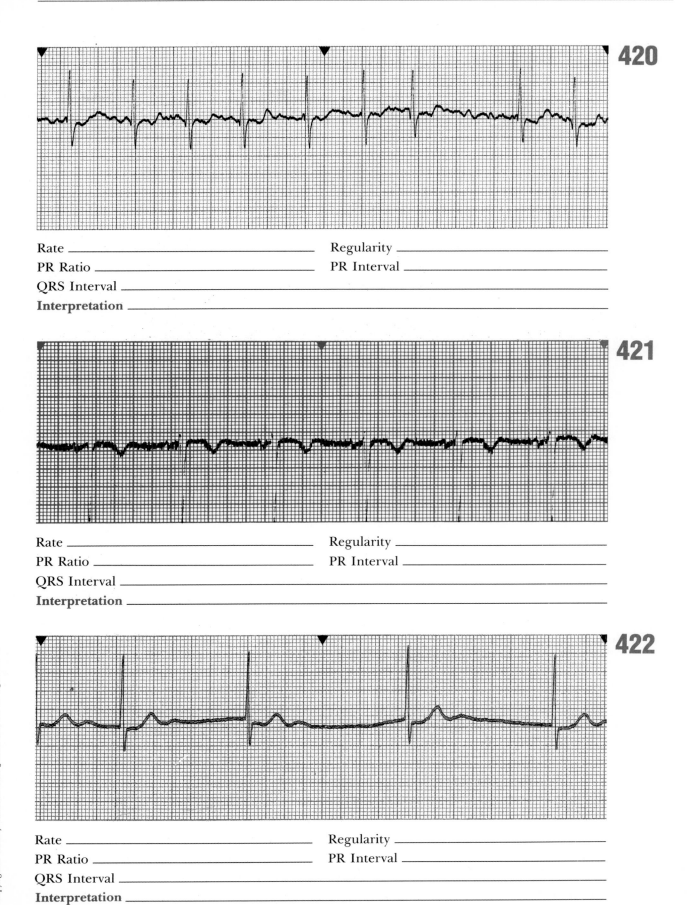

420

Rate _____   Regularity _____
PR Ratio _____   PR Interval _____
QRS Interval _____
Interpretation _____

421

Rate _____   Regularity _____
PR Ratio _____   PR Interval _____
QRS Interval _____
Interpretation _____

422

Rate _____   Regularity _____
PR Ratio _____   PR Interval _____
QRS Interval _____
Interpretation _____

423

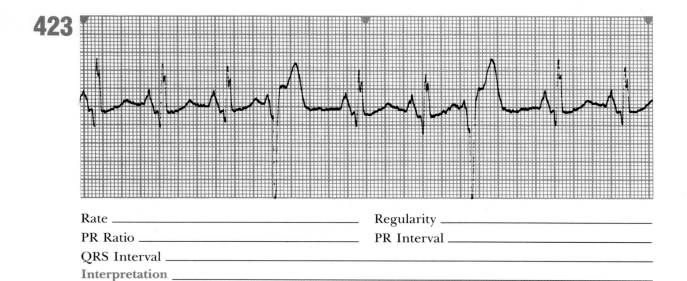

Rate _____ Regularity _____

PR Ratio _____ PR Interval _____

QRS Interval _____

Interpretation _____

424

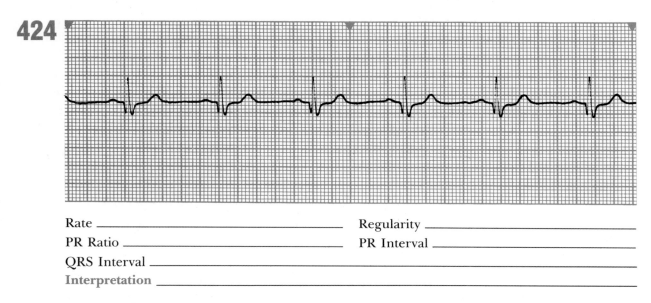

Rate _____ Regularity _____

PR Ratio _____ PR Interval _____

QRS Interval _____

Interpretation _____

425

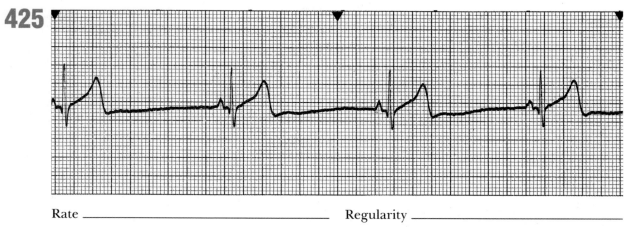

Rate _____ Regularity _____

PR Ratio _____ PR Interval _____

QRS Interval _____

Interpretation _____

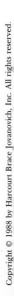

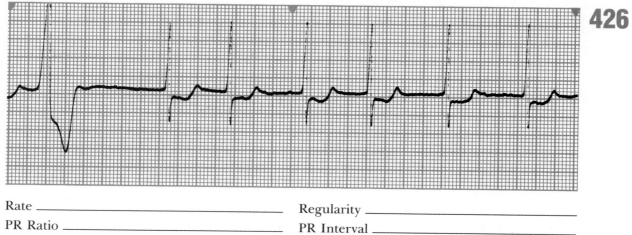

426

Rate _____   Regularity _____

PR Ratio _____   PR Interval _____

QRS Interval _____

Interpretation _____

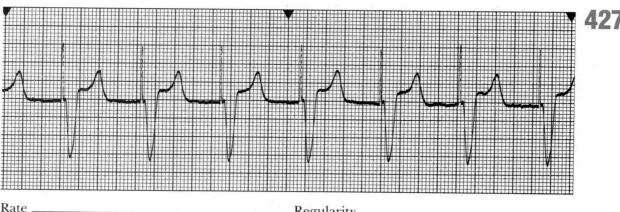

427

Rate _____   Regularity _____

PR Ratio _____   PR Interval _____

QRS Interval _____

Interpretation _____

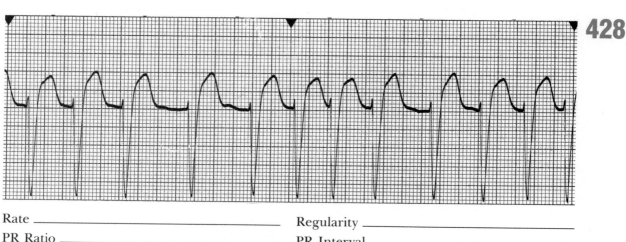

428

Rate _____   Regularity _____

PR Ratio _____   PR Interval _____

QRS Interval _____

Interpretation _____

429

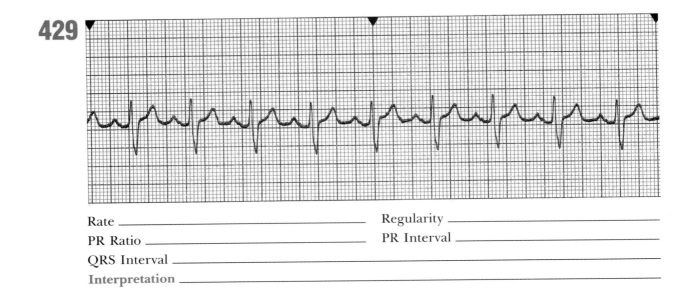

Rate _____   Regularity _____

PR Ratio _____   PR Interval _____

QRS Interval _____

Interpretation _____

Advanced EKG Rhythms

The following EKGs are more complex. They are inherently more subject to difference of opinion.

Keep an open, humble mind while interpreting them.

430

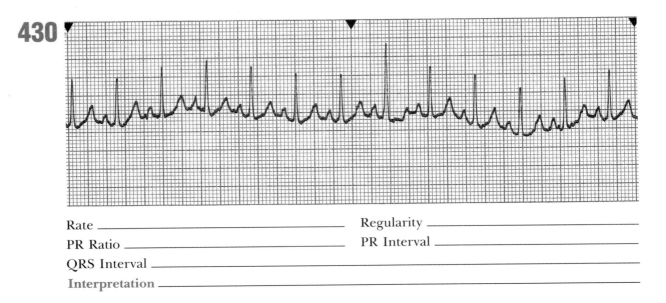

Rate _____   Regularity _____

PR Ratio _____   PR Interval _____

QRS Interval _____

Interpretation _____

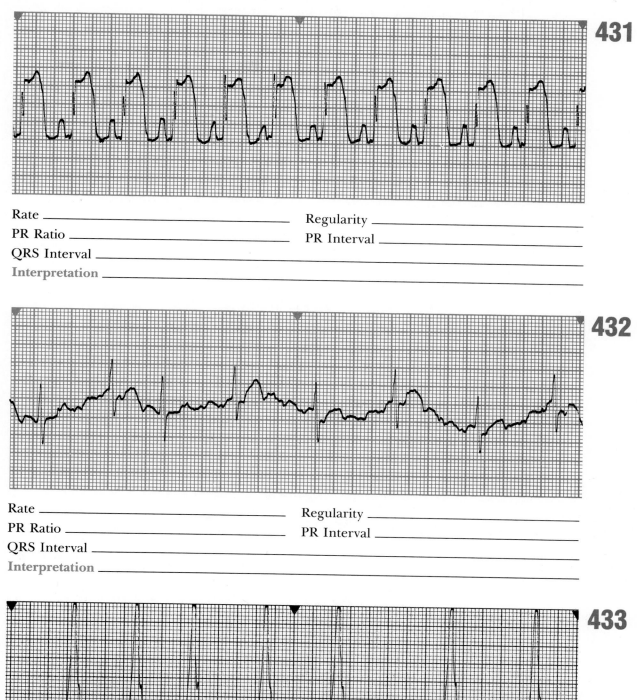

431

Rate _____   Regularity _____

PR Ratio _____   PR Interval _____

QRS Interval _____

Interpretation _____

432

Rate _____   Regularity _____

PR Ratio _____   PR Interval _____

QRS Interval _____

Interpretation _____

433

Rate _____   Regularity _____

PR Ratio _____   PR Interval _____

QRS Interval _____

Interpretation _____

434

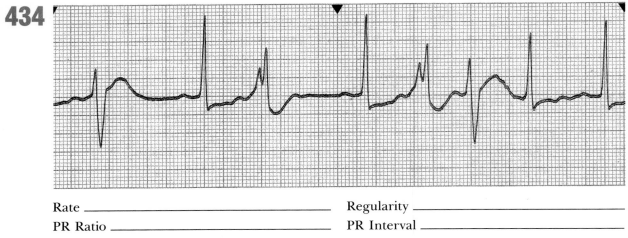

Rate _____ Regularity _____

PR Ratio _____ PR Interval _____

QRS Interval _____

Interpretation _____

435

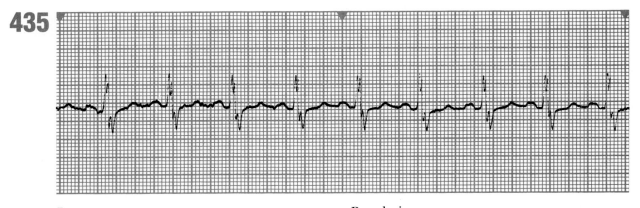

Rate _____ Regularity _____

PR Ratio _____ PR Interval _____

QRS Interval _____

Interpretation _____

436

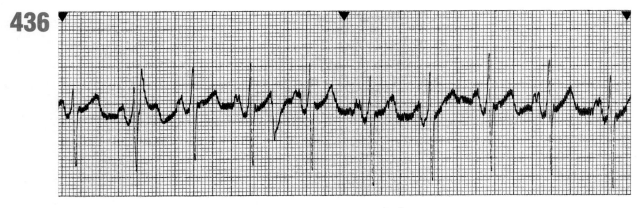

Rate _____ Regularity _____

PR Ratio _____ PR Interval _____

QRS Interval _____

Interpretation _____

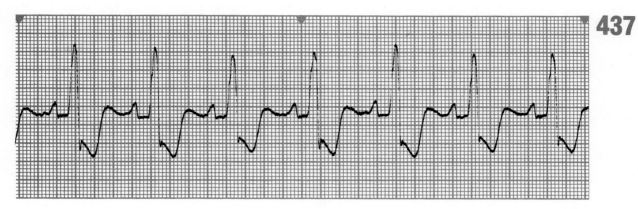

437

Rate _____ Regularity _____

PR Ratio _____ PR Interval _____

QRS Interval _____

Interpretation _____

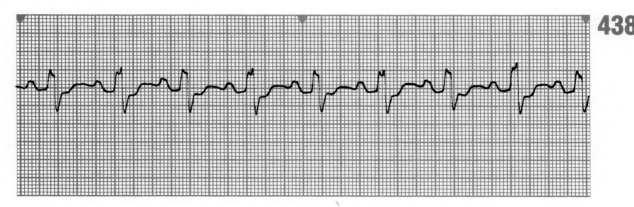

438

Rate _____ Regularity _____

PR Ratio _____ PR Interval _____

QRS Interval _____

Interpretation _____

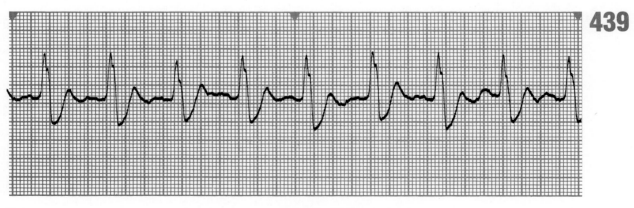

439

Rate _____ Regularity _____

PR Ratio _____ PR Interval _____

QRS Interval _____

Interpretation _____

440

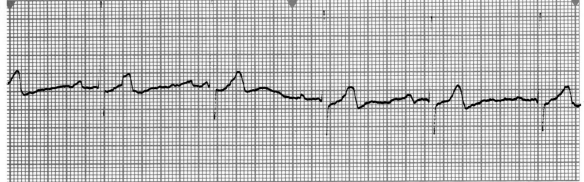

Rate _____ Regularity _____

PR Ratio _____ PR Interval _____

QRS Interval _____

Interpretation _____

441

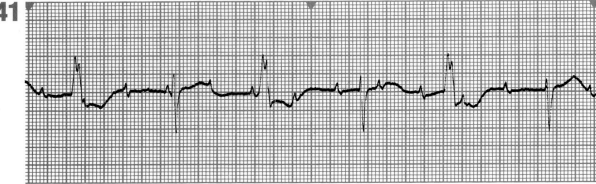

Rate _____ Regularity _____

PR Ratio _____ PR Interval _____

QRS Interval _____

Interpretation _____

442

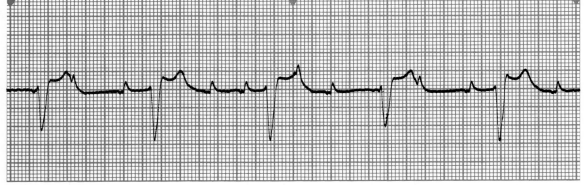

Rate _____ Regularity _____

PR Ratio _____ PR Interval _____

QRS Interval _____

Interpretation _____

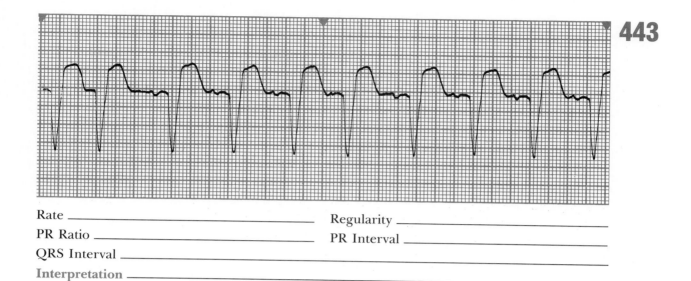

443

Rate _____ Regularity _____

PR Ratio _____ PR Interval _____

QRS Interval _____

Interpretation _____

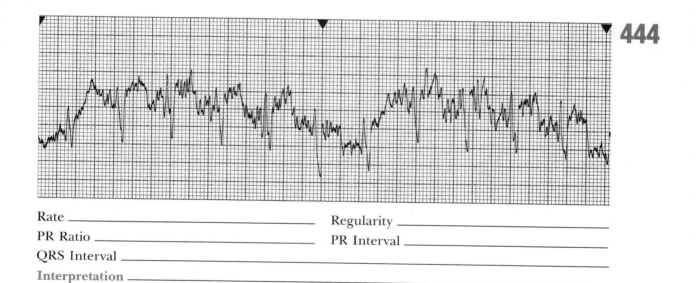

444

Rate _____ Regularity _____

PR Ratio _____ PR Interval _____

QRS Interval _____

Interpretation _____

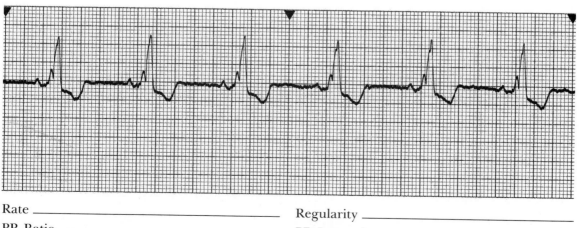

Rate _____ Regularity _____

PR Ratio _____ PR Interval _____

QRS Interval _____

Interpretation _____

446

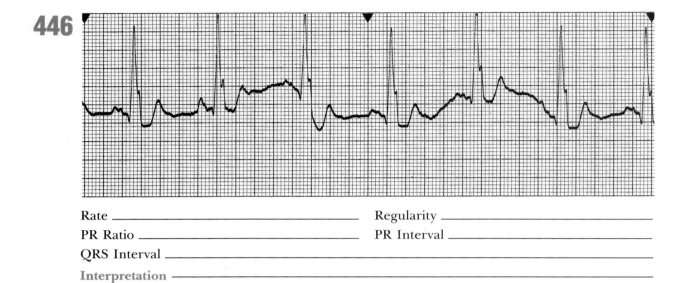

Rate _____ Regularity _____

PR Ratio _____ PR Interval _____

QRS Interval _____

Interpretation _____

447

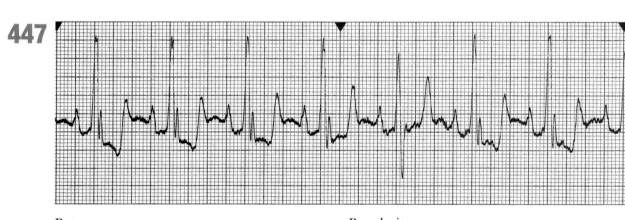

Rate _____ Regularity _____

PR Ratio _____ PR Interval _____

QRS Interval _____

Interpretation _____

448

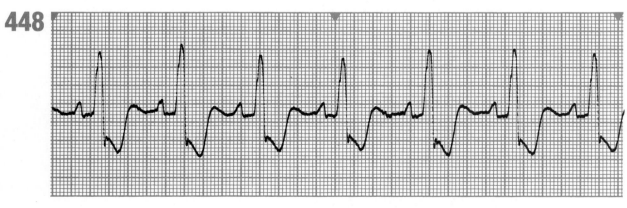

Rate _____ Regularity _____

PR Ratio _____ PR Interval _____

QRS Interval _____

Interpretation _____

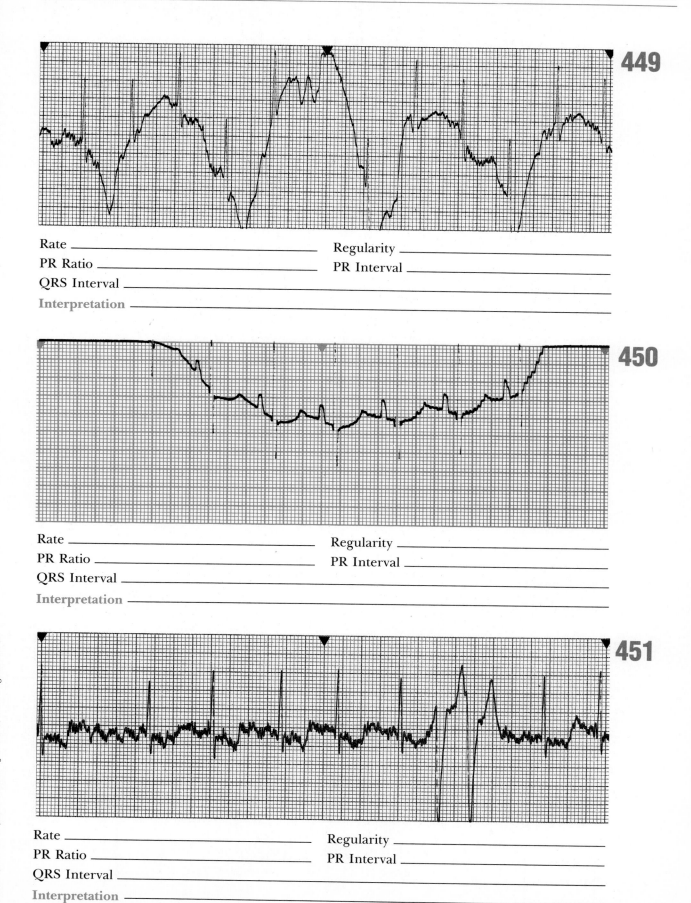

449

Rate _____   Regularity _____

PR Ratio _____   PR Interval _____

QRS Interval _____

Interpretation _____

450

Rate _____   Regularity _____

PR Ratio _____   PR Interval _____

QRS Interval _____

Interpretation _____

451

Rate _____   Regularity _____

PR Ratio _____   PR Interval _____

QRS Interval _____

Interpretation _____

452

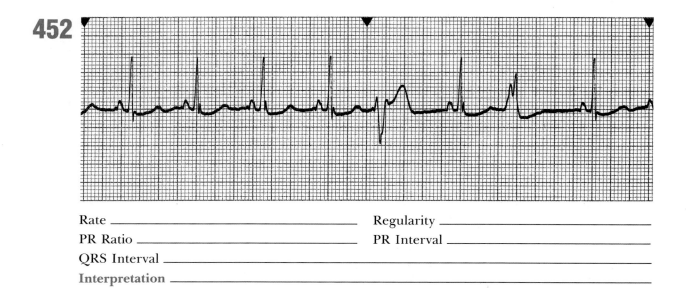

Rate _____   Regularity _____
PR Ratio _____   PR Interval _____
QRS Interval _____
Interpretation _____

453

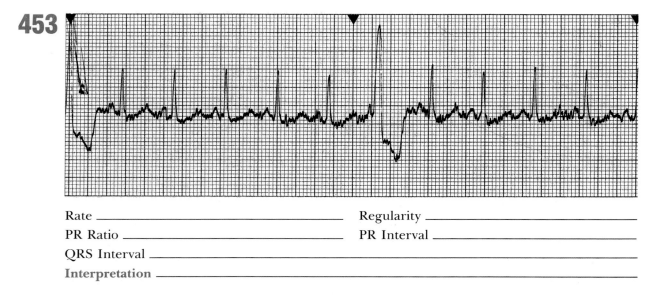

Rate _____   Regularity _____
PR Ratio _____   PR Interval _____
QRS Interval _____
Interpretation _____

454

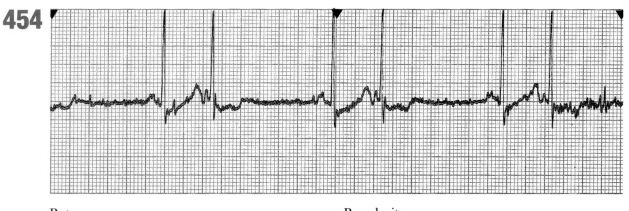

Rate _____   Regularity _____
PR Ratio _____   PR Interval _____
QRS Interval _____
Interpretation _____

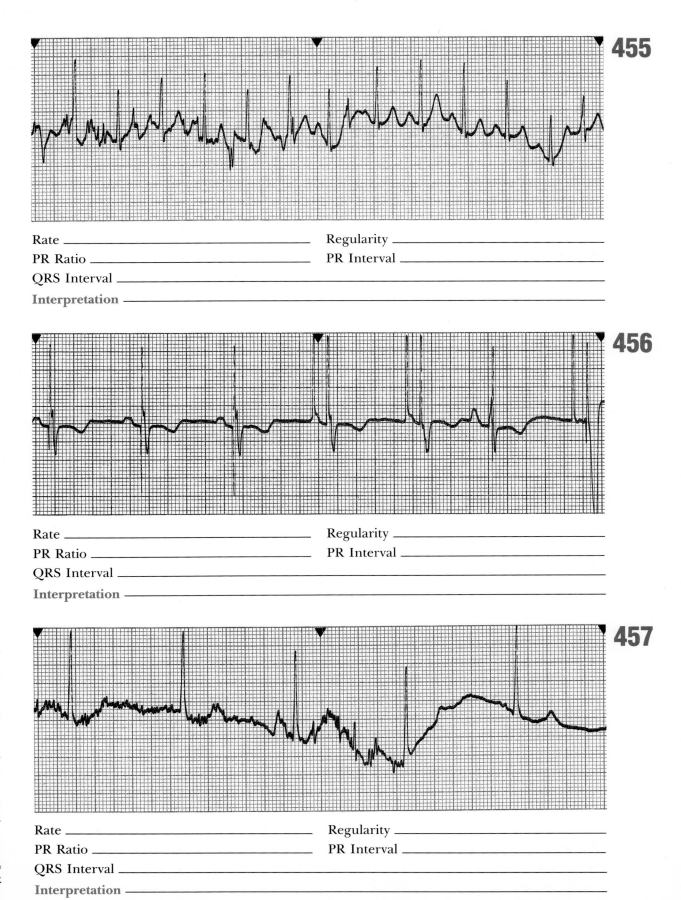

455

Rate _____ Regularity _____

PR Ratio _____ PR Interval _____

QRS Interval _____

Interpretation _____

456

Rate _____ Regularity _____

PR Ratio _____ PR Interval _____

QRS Interval _____

Interpretation _____

457

Rate _____ Regularity _____

PR Ratio _____ PR Interval _____

QRS Interval _____

Interpretation _____

458

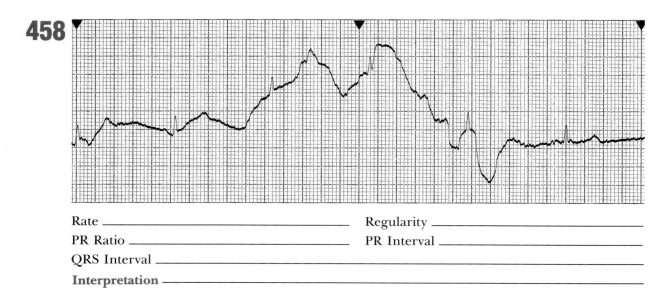

Rate _____   Regularity _____

PR Ratio _____   PR Interval _____

QRS Interval _____

Interpretation _____

459

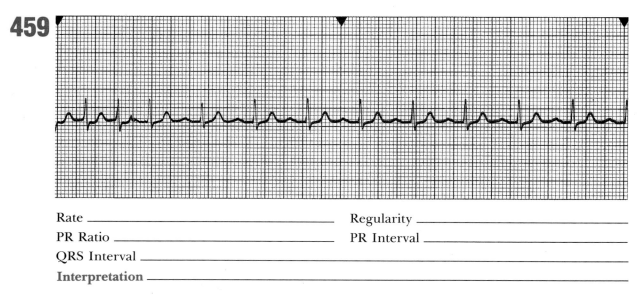

Rate _____   Regularity _____

PR Ratio _____   PR Interval _____

QRS Interval _____

Interpretation _____

460

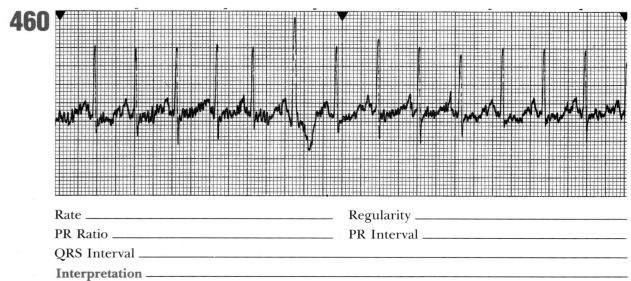

Rate _____   Regularity _____

PR Ratio _____   PR Interval _____

QRS Interval _____

Interpretation _____

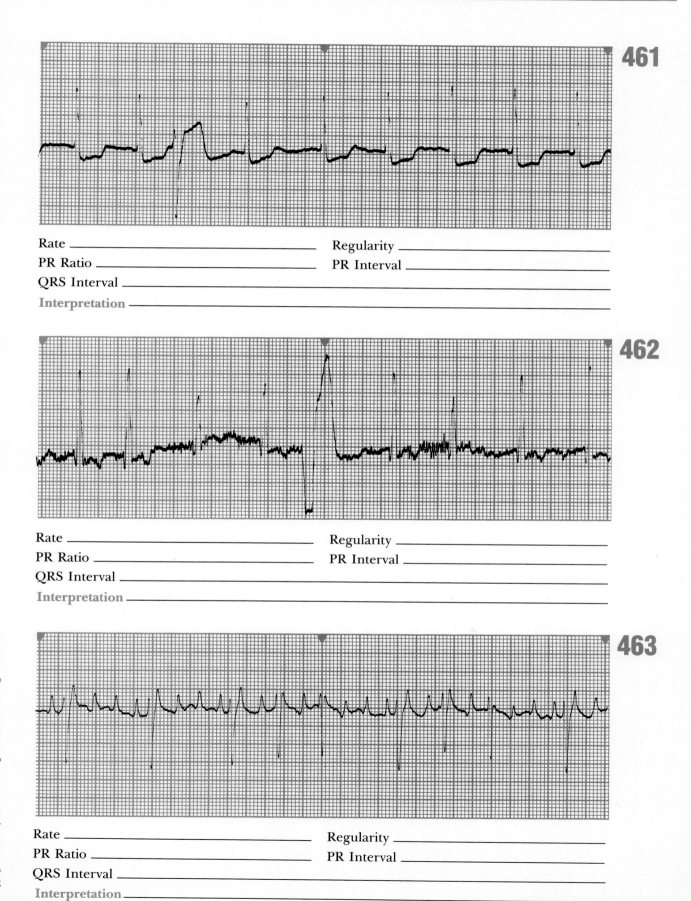

461

Rate _____   Regularity _____

PR Ratio _____   PR Interval _____

QRS Interval _____

Interpretation _____

462

Rate _____   Regularity _____

PR Ratio _____   PR Interval _____

QRS Interval _____

Interpretation _____

463

Rate _____   Regularity _____

PR Ratio _____   PR Interval _____

QRS Interval _____

Interpretation _____

464

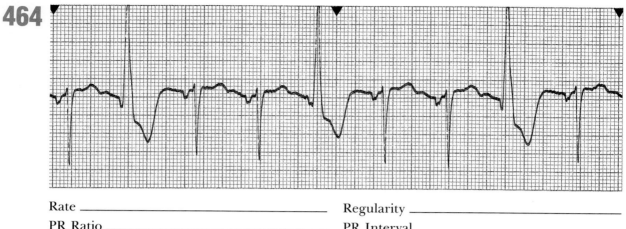

Rate _____   Regularity _____

PR Ratio _____   PR Interval _____

QRS Interval _____

Interpretation _____

465

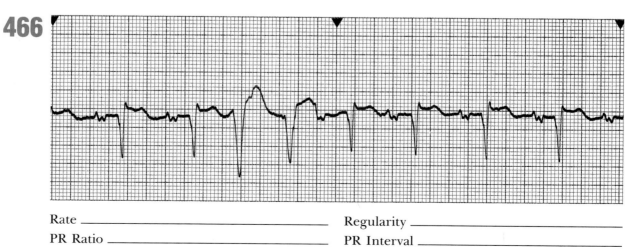

Rate _____   Regularity _____

PR Ratio _____   PR Interval _____

QRS Interval _____

Interpretation _____

466

Rate _____   Regularity _____

PR Ratio _____   PR Interval _____

QRS Interval _____

Interpretation _____

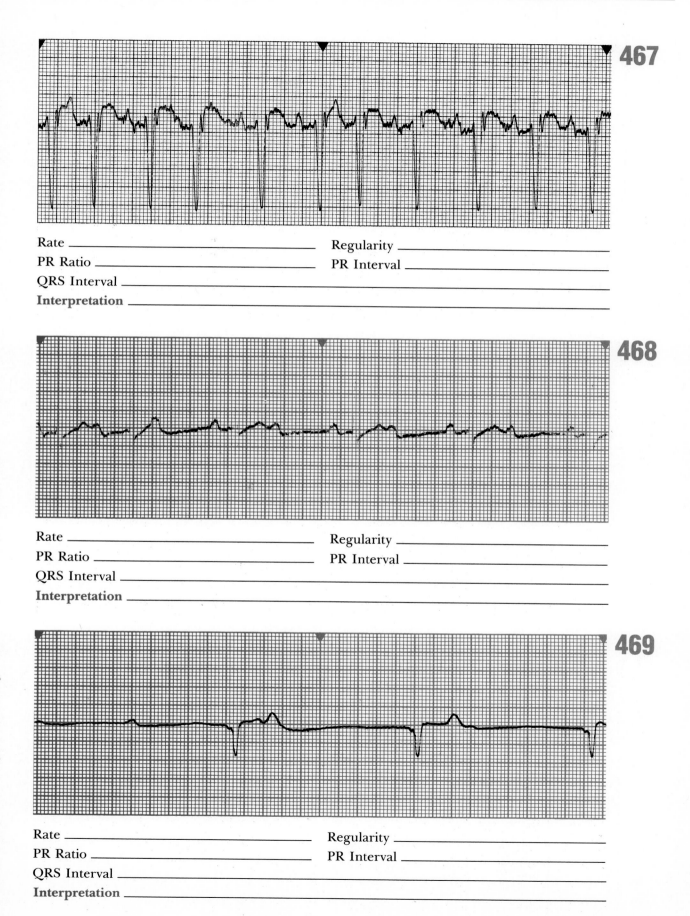

467

Rate _____   Regularity _____

PR Ratio _____   PR Interval _____

QRS Interval _____

Interpretation _____

468

Rate _____   Regularity _____

PR Ratio _____   PR Interval _____

QRS Interval _____

Interpretation _____

469

Rate _____   Regularity _____

PR Ratio _____   PR Interval _____

QRS Interval _____

Interpretation _____

470

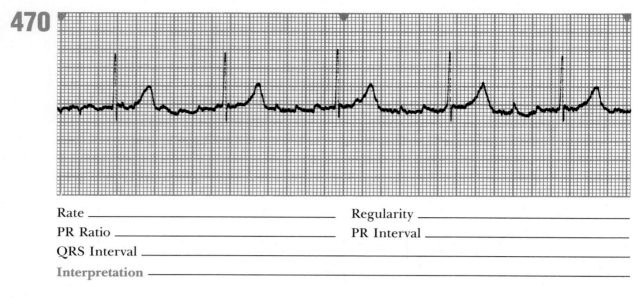

Rate _____   Regularity _____

PR Ratio _____   PR Interval _____

QRS Interval _____

Interpretation _____

471

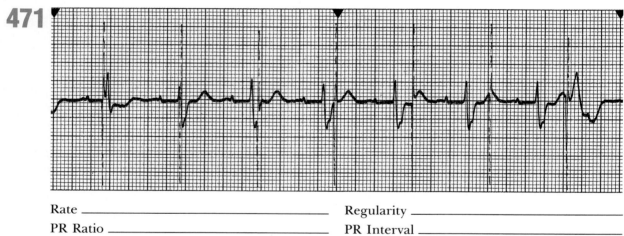

Rate _____   Regularity _____

PR Ratio _____   PR Interval _____

QRS Interval _____

Interpretation _____

Answer Key to Practice EKG Rhythms

1. Normal sinus rhythm.
2. Sinus tachycardia.
3. Regular sinus rhythm with premature ventricular contractions.
4. Atrial fibrillation.
5. Atrial fibrillation with premature junctional contractions.
6. Junctional rhythm.
7. Normal sinus rhythm.
8. Atrial fibrillation with premature ventricular contractions.
9. Wenckebach block.
10. Regular sinus rhythm with premature junctional contractions.
11. Normal sinus rhythm.
12. Regular sinus rhythm with trigeminal premature ventricular contractions.
13. Atrial fibrillation.
14. Normal sinus rhythm.
15. Artifact.
16. Regular sinus rhythm with premature junctional contractions.
17. Normal sinus rhythm.
18. Pacemaker rhythm.
19. Regular sinus rhythm with premature ventricular contractions and artifact.
20. Atrial fibrillation.
21. Junctional rhythm.
22. Regular sinus rhythm with premature junctional contractions.
23. Normal sinus rhythm with artifact.
24. Normal sinus rhythm.
25. Sinus bradycardia with artifact.
26. Artifact (possibly seizure).
27. Atrial fibrillation.
28. Regular sinus rhythm with premature junctional contractions.
29. Normal sinus rhythm.
30. Sinus tachycardia.
31. Normal sinus rhythm.
32. Sinus bradycardia with multifocal premature ventricular contractions.
33. Sinus tachycardia.
34. Sinus bradycardia.
35. Sinus arrhythmia.
36. Normal sinus rhythm.
37. Atrial fibrillation.
38. Regular sinus rhythm with artifact.
39. Sinus tachycardia with (fusion) premature ventricular contractions.
40. Junctional rhythm.
41. Regular sinus rhythm with multifocal premature ventricular contractions.
42. Sinus tachycardia.
43. First degree heart block.
44. Pacemaker rhythm.
45. Normal sinus rhythm.
46. Regular sinus rhythm with (interpolated) premature ventricular contractions.
47. Sinus bradycardia.
48. Regular sinus rhythm with premature ventricular contractions.
49. Atrial fibrillation.
50. Regular sinus rhythm with bigeminal premature ventricular contractions.
51. Normal sinus rhythm.
52. Sinus tachycardia.
53. Sinus bradycardia with depressed P waves.
54. Regular sinus rhythm with premature junctional contractions.
55. Regular sinus rhythm with bigeminal premature ventricular contractions.
56. Normal sinus rhythm with artifact.
57. Regular sinus rhythm with artifact.
58. Atrial fibrillation.
59. Regular sinus rhythm with premature ventricular contractions.
60. Normal sinus rhythm.
61. Sinus tachycardia.
62. First degree heart block.
63. Atrial fibrillation with premature ventricular contraction.
64. Sinus bradycardia.
65. Normal sinus rhythm.
66. Regular sinus rhythm with premature ventricular contractions and artifact.
67. Pacemaker rhythm.
68. Regular sinus rhythm with multifocal premature ventricular contractions.
69. Regular sinus rhythm with premature junctional contractions.
70. Atrial fibrillation.

71. Normal sinus rhythm.
72. Sinus arrhythmia.
73. Normal sinus rhythm.
74. Sinus bradycardia.
75. Pacemaker rhythm.
76. First degree heart block.
77. Pacemaker rhythm.
78. Regular sinus rhythm with (patient movement) artifact.
79. Regular sinus rhythm with premature junctional contractions.
80. Normal sinus rhythm.
81. Sinus tachycardia.
82. Agonal rhythm.
83. Sinus arrhythmia.
84. Normal sinus rhythm.
85. Regular sinus rhythm with (fusion) premature ventricular contractions.
86. Sinus bradycardia.
87. Pacemaker rhythm.
88. First degree heart block.
89. Regular sinus rhythm with premature atrial contractions.
90. Sinus tachycardia.
91. Pacemaker rhythm.
92. Atrial flutter.
93. First degree heart block.
94. Sinus bradycardia.
95. Sinus tachycardia.
96. Third degree heart block.
97. Atrial fibrillation.
98. Regular sinus rhythm with premature junctional contractions.
99. First degree heart block.
100. Pacemaker rhythm.
101. Normal sinus rhythm.
102. Regular sinus rhythm with premature junctional contractions.
103. Sinus bradycardia.
104. Regular sinus rhythm with artifact.
105. Regular sinus rhythm with premature junctional contractions.
106. Atrial fibrillation.
107. Normal sinus rhythm.
108. Sinus arrhythmia.
109. Idioventricular rhythm with artifact.
110. Third degree heart block.
111. Atrial flutter.
112. Sinus tachycardia.
113. Regular sinus rhythm with aberrant premature atrial contractions.
114. AV synchronous pacemaker rhythm.
115. First degree heart block.
116. Regular sinus rhythm with premature ventricular contractions.
117. First degree heart block with artifact.
118. Sinus bradycardia.
119. Regular sinus rhythm with premature ventricular contractions.
120. Pacemaker rhythm.
121. Regular sinus rhythm with (patient movement) artifact.
122. Atrial fibrillation.
123. Pacemaker rhythm.
124. Normal sinus rhythm.
125. Regular sinus rhythm with bigeminal premature ventricular contractions.
126. Sinus bradycardia.
127. First degree heart block with aberrancy.
128. Sinus bradycardia.
129. Pacemaker rhythm.
130. Sinus bradycardia.
131. Atrial fibrillation.
132. Regular sinus rhythm with premature ventricular contractions.
133. Regular sinus rhythm with premature junctional contractions.
134. Atrial fibrillation.
135. Normal sinus rhythm.
136. Pacemaker rhythm.
137. Regular sinus rhythm with artifact.
138. First degree heart block with bigeminal premature ventricular contractions.
139. First degree heart block.
140. Regular sinus rhythm with premature ventricular contractions.
141. Normal sinus rhythm.
142. Regular sinus rhythm with premature ventricular contractions.
143. Sinus bradycardia.
144. Wenckebach heart block.
145. Regular sinus rhythm with artifact.
146. Sinus arrhythmia.
147. Normal sinus rhythm with artifact.
148. Atrial fibrillation
149. Sinus bradycardia with artifact.
150. Regular sinus rhythm with premature ventricular contractions.
151. Sinus bradycardia.
152. Pacemaker rhythm.
153. Mobitz II heart block.
154. Regular sinus rhythm with artifact.
155. Regular sinus rhythm with bigeminal premature ventricular contractions.
156. Normal sinus rhythm.
157. Wenckebach heart block

158. Regular sinus rhythm with premature junctional contractions.
159. Sinus arrhythmia with artifact.
160. Atrial fibrillation.
161. Artifact.
162. Regular sinus rhythm with premature ventricular contractions and artifact.
163. Pacemaker rhythm.
164. Wenckebach heart block.
165. Pacemaker rhythm.
166. Normal sinus rhythm with artifact.
167. Normal sinus rhythm.
168. Atrial fibrillation.
169. Regular sinus rhythm with premature ventricular contractions.
170. AV synchronous pacemaker rhythm.
171. Normal sinus rhythm.
172. Normal sinus rhythm with 60 cycle artifact.
173. First degree heart block with premature junctional contractions.
174. Regular sinus rhythm with bigeminal premature ventricular contractions.
175. Regular sinus rhythm with artifact.
176. Third degree heart block.
177. Sinus bradycardia.
178. Sinus tachycardia.
179. Atrial fibrillation.
180. Third degree heart block with ventricular escape beat.
181. Junctional rhythm.
182. Pacemaker rhythm.
183. Ventricular tachycardia.
184. Atrial fibrillation.
185. Sinus tachycardia rhythm with artifact.
186. Regular sinus rhythm with bigeminal premature ventricular contractions.
187. Normal sinus rhythm.
188. Atrial fibrillation.
189. Regular sinus rhythm with artifact.
190. Sinus bradycardia.
191. Regular sinus rhythm with trigeminal premature ventricular contractions.
192. Atrial flutter.
193. Normal sinus rhythm.
194. Atrial fibrillation.
195. Regular sinus rhythm with premature ventricular contractions.
196. First degree heart block.
197. Atrial fibrillation.
198. Sinus bradycardia.
199. Normal sinus rhythm.
200. First degree heart block.
201. Sinus bradycardia.

202. Idioventricular rhythm.
203. Junctional tachycardia.
204. Atrial flutter.
205. First degree heart block.
206. Regular sinus rhythm with bigeminal premature ventricular contractions.
207. Sinus bradycardia with artifact.
208. Regular sinus rhythm with (patient movement) artifact.
209. Normal sinus rhythm.
210. Third degree heart block.
211. Regular sinus rhythm with premature atrial contractions.
212. Sinus bradycardia with artifact.
213. Normal sinus rhythm.
214. Ventricular tachycardia.
215. Pacemaker rhythm.
216. Regular sinus rhythm with premature ventricular contractions.
217. First degree heart block.
218. Pacemaker rhythm.
219. Regular sinus rhythm with premature ventricular contractions.
220. Regular sinus rhythm with (patient movement) artifact.
221. Atrial fibrillation.
222. Regular sinus rhythm with premature ventricular contractions.
223. Sinus tachycardia.
224. Regular sinus rhythm with premature atrial contractions.
225. AV synchronous pacemaker rhythm.
226. Sinus bradycardia.
227. Third degree heart block.
228. Idioventricular rhythm.
229. Atrial fibrillation.
230. Regular sinus rhythm with premature ventricular contractions.
231. Sinus arrhythmia.
232. Normal sinus rhythm.
233. AV synchronous pacemaker rhythm.
234. Atrial flutter.
235. Accelerated idioventricular rhythm with artifact.
236. Third degree heart block.
237. Junctional rhythm.
238. Sinus bradycardia with artifact.
239. Third degree heart block.
240. Sinus tachycardia.
241. Normal sinus rhythm.
242. Wenckebach heart block
243. Regular sinus rhythm with premature ventricular contractions.

244. Pacemaker rhythm.
245. Atrial fibrillation.
246. Ventricular tachycardia.
247. Regular sinus rhythm with premature atrial contractions.
248. Regular sinus rhythm with premature ventricular contractions.
249. Regular sinus rhythm with artifact.
250. Pacemaker rhythm.
251. Wenckebach heart block.
252. Regular sinus rhythm with bigeminal premature ventricular contractions.
253. Accelerated junctional rhythm.
254. Normal sinus rhythm.
255. Atrial flutter.
256. Regular sinus rhythm with premature ventricular contractions.
257. Third degree heart block.
258. Regular sinus rhythm with artifact.
259. Regular sinus rhythm with premature junctional contractions.
260. Atrial fibrillation.
261. Regular sinus rhythm with premature ventricular contractions.
262. Normal sinus rhythm with 60 cycle artifact.
263. Atrial fibrillation.
264. Regular sinus rhythm with premature atrial contractions.
265. Agonal rhythm.
266. Normal sinus rhythm.
267. Regular sinus rhythm with premature ventricular contractions.
268. Atrial fibrillation.
269. Agonal rhythm.
270. AV synchronous pacemaker rhythm.
271. Sinus bradycardia.
272. Wenckebach heart block.
273. Normal sinus rhythm.
274. Atrial fibrillation with aberrancy.
275. Regular sinus rhythm with premature ventricular contractions.
276. Third degree heart block.
277. Regular sinus rhythm with trigeminal premature ventricular contractions.
278. Atrial fibrillation.
279. Pacemaker rhythm.
280. Agonal rhythm.
281. Normal sinus rhythm.
282. Wenckebach heart block.
283. Regular sinus rhythm with premature ventricular contractions.
284. Atrial fibrillation.
285. Atrial tachycardia.
286. Regular sinus rhythm with trigeminal premature junctional contractions.
287. Regular sinus rhythm with bigeminal premature ventricular contractions.
288. Atrial fibrillation.
289. Regular sinus rhythm with 60 cycle artifact.
290. Normal sinus rhythm.
291. Sinus bradycardia.
292. Atrial fibrillation.
293. Atrial tachycardia.
294. Atrial fibrillation.
295. Wenckebach heart block.
296. Regular sinus rhythm with bigeminal premature ventricular contractions.
297. Atrial flutter.
298. First degree heart block.
299. Regular sinus rhythm with multifocal couplet of premature ventricular contractions.
300. Normal sinus rhythm.
301. Sinus tachycardia with (interpolated) premature ventricular contractions.
302. Pacemaker rhythm.
303. Sinus bradycardia.
304. Regular sinus rhythm with bigeminal premature atrial contractions.
305. Sinus bradycardia.
306. Regular sinus rhythm with trigeminal premature ventricular contractions.
307. Normal sinus rhythm.
308. Atrial fibrillation.
309. Regular sinus rhythm with bigeminal premature ventricular contractions.
310. Sinus bradycardia.
311. Atrial flutter.
312. Normal sinus rhythm.
313. Atrial tachycardia.
314. Sinus bradycardia.
315. AV synchronous pacemaker rhythm.
316. Regular sinus rhythm with a premature ventricular contraction.
317. First degree heart block.
318. Atrial flutter.
319. Atrial tachycardia.
320. Normal sinus rhythm.
321. Junctional rhythm.
322. Normal sinus rhythm.
323. Sinus tachycardia.
324. AV synchronous pacemaker rhythm.
325. Agonal rhythm.
326. Normal sinus rhythm.
327. Wenckebach heart block.
328. Pacemaker rhythm.
329. Sinus bradycardia.

330. Atrial tachycardia.

331. Atrial flutter.

332. Regular sinus rhythm with (patient movement) artifact.

333. Regular sinus rhythm with premature ventricular contractions.

334. Artifact.

335. Atrial fibrillation.

336. Mobitz II heart block.

337. Atrial fibrillation.

338. Normal sinus rhythm.

339. AV synchronous pacemaker rhythm.

340. Junctional rhythm.

341. Regular sinus rhythm with premature atrial contractions.

342. Pacemaker rhythm.

343. Regular sinus rhythm with trigeminal premature ventricular contractions.

344. Normal sinus rhythm.

345. Regular sinus rhythm with a run of ventricular tachycardia.

346. Normal sinus rhythm.

347. First degree heart block.

348. Regular sinus rhythm with artifact.

349. Normal sinus rhythm.

350. Atrial fibrillation.

351. Regular sinus rhythm with premature ventricular contractions and artifact.

352. Sinus tachycardia.

353. First degree heart block.

354. Atrial fibrillation.

355. Pacemaker rhythm.

356. Mobitz II heart block.

357. Pacemaker rhythm.

358. Atrial fibrillation.

359. Regular sinus rhythm with bigeminal premature ventricular contractions.

360. Atrial fibrillation.

361. Ventricular fibrillation.

362. Normal sinus rhythm.

363. Regular sinus rhythm with premature ventricular contractions.

364. Sinus bradycardia.

365. Regular sinus rhythm with premature atrial contractions.

366. Junctional rhythm.

367. Pacemaker rhythm.

368. Regular sinus rhythm with multifocal premature ventricular contractions.

369. Pacemaker rhythm.

370. Sinus tachycardia.

371. First degree heart block.

372. Normal sinus rhythm.

373. Regular sinus rhythm with multifocal premature ventricular contractions.

374. Wenckebach heart block.

375. Ventricular tachycardia.

376. Regular sinus rhythm with premature ventricular contractions.

377. Sinus bradycardia.

378. Normal sinus rhythm.

379. Pacemaker rhythm.

380. Regular sinus rhythm with (fusion) premature ventricular contractions.

381. Atrial flutter (with variable block).

382. Regular sinus rhythm with premature ventricular contractions.

383. Normal sinus rhythm.

384. Pacemaker rhythm.

385. Third degree heart block.

386. Normal sinus rhythm.

387. Regular sinus rhythm with bigeminal premature atrial contractions.

388. Regular sinus rhythm with premature ventricular contractions.

389. Wenckebach heart block.

390. Regular sinus rhythm with artifact.

391. Normal sinus rhythm.

392. Regular sinus rhythm with premature atrial contractions.

393. Regular sinus rhythm with multifocal premature ventricular contractions.

394. Atrial fibrillation.

395. Sinus bradycardia.

396. Pacemaker rhythm.

397. Atrial fibrillation.

398. Atrial fibrillation aberrancy and multifocal premature ventricular contractions.

399. Normal sinus rhythm.

400. Sinus bradycardia.

401. Normal sinus rhythm with artifact.

402. Ventricular tachycardia.

403. Atrial fibrillation with aberrancy.

404. Regular sinus rhythm with multifocal premature junctional contractions.

405. Regular sinus rhythm with premature ventricular contractions.

406. Atrial flutter (with variable block).

407. Normal sinus rhythm.

408. Ventricular tachycardia.

409. Normal sinus rhythm.

410. Atrial fibrillation with premature ventricular contractions.

411. Atrial fibrillation.

412. Regular sinus rhythm with bigeminal premature junctional contractions.

413. Sinus arrhythmia.

414. Atrial fibrillation.

415. Sinus tachycardia with premature ventricular contractions.

416. Normal sinus rhythm.

417. Pacemaker rhythm.

418. Sinus bradycardia.

419. Regular sinus rhythm with premature ventricular contractions.

420. Atrial fibrillation.

421. Regular sinus rhythm with artifact.

422. Atrial fibrillation.

423. Regular sinus rhythm with premature ventricular contractions.

424. Normal sinus rhythm.

425. Sinus bradycardia.

426. Atrial fibrillation with premature ventricular contractions.

427. Pacemaker rhythm.

428. Atrial fibrillation.

429. Normal sinus rhythm.

Answer Key to Advanced EKG Rhythms

430. Atrial tachycardia (rate is a sinus rate, but the P waves are multifocal indicating an atrial origin).

431. Sinus tachycardia with a possible ST elevation.

432. Atrial fibrillation with artifact.

433. Atrial fibrillation with aberrant ventricular conduction.

434. Regular sinus rhythm with multifocal PVCs.

435. Regular sinus rhythm with aberrant ventricular conduction (RR′SS′).

436. Normal sinus rhythm with artifact.

437. Regular sinus rhythm with aberrant ventricular conduction.

438. First degree block with aberrancy (RR′ with wide QRS).

439. Wandering atrial pacemaker with aberrant ventricular conduction.

440. Wandering atrial pacemaker.

441. Third degree heart block with bigeminal ventricular escape beats.

442. Third degree heart block with irregular PP (exception to rule).

443. Accelerated junctional rhythm with ventricular aberrancy and slight irregularity.

444. Sinus tachycardia with artifact.

445. Regular sinus rhythm with aberrant ventricular conduction (RR′R″).

446. Regular sinus rhythm with aberrancy and (wandering baseline) artifact.

447. Regular sinus rhythm with aberrancy and artifact.

448. Regular sinus rhythm with aberrancy.

449. Normal sinus rhythm with (wandering baseline) artifact.

450. Normal sinus rhythm with (wandering baseline) artifact.

451. Coarse atrial fibrillation with baseline artifact and a PVC couplet.

452. Regular sinus rhythm with multifocal interpolated PVCs.

453. Sinus tachycardia with PJCs.

454. Regular sinus rhythm with bigeminal PJCs and artifact.

455. Sinus tachycardia with PAC and baseline artifact.

456. Sinus bradycardia with fixed rate pacemaker.

457. Sinus bradycardia with artifact.

458. Sinus bradycardia with wandering baseline artifact.

459. Atrial tachycardia convert to sinus tachycardia.

460. Sinus tachycardia with artifact.

461. Atrial fibrillation with a P.V.C.

462. Atrial fibrillation with baseline artifact and a PVC.

463. Atrial flutter with variable block (4:1 and 2:1).

464. Junctional rhythm with trigeminal interpolated PVCs.

465. Accelerated junctional rhythm (with inverted P waves).

466. First degree heart block with couplet of PVCs.

467. First degree heart block with PACs and artifact (first reaction becomes atrial fibrillation).

468. Wenckebach converting to Mobitz II.

469. Third degree heart block with irregular atrial response.

470. Third degree heart block with artifact.

471. Pacemaker rhythm (in fixed-rate mode) and first degree heart block. Three pacer spikes were captured.

A 7
B 8
C 9
D 0
E 1
F 2
G 3
H 4
I 5
J 6

Flash Cards

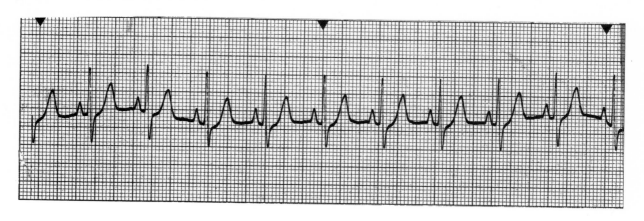

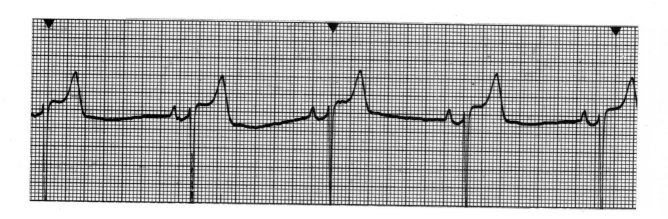

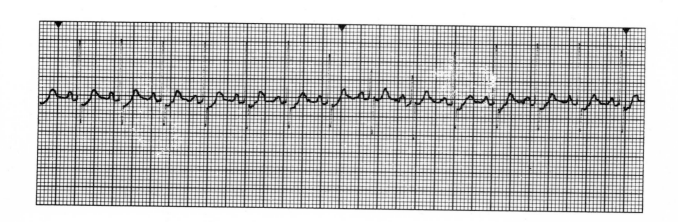

Normal Sinus Rhythm ━━━━━━━━━━

Primary Differential Criteria

1. Rate   *normocardic*
2. Regularity   *regular*
3. P:R Ratio   *1:1*
4. PR Interval   *normal*
5. QRS Interval   *normal*

Interpretation

Regular, with normal QRS interval.

- -

Sinus Bradycardia ━━━━━━━━━━

Primary Differential Criteria

1. Rate   *bradycardic*
2. Regularity   *regular*
3. P:R Ratio   *1:1*
4. PR Interval   *normal*
5. QRS Interval   *normal*

Interpretation

Looks like normal sinus rhythm, with a slow rate.

- -

Sinus Tachycardia ━━━━━━━━━━

Primary Differential Criteria

1. Rate   *100 to 150 bpm*
2. Regularity   *regular*
3. P:R Ratio   *1:1*
4. PR Interval   *normal (P may be on preceding T)*
5. QRS Interval   *normal*

Interpretation

Looks like normal sinus rhythm, but faster.

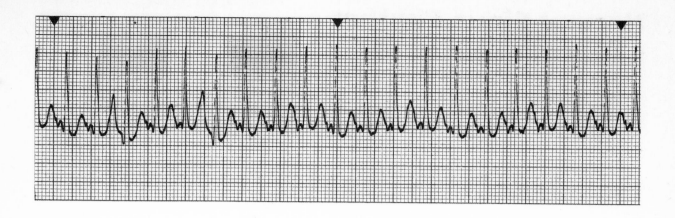

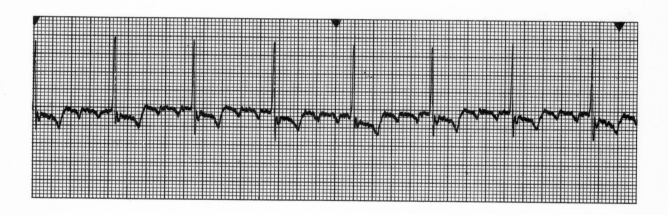

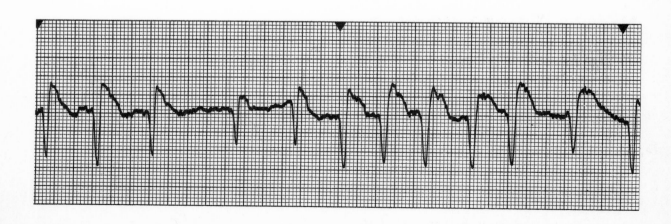

Atrial Tachycardia

Primary Differential Criteria

1. Rate   *150–250 bpm*
2. Regularity   *regular*
3. P:R Ratio   *1:1*
4. PR Interval   *normal (P is commonly on preceding T)*
5. QRS Interval   *normal*

Interpretation

Looks like normal sinus rhythm and sinus tachycardia, but faster.

Atrial Flutter

Primary Differential Criteria

1. Rate   *atrial 250–350 bpm (ventricular varies widely)*
2. Regularity   *usually very regular—may have variable block*
3. P:R Ratio   *2:1 or >2:1*
4. PR Interval   *regular*
5. QRS Interval   *normal*

Interpretation

Regular R to R interval with saw-toothed baseline.

Atrial Fibrillation

Primary Differential Criteria

1. Rate   *variable from bradycardic to tachycardic*
2. Regularity   *irregularly irregular*
3. P:R Ratio   *0:1 (no P waves)*
4. PR Interval   *no regular measurable interval*
5. QRS Interval   *normal*

Interpretation

Irregularly irregular: wavy or flat baseline.

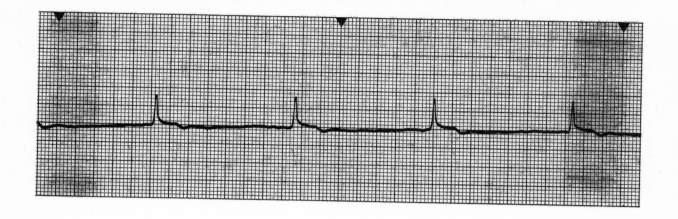

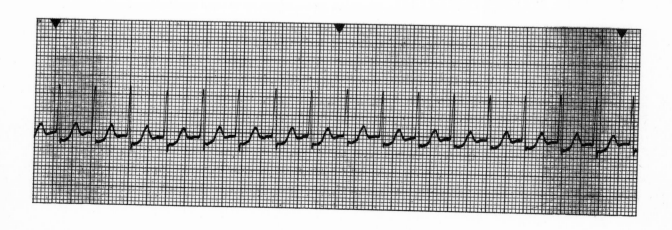

Junctional Rhythm ━━━━━━━━━━━━━━━

Primary Differential Criteria

1. Rate   *40 to 60 bpm*
2. Regularity   *very regular*
3. P:R Ratio   *1:1 (or 0:1 with normal, regular QRS interval)*
4. PR Interval   *abnormal (abbreviated, retrograde, inverted, or absent)*
5. QRS Interval   *usually normal*

Interpretation

Slow, very regular rhythm with absent or abnormal P waves.

- -

Accelerated Junctional Rhythm ━━━━━━━

Primary Differential Criteria

1. Rate   *60 to 100 bpm*
2. Regularity   *very regular*
3. P:R Ratio   *1:1 (or 0:1 with normal, regular QRS interval)*
4. PR Interval   *abnormal (abbreviated, retrograde, inverted, or absent)*
5. QRS Interval   *usually normal*

Interpretation

Looks like junctional rhythm, but faster.

- -

Junctional Tachycardia ━━━━━━━━━━━

Primary Differential Criteria

1. Rate   *>100 bpm*
2. Regularity   *very regular*
3. P:R Ratio   *1:1 (or 0:1 with normal, regular QRS interval)*
4. PR Interval   *abnormal (abbreviated, retrograde, inverted, or absent)*
5. QRS Interval   *usually normal*

Interpretation

Looks like junctional rhythm, but faster.

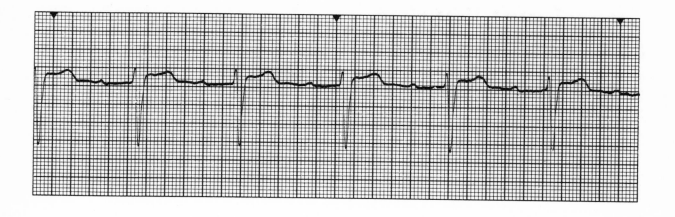

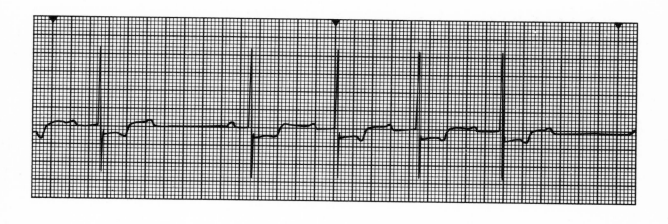

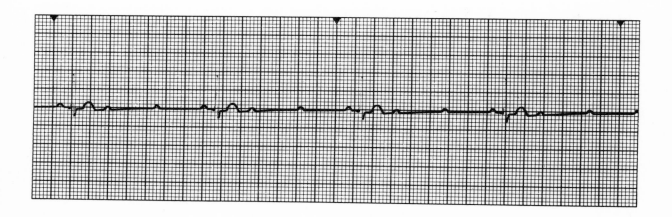

First Degree Heart Block ━━━━━━━

Primary Differential Criteria

1. Rate   *normocardic or bradycardic*
2. Regularity   *very regular*
3. P:R Ratio   *1:1*
4. PR Interval   *elongated (or "prolonged") and regular*
5. QRS Interval   *normal*

Interpretation

Looks like normal sinus rhythm, with a long PR interval. It may be bradycardic.

Wenckebach (Mobitz I) Heart Block ━━━━

Primary Differential Criteria

1. Rate   *normal to bradycardic*
2. Regularity   *regularly irregular (RR interval & PR interval get shorter in group)*
3. P:R Ratio   *>1:1 but <2:1*
4. PR Interval   *irregular (progressively longer in groups)*
5. QRS Interval   *normal*

Interpretation

Groups of QRS complexes: irregular PR intervals that get longer within each group.

Mobitz II Heart Block ━━━━━━━━

Primary Differential Criteria

1. Rate   *normal to bradycardic*
2. Regularity   *very regular*
3. P:R Ratio   *2:1 or >2:1*
4. PR Interval   *regular, may be abnormal*
5. QRS Interval   *normal (occasionally wide)*

Interpretation

Looks like normal sinus rhythm with more than one P wave per QRS complex.

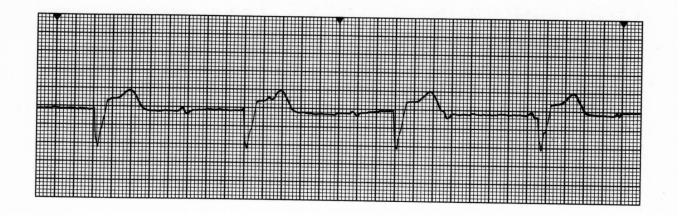

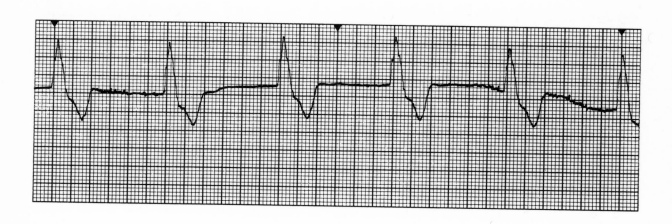

Third Degree (Complete) Heart Block ___

Primary Differential Criteria

1. Rate   *45 bpm or less (rate >45 is probably AV dissociation)*
2. Regularity   *PP interval regular: RR interval regular: PR interval irregular*
3. P:R Ratio   *>1:1 (also irregular)*
4. PR Interval   *irregularly irregular*
5. QRS Interval   *wide (may be normal)*

Interpretation

Very slow rhythm with irregularly irregular PR interval.

Idioventricular Rhythm ___

Primary Differential Criteria

1. Rate   *40 bpm or less*
2. Regularity   *very regular*
3. P:R Ratio   *0:1*
4. PR Interval   *none*
5. QRS Interval   *wide*

Interpretation

Looks like junctional rhythm only slower with wide QRS complexes.

Ventricular Tachycardia ___

Primary Differential Criteria

1. Rate   *>100 bpm*
2. Regularity   *regular*
3. P:R Ratio   *0:1*
4. PR Interval   *none*
5. QRS Interval   *wide*

Interpretation

Very fast rhythm with wide complexes and no recognizable P waves: patient may be pulseless.

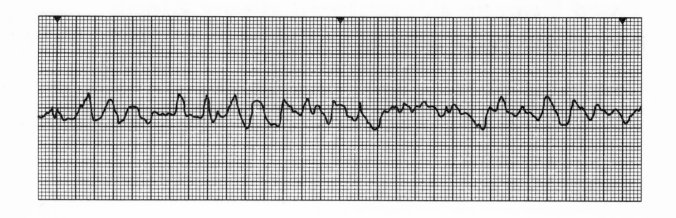

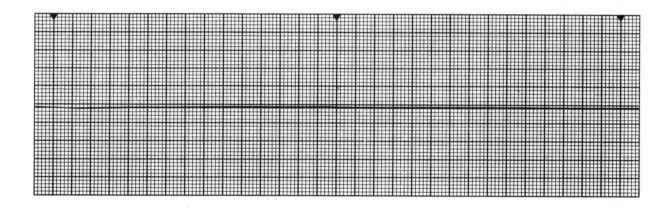

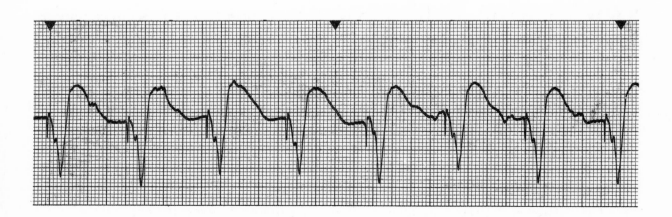

Ventricular Fibrillation

Primary Differential Criteria

1. Rate   *none*
2. Regularity   *grossly irregular*
3. P:R Ratio   *none*
4. PR Interval   *none*
5. QRS Interval   *no QRS complexes*

Interpretation

Wavy line: patient is pulseless and apneic.

Asystole

Primary Differential Criteria

1. Rate   *none*
2. Regularity   *regular*
3. P:R Ratio   *none*
4. PR Interval   *none*
5. QRS Interval   *none*

Interpretation

Flat or mildly flat, depending on calibration line.

Pacemaker Rhythm

Primary Differential Criteria

1. Rate   *minimum is usually 70*
2. Regularity   *depends on underlying rhythm*
3. P:R Ratio   *depends on underlying rhythm*
4. PR Interval   *depends on underlying rhythm*
5. QRS Interval   *regular (with spike when rate is below 70)*

Interpretation

Pacemaker spike is present. Spike may be absent during periods of normal (natural heart) rate.

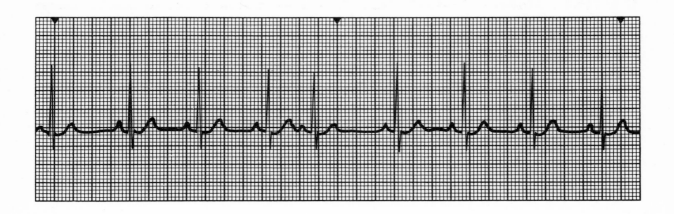

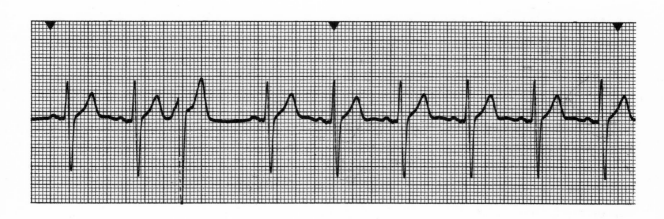

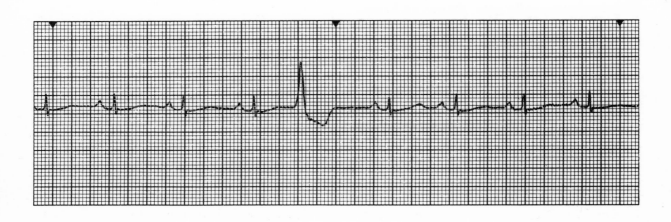

Premature Atrial Contraction (PAC) ___

Primary Differential Criteria

1. P Wave   *within normal limits*
2. QRS Interval   *within normal limits (≤.10)*
3. Pause   *non-compensatory*

Interpretation

Premature complex with a normal PR interval.

Premature Junctional Contraction (PJC)

Primary Differential Criteria

1. P Wave   *absent or abnormal*
2. QRS Interval   *within normal limits (≤.10)*
3. Pause   *either/or*

Interpretation

Premature complex with an abnormal PR interval (or absent P wave and normal QRS interval).

Premature Ventricular Contraction (PVC)

Primary Differential Criteria

1. P Wave   *absent*
2. QRS Interval   *wide and bizarre (≥.12 sec)*
3. Pause   *compensatory*

Interpretation

Premature complex with an absent P wave and wide QRS complex.

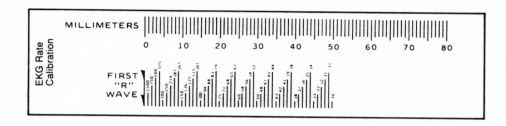

Cut out rulers for use

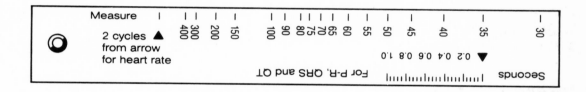